Molecular Cardiology

METHODS IN MOLECULAR MEDICINE™

John M. Walker, SERIES EDITOR

METHODS IN MOLECULAR MEDICINE™

Molecular Cardiology

Methods and Protocols

Edited by

Zhongjie Sun

Departments of Medicine and Physiology and Functional Genomics, College of Medicine, University of Florida, Gainesville, FL

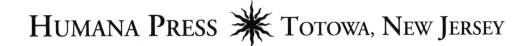

HUMANA PRESS ✴ TOTOWA, NEW JERSEY

© 2005 Humana Press Inc.
999 Riverview Drive, Suite 208
Totowa, New Jersey 07512

www.humanapress.com

For additional copies, pricing for bulk purchases, and/or information about other Humana titles, contact Humana at the above address or at any of the following numbers: Tel.: 973-256-1699; Fax: 973-256-8341; E-mail: humana@humanapr.com; or visit our Website: www.humanapress.com

This publication is printed on acid-free paper. ∞
ANSI Z39.48-1984 (American Standards Institute) Permanence of Paper for Printed Library Materials.

Production Editor: Nicole E. Furia
Cover design by Patricia F. Cleary
Cover Illustration: Figure 1 from Chapter 11, "Autologous Mesenchymal Stem Cells for Post-Ischemic Myocardial Repair," by Yao Liang Tang.

Photocopy Authorization Policy:
Authorization to photocopy items for internal or personal use, or the internal or personal use of specific clients, is granted by Humana Press Inc., provided that the base fee of US $25.00 per copy is paid directly to the Copyright Clearance Center at 222 Rosewood Drive, Danvers, MA 01923. For those organizations that have been granted a photocopy license from the CCC, a separate system of payment has been arranged and is acceptable to Humana Press Inc. The fee code for users of the Transactional Reporting Service is: [1-58829-363-7/05 $25.00].

Printed in the United States of America. 10 9 8 7 6 5 4 3 2 1

eISBN 1-59259-879-X
ISSN 1543-1894

Library of Congress Cataloging-in-Publication Data

Molecular cardiology : methods and protocols / edited by Zhongjie Sun.
  p. ; cm. — (Methods in molecular medicine ; 112)
 Includes bibliographical references and index.
 ISBN 1-58829-363-7 (hardcover : alk. paper)
 1. Heart—Diseases—Molecular aspects—Laboratory manuals. 2.
Heart—Molecular aspects—Laboratory manuals.
 [DNLM: 1. Cardiovascular Diseases—therapy. 2. Gene Therapy. 3. Gene
Transfer Techniques. 4. Heart—physiopathology. WG 166 M718 2005] I. Sun,
Zhongjie. II. Series.
 RC682.9. M648 2005
 616.1'2042—dc22
                    2004012780

Preface

The aim of *Molecular Cardiology: Methods and Protocols* is to document state-of-the-art molecular and genetic techniques in the area of cardiology. These modern approaches enable researchers to readily study heart diseases at the molecular level and will promote the development of new therapeutic strategies. Methods for genetic dissection, signal transduction, and microarray analysis are excellent tools for the study of the molecular mechanisms of cardiovascular diseases. Protocols for transgenesis take advantage of recent advances in many areas of molecular and cell biology. Transgenic models of heart diseases (cardiac hypertrophy, cardiac dysfunction, and so on.) are powerful tools for the study of heart disease pathogenesis. Methods for gene transfer to heart tissue using viral and nonviral vectors form the basis of gene therapy for heart diseases. Heart-specific promoters containing a hypoxia-inducible cardioprotective gene switch are key for protection of the heart from ischemia. Gene and stem cell therapies open novel and exciting avenues for the prevention and treatment of heart diseases.

Molecular Cardiology: Methods and Protocols consists of 26 chapters dealing with various aspects of molecular cardiology, including gene transfer and gene therapy for cardiovascular disease, stem cell therapy for cardiovascular disease, gene analysis in the injured and hypertrophied heart, and transgenesis in cardiovascular research. This book provides step-by-step methods for the successful completion of experimental procedures, and would be useful for both experienced and new investigators in the field of molecular cardiology. The "Notes" section in each chapter contains the most critical information and provides valuable troubleshooting guides to help develop protocols for your research. This book, however, is not all-inclusive owing to the broad range and fast advances in molecular biological technology.

Molecular Cardiology: Methods and Protocols should be of general interest to both basic and clinical researchers and of special interest to cardiovascular researchers, cardiologists, and molecular biologists.

I have been very fortunate to enlist a group of renowned experts in molecular cardiology for this book. I would like to thank them for their dedication and contribution. I very much appreciate the constant guidance and support from Dr. John Walker, the series editor. Many thanks also go to Thomas Lanigan and Craig Adams at the Humana Press for their professional assistance in the successful completion of this book.

Zhongjie Sun

Contents

Contributors

NATALIA ALENINA • *Max-Delbrück-Center for Molecular Medicine, Berlin-Buch, Germany*

HIROKI AOKI • *Department of Molecular Cardiovascular Biology, Yamaguchi University School of Medicine, Ube, Yamaguchi, Japan*

TAKAYUKI ASAHARA • *Department of Regenerative Medicine, Institute of Biomedical Research and Innovation, RIKEN Kobe Center for Developmental Biology, Kobe, Japan*

GOPAL J. BABU • *Department of Physiology and Cell Biology, The Ohio State University, Columbus, OH*

MICHAEL BADER • *Max-Delbrück-Center for Molecular Medicine, Berlin-Buch, Germany*

MARCOS E. BARBOSA • *Max-Delbrück-Center for Molecular Medicine, Berlin-Buch, Germany*

LUBOS BOHUNEK • *The James Hogg iCAPTURE Centre for Cardiovascular and Pulmonary Research, Department of Pathology and Laboratory Medicine, St. Paul's Hospital–University of British Columbia, Vancouver, British Columbia, Canada*

ROBERT CADE • *Departments of Medicine and Physiology and Functional Genomics, College of Medicine, University of Florida, Gainesville, FL*

KEITH M. CHANNON • *Department of Cardiovascular Medicine University of Oxford, Oxford, United Kingdom*

JONATHAN C. CHOY • *Department of Pathology and Laboratory Medicine, James Hogg iCAPTURE Centre for Cardiovascular and Pulmonary Research, St. Paul's Hospital, University of British Columbia, Vancouver, British Columbia, Canada*

THERESA A. DEISHER • *Vascular Biology, Amgen Inc., Thousand Oaks, CA*

CHRISTIAN F. DESCHEPPER • *Experimental Cardiovascular Biology Research Unit, Institut de recherches cliniques de Montréal, Montréal, Québec, Canada*

SHARON ETZION • *Neufeld Cardiac Research Institute, Tel-Aviv University, Sheba Medical Center, Tel-Hashomer, Israel*

PAUL N. EPSTEIN • *Departments of Pediatrics and Pharmacology and Toxicology, School of Medicine, University of Louisville, Louisville, KY*

ROBERTA A. GOTTLIEB • *Department of Molecular and Experimental Medicine, The Scripps Research Institute, La Jolla, CA*

DAVID J. GRANVILLE • *James Hogg iCAPTURE Centre for Cardiovascular and Pulmonary, Research St. Paul's Hospital, Department of Pathology and Laboratory Medicine, University of British Columbia, Vancouver, British Columbia, Canada*

ÅSA B. GUSTAFSSON • *Department of Molecular and Experimental Medicine, The Scripps Research Institute, La Jolla, CA*

HEATHER L. HEINE • *The James Hogg iCAPTURE Center for Cardiovascular and Pulmonary Research/MRL, Department of Pathology and Laboratory Medicine, University of British Columbia–St. Paul's Hospital, Vancouver, British Columbia, Canada*

SIGRID HOFFMANN • *Medical Research Center, Faculty for Clinical Medicine Mannheim, University of Heidelberg, Mannheim, Germany*

RADKA HOLBOVA • *Neufeld Cardiac Research Institute, Tel-Aviv University, Sheba Medical Center, Tel-Hashomer, Israel*

ARWEN L. HUNTER • *Department of Pathology and Laboratory Medicine, James Hogg iCAPTURE Centre for Cardiovascular and Pulmonary Research, St. Paul's Hospital, University of British Columbia, Vancouver, British Columbia, Canada*

HIDEKI IWAGURO • *Department of Regenerative Medicine, Division of Basic Clinical Science, Tokai University School of Medicine, Kanagawa, Japan*

RADHAKRISHNAN JEEJABAI • *Center for Advanced Studies in Functional Genomics, Department of Biochemistry, School of Biological Sciences, Madurai Kamaraj University, Madurai, India*

J. MARK JONES • *Department of Cardiac Surgery, Royal Victoria Hospital, Belfast, United Kingdom; formerly Department of Surgery, Duke University Medical Center, Durham, NC*

HIDEKO KASAHARA • *Department of Physiology and Functional Genomics, University of Florida College of Medicine, Gainesville, FL*

ALEXANDRA KERJNER • *The James Hogg iCAPTURE Centre for Cardiovascular and Pulmonary Research, Department of Pathology and Laboratory Medicine, St. Paul's Hospital–University of British Columbia, Vancouver, British Columbia, Canada*

WALTER J. KOCH • *Center for Translational Medicine, Thomas Jefferson University, Philadelphia, PA*

HON SING LEONG • *The James Hogg iCAPTURE Center for Cardiovascular and Pulmonary Research/MRL, Department of Pathology and Laboratory Medicine, University of British Columbia–St. Paul's Hospital, Vancouver, British Columbia, Canada*

JONATHAN LEOR • *Neufeld Cardiac Research Institute, Tel-Aviv University, Sheba Medical Center, Tel-Hashomer, Israel*

BASTIEN LLAMAS • *Experimental Cardiovascular Biology Research Unit, Institut de recherches cliniques de Montréal, Montréal, Québec, Canada*

YI-FAN LI • *Department of Physiology and Biophysics, University of Nebraska Medical Center, Omaha, NE*

HONGLIN LUO • *The James Hogg iCAPTURE Centre for Cardiovascular and Pulmonary Research, Department of Pathology and Laboratory Medicine, St. Paul's Hospital/Providence Health Care–University of British Columbia, Vancouver, British Columbia, Canada*

BRUCE M. MCMANUS • *The James Hogg iCAPTURE Centre for Cardiovascular and Pulmonary Research, Department of Pathology and Laboratory Medicine, St. Paul's Hospital/Providence Health Care–University of British Columbia, and Institute of Circulatory and Respiratory Health, Canadian Institutes of Health Research, Vancouver, British Columbia, Canada*

CLAUDINE MÉNARD • *Centre de Recherches de Biochimie Macromoléculaire, CNRS, Montpellier, France*

ANNABELLE MERY • *Centre de Recherches de Biochimie Macromoléculaire, CNRS, Montpellier, France*

NAIRA S. METREVELI • *Department of Pediatrics, University of Louisville School of Medicine, Louisville, KY*

LIRON MILLER • *Neufeld Cardiac Research Institute, Tel-Aviv University, Sheba Medical Center, Tel-Hashomer, Israel*

RAYMOND NG • *The James Hogg iCAPTURE Centre for Cardiovascular and Pulmonary Research, Department of Pathology and Laboratory Medicine, St. Paul's Hospital/Providence Health Care–University of British Columbia, Vancouver, British Columbia, Canada*

EVANGELIA PAPADIMOU • *Centre de Recherches de Biochimie Macromoléculaire, CNRS, Montpellier, France*

KAUSHIK P. PATEL • *Department of Physiology and Biophysics, University of Nebraska Medical Center, Omaha, NE*

MUTHU PERIASAMY • *Department of Physiology and Cell Biology, The Ohio State University, Columbus, OH*

THOMAS J. PODOR • *The James Hogg iCAPTURE Centre for Cardiovascular and Pulmonary Research, Department of Pathology and Laboratory Medicine, St. Paul's Hospital–University of British Columbia, Vancouver, British Columbia, Canada*

MICHEL PUCÉAT • *Centre de Recherches de Biochimie Macromoléculaire, CNRS, Montpellier, France*

MAZIAR RAHMANI • *The James Hogg iCAPTURE Centre for Cardiovascular and Pulmonary Research, Department of Pathology and Laboratory Medicine, St. Paul's Hospital/Providence Health Care–University of British Columbia, Vancouver, British Columbia, Canada*

CHELLAM RAJAMANICKAM • *Center for Advanced Studies in Functional Genomics, Department of Biochemistry, School of Biological Sciences, Madurai Kamaraj University, Madurai, India*

NANA REZAI • *The James Hogg iCAPTURE Centre for Cardiovascular and Pulmonary Research, Department of Pathology and Laboratory Medicine, St. Paul's Hospital–University of British Columbia, Vancouver, British Columbia, Canada*

HOWARD A. ROCKMAN • *Departments of Medicine, Cell Biology, and Molecular Genetics, Duke University Medical Center, Durham, NC*

FABIO M.V. ROSSI • *Biomedical Research Centre, Department of Medical Genetics, University of British Columbia, Vancouver British Columbia, Canada*

GEORGE F. SCHREINER • *SCIOS Inc., Fremont, CA*

HAROLD D. SCHULTZ • *Department of Physiology and Biophysics, University of Nebraska Medical Center, Omaha, NE*

XIA SHEN • *Departments of Pediatrics and Pharmacology and Toxicology, School of Medicine, University of Louisville, Louisville, KY*

XIAONING SI • *The James Hogg iCAPTURE Centre for Cardiovascular and Pulmonary Research, Department of Pathology and Laboratory Medicine, St. Paul's Hospital/Providence Health Care–University of British Columbia, Vancouver, British Columbia, Canada*

ZHONGJIE SUN • *Departments of Medicine and Physiology and Functional Genomics, College of Medicine, University of Florida, Gainesville, FL*

HIDEO TACHIBANA • *Pharmaceutical Development Division, Takeda Chemical Industries, Ltd., Chuo-ku, Osaka, Japan*

YAO LIANG TANG • *Department of Pediatrics, All Children's Hospital, University of South Florida, St. Petersburg, FL*

YI TANG • *Department of Surgery, Stanford University, Stanford, CA*

LYDIA TAYLOR • *The James Hogg iCAPTURE Centre for Cardiovascular and Pulmonary Research, Department of Pathology and Laboratory Medicine, St. Paul's Hospital/Providence Health Care–University of British Columbia, Vancouver, British Columbia, Canada*

TIMOTHY J. TRICHE • *Children's Hospital Los Angeles, University of Southern California, CA*

HUBERT WALINSKI • *The James Hogg iCAPTURE Centre for Cardiovascular and Pulmonary Research, Department of Pathology and Laboratory Medicine, St. Paul's Hospital–University of British Columbia, Vancouver, British Columbia, Canada*

XIUQING WANG • *Department of Medicine, College of Medicine, University of Florida, Gainesville, FL*

Yu Wang • *Department of Physiology and Biophysics, University of Nebraska Medical Center, Omaha, NE*

Matthew J. Wolf • *Department of Medicine, Duke University Medical Center, Durham, NC*

Bobby Yanagawa • *The James Hogg iCAPTURE Centre for Cardiovascular and Pulmonary Research, Department of Pathology and Laboratory Medicine, St. Paul's Hospital/Providence Health Care–University of British Columbia, Vancouver, British Columbia, Canada*

Decheng Yang • *The James Hogg iCAPTURE Centre for Cardiovascular and Pulmonary Research, Department of Pathology and Laboratory Medicine, St. Paul's Hospital/Providence Health Care–University of British Columbia, Vancouver, British Columbia, Canada*

Gang Ye • *Department of Pediatrics, University of Louisville School of Medicine, Louisville, KY*

Ji Yuan • *The James Hogg iCAPTURE Centre for Cardiovascular and Pulmonary Research, Department of Pathology and Laboratory Medicine, St. Paul's Hospital/Providence Health Care–University of British Columbia, Vancouver, British Columbia, Canada*

Dana Zeineddine • *Centre de Recherches de Biochimie Macromoléculaire, Montpellier, France*

Irving H. Zucker • *Department of Physiology and Biophysics, University of Nebraska Medical Center, Omaha, NE*

I

INTRODUCTION

1

Introduction to Methods in Molecular Cardiology

Zhongjie Sun

Summary

Molecular cardiology is a new area of cardiovascular medicine that aims to apply molecular biological techniques for the mechanistic investigation, diagnosis, prevention, and treatment of cardiovascular disease. As an emerging discipline, it has changed our conceptual thinking of cardiovascular development, disease etiology, and pathophysiology. Although molecular cardiology is still at a very early stage, it has opened a promising avenue for understanding and controlling cardiovascular disease. With the rapid development and application of molecular biological techniques, scientists and clinicians are closer to curing heart diseases that were thought to be incurable 20 yr ago. There clearly is a need for a more thorough understanding of the molecular mechanisms of cardiovascular diseases to promote the advancement of cell and gene therapy for heart diseases. This chapter briefly reviews state-of-the-art techniques in the area of molecular cardiology.

Key Words: Molecular cardiology; genetic cardiology; heart; cardiovascular disease; cardiac hypertrophy; myocardial infarction; cloning; cDNA; vector; molecular biology; gene therapy; molecular genetics; stem cell; cell therapy; genotype; phenotype; cardiovascular genetics; transgene; RNAi; gene silencing.

1. Introduction

Rapid advances in molecular biology in the last decade have changed the classical practice of clinical cardiology in many ways, increasing our understanding of molecular mechanisms of cardiovascular disease and providing new diagnostic and therapeutic tools. It is expected that our knowledge of molecu-

From: *Methods in Molecular Medicine, vol. 112: Molecular Cardiology: Methods and Protocols*
Edited by: Z. Sun © Humana Press Inc., Totowa, NJ

lar cardiology will grow exponentially in the next few years. Molecular and genetic cardiology has increased our awareness of the inheritance of defective genes and their impact on cardiovascular disease. Numerous attempts to apply this new knowledge at the bedside have already been made. However, routine molecular genetic testing or DNA analysis is still a specialized laboratory procedure that is not available in most hospitals or clinical chemistry laboratories. In addition, few powerful molecular biological tests and gene therapy protocols have been established for treating cardiovascular diseases, mainly because of a lack of dependable techniques in molecular cardiology. Cardiac disease represents an enormous clinical challenge in need of effective therapeutic approaches. Thus, there is an urgent demand for the development of efficient and dependable molecular cardiology techniques.

The development of molecular cardiology depends on the availability of established molecular biology techniques. Several major advances in the area of molecular biology have contributed significantly to the field of molecular cardiology: (1) the discovery and application of specific restriction endonucleases and reverse transcriptase, (2) the development of cloning techniques, (3) the availability of rapid DNA sequencing, (4) the improvement in vector technology, and (5) the completion or near completion of human and animal genomes. These advances will allow us (1) to understand the gene regulation of cardiac and vascular growth, (2) to identify genes responsible for cardiovascular diseases, (3) to perform diagnostic *in situ* hybridization, and (4) to develop gene therapy approaches to cardiovascular diseases.

This review covers the following four areas: gene transfer and gene therapy for cardiovascular disease, stem cell therapy for cardiovascular disease, gene analysis in the injured and hypertrophied heart, and transgenic techniques in cardiovascular research.

2. Gene Transfer and Gene Therapy for Cardiovascular Disease

Although drug therapy is available for the treatment of cardiovascular disease, cardiovascular morbidity and mortality are poorly controlled throughout the world. Many of the pharmacological agents used to treat cardiovascular disease are expensive and therefore unavailable to poor segments of all societies. The available drugs are transient or short lasting in effect (usually <24 h), have adverse side effects, and are not highly specific. Pharmacological therapy only partly mitigates cardiovascular complications. In addition, repeated doses and increased doses are required for long-term and chronic control of hypertension and related cardiovascular disease. Most cardiovascular disease (hypertension, cardiac hypertrophy, and so on) is multifactorial and multigenic; however, the drugs used for controlling the disease are aimed at relatively few targets. Most patients with heart diseases are excluded from consideration for cardiac transplantation because of their medical complications and the short-age of donors. Clearly, it is imperative to develop new approaches to the treat-ment of cardiovascular disease. Gene therapy offers the possibility of producing longer lasting effects with precise specificity based on the genetic design. Indeed, gene therapy opens a promising and novel avenue, although this new approach is in its early, experimental, stage and so far has been short on clini-cal success.

2.1. Considerations for Gene Therapy

2.1.1. The Vector System

An effective and efficient vector system is essential for delivering therapeu-tic genes. Gene therapy uses a variety of gene transfer techniques. Some gene therapy approaches to cardiovascular disease are reviewed in Chapter 2. Advantages and disadvantages of some of the virus- and nonvirus-mediated gene delivery methods are discussed in this chapter. A vector is chosen accord-ing to its delivering efficiency, size, safety, and stability. Of note, only a few of the currently available viral vectors achieve efficient, high-level transgene ex-pression in postmitotic cells, such as cardiomyocytes. These include recombi-nant adenovirus *(1)*, adeno-associated virus *(2)*, and lentivirus *(3)*. To illustrate, if one compares the vector with computer hardware, the software would be the therapeutic gene with its regulatory gene sequence. The latter gives scientists the opportunity to design an efficient therapeutic gene for a specific disease.

Hypoxia-inducible double plasmids represent an exemplary gene-engineer-ing design (Chapter 3), which can switch on protective genes either to depress the metabolic rate or to increase blood supply to the ischemic tissue when the tissue oxygen level decreases to a dangerous level. Adenovirus is not safe as a vector for human gene therapy *(4)* because of its propensity to initiate inflam-mation in the host. However, adenovirus is still widely used in the laboratory because of its high transduction efficiency, easy and fast packaging, transduc-tion of both dividing and nondividing cells, and success in delivering genes to cells and animals. The ability to clone transgenes as large as 8 kb into replica-tion-deficient adenoviral vectors has resulted in more efficient transgene expression in cardiac and vascular tissues.

The construction and packaging of adenoviruses with human endothelial nitric oxide synthase (eNOS) is described in Chapter 7. The authors demon-strate that human eNOS can be expressed in both human aortic endothelial cells and rat heart cells, providing an interesting and promising approach for testing human gene expression in animals *(5)*.

RNA interference (RNAi) is emerging as an important biological strategy for gene silencing and potentially could be a powerful tool for gene therapy.

Small interfering RNA (siRNA)-mediated reduction in gene expression has been accomplished in mammalian cell culture by transfecting synthetic RNA oligonucleotides or plasmids, with the requirement that fragments be <30 bp to ensure specificity. Application of siRNA to in vivo gene silencing in mammalian tissues would require expression from intracellular transcription rather than transient transfection of dsRNA. Virus-mediated delivery of siRNA has been shown to be effective in reducing expression of targeted genes specifically in various cell types, both in vitro and in vivo *(6)*.

2.1.2. Vector Delivery

The vector must be delivered, directly or indirectly, to the target organ or tissue, such as the heart. Employment of tissue-specific promoter is an ideal approach to achieve tissue-specific gene expression or inhibition. For example, the use of α-MHC promoter will allow target gene expression and inhibition specifically in the heart. Chapters 2 and 4 describe gene delivery approaches relevant to cardiovascular therapy.

2.1.3. Regulatory Mechanism

A regulatory mechanism (sequence) should be incorporated into the vector to control transgene expression or inhibition, for optimal treatment. The ideal promoter should be specific for the target cell type in the tissue and should be active for prolonged periods to maintain consistent levels of transgene expression. Thus, the promoter needs mechanisms to switch them on or off as required by pathological conditions. This hypothesis is being tested with the tetracycline transactivator system, by which a transgene can be switched on or off in the presence or absence of tetracycline *(7)*. However, the tetracycline regulatory mechanism is leaky and therefore unsatisfactory. Obviously, a successful and reliable regulatory mechanism is needed before virus-mediated gene therapy can be used in humans. This is a weak area that requires significant advances.

2.1.4. Reporter Genes

Reporter genes should be employed to monitor real-time, tissue-specific transgene expression. Strategies for using conditional gene expression in myocardium are reviewed in Chapter 8.

Finally, bridging the gap between these basic investigative studies and clinical gene therapy is a formidable but not insurmountable task. Experimental proof in rodents will need to be extended to large-animal models with clinical grade vectors and delivery systems to assess both efficacy and safety.

3. Stem Cell Therapy for Cardiovascular Disease

The adult mammalian heart lacks the potential for effective regeneration. The infarcted myocardium is usually transformed into a noncontractile fibrous scar. This remodeling process leads to expansion of the initial infarcted area and dilatation of the left ventricular lumen *(8)*. A novel and attractive approach to the cure of ischemic heart disease is the use of stem cells *(9–13)*. Pluripotent stem cells are cells that have not taken on the identity of any specific cell type and are not yet committed to any dedicated function; they can divide indefinitely and may be induced to give rise to one or more specialized cell types. Murry et al. *(14)* and Balsam et al. *(15)* recently reported that hematopoietic stem cells failed to transdifferentiate into cardiac myocytes in myocardial infarcts. The stem cells, however, developed into different blood cell types, despite being in the heart. Thus, for physicians, the use of stem cell therapy in treating cardiac-muscle diseases remains a worthy, but perhaps long-term, goal. For scientists, how to effectively induce stem cells to differentiate into specific cell types is the key to the success of stem cell therapy. Although there is proof of concept that transplantation of muscle cell progenitors may improve function after a heart attack, the task is to find the ideal source of cells. Therefore, it may be necessary to search for naturally occurring, authentic cardiac progenitors and to identify and dissect the signals that guide their migration and differentiation. An understanding of the biology of embryonic cardiac progenitors during development may offer new clues to cardiac stem cell therapy.

Chapter 15 describes an exemplary approach to the study of endothelial progenitor cells in the regeneration of vascular endothelial cells. Since stem cell therapy is still in its experimental stage, there is a distinct advantage to evaluating many different types of stem cells, which will eventually lead to successful selection of optimal cells for cardiac stem cell therapy. Chapters 10 and 13 offer protocols for myocardial repair using embryonic stem cells and fetal cardiac myocytes. It has been reported that fetal heart cells might be optimal for heart-cell transplantation therapy *(16)* because they graft easily, adopt the identity of an adult cardiac cell without fusion, and are electrically coupled. However, the ethical controversy that surrounds their use in scientific research means that fetal stem cells may not be used in clinical studies, at least for the foreseeable future. Protocols for autologous mesenchymal stem cells and skeletal myoblasts for myocardial repair are provided in Chapters 11 and 12. It has been reported that mesenchymal stem cells modified with Akt prevent remodeling and restore performance of infarcted hearts *(17)*. Therefore, the use of stem cells genetically engineered with the desired genes increases the potential of stem cell therapy.

4. Gene Analysis in the Injured and Hypertrophied Heart

Accumulating evidence indicates that cardiovascular diseases are associated with changes in gene expression. Identification of new candidate genes involved in heart disease will provide the molecular basis for diagnosis, prevention, and intervention. It is important to determine whether the changes in gene expression cause heart diseases or are secondary to heart diseases.

Cardiac hypertrophy is the most common risk factor contributing to cardiovascular mortality and morbidity. The pathogenesis of cardiac hypertrophy is multifactorial, with genetic background and environmental stress as two critical components. In some cases, the development of cardiac hypertrophy is the result of compensatory responses of the heart to increased hemodynamic load. However, some forms of cardiac hypertrophy are independent of pressure overload *(18,19)*. Endocrine factors (catecholamines, angiotensin II, thyroxine hormone, cytokines, and so on) or primary genetic abnormalities can cause cardiac hypertrophy. It is possible that cardiac hypertrophy is a multigenic disease.

It is interesting that different mutations inducing hypertrophic cardiomyopathy are associated with different prognoses and survival times. With respect to the genetic diagnosis of cardiac diseases such as hypertrophic cardiomyopathy or the long QT syndrome, it has become possible to characterize genetic mutations responsible for some heart diseases. Chapters 16 and 17 provide protocols for delineating and evaluating genes involved in cardiac hypertrophy in response to pressure overload. Perhaps a better way to determine the role of a specific gene in pressure-overload hypertrophy is to evaluate the hypertrophic response of rodents lacking or overexpressing this gene (Chapter 22). Angiotensinogen gene knockout did not affect the development of cardiac hypertrophy in cold-exposed mice *(19)*, suggesting that the renin–angiotensin system (RAS) is not involved in cold-induced cardiac hypertrophy, which is independent of pressure overload. Similarly, mice lacking AT_{1A} receptors develop cardiac hypertrophy to the same extent as wild-type mice do in response to aortic banding or chronic cold exposure *(20,21)*, indicating that AT_{1A} receptors do not play a role in these models of cardiac hypertrophy. However, the RAS and AT_{1A} receptors have been reported to play a role in some forms of cardiac hypertrophy *(22,23)*. Upregulation of the AT_1 receptor gene may be involved in human cardiac hypertrophy *(24)*. Thus, molecular mechanisms mediating hypertrohpic responses vary with models of cardiac hypertrophy.

Microarray analysis of gene expression is a useful tool for mapping gene expression profiles in the injured or hypertrophied heart. Chapter 20 provides technical information and experimental protocols for using Affymetrix oligonucleotide analysis of gene expression. Several intracellular signaling pathways are known to be involved in the pathogenesis of cardiac hypertrophy.

Methods for detecting cardiac signaling in the hypertrophied heart are detailed in Chapter 19.

Chapter 18 documents widely used protocols for detecting and quantifying apoptosis in cardiovascular tissues. Knowledge of the role of apoptosis in cardiac diseases will help in the development of approaches to the control of apoptosis, which is believed to be involved in cardiovascular abnormalities such as cardiac hypertrophy, myocardial infarction, and atherosclerosis. Altered β-adrenergic receptor gene regulation and signaling can result in cardiac malfunctions. The β-adrenergic receptor is a well-known therapeutic target for cardiac dysfunction. Methods for the detection of altered β-adrenergic signaling pathways in hypertrophied hearts are provided in Chapter 23. The proto-oncogene c-*myc* mediates cell growth and proliferation in many cell types. Inducible activation of c-*myc* in adult myocardium in vivo provokes cardiac myocyte hypertrophy and reactivation of DNA synthesis *(25)*. Enhanced expression of c-*myc*, c-*fos*, and H-*ras* genes are found in cardiac hypertrophy and cardiac dilation in patients *(26)*. Thus, biomechanical stress-induced cardiac myocyte hypertrophy is accompanied by changes in several intracellular signals, including oncogene expression.

5. Transgenic Techniques in Cardiovascular Research

Rapid advances in molecular genetics have heralded a new era of genetic cardiology to study cardiovascular function and disease at the molecular level. Since the first cardiac-specific transgenic mouse was created in 1988 *(27)*, hundreds of transgenic or gene-targeted murine models have been generated for the overexpression, genetic ablation, or site-specific mutation of key proteins governing cardiac structure and function. Transgenic techniques are powerful and valuable tools for cardiovascular research whereby transgenic animal models are produced to mimic human cardiovascular diseases. This has provided scientists with a unique approach to the study of the role of a particular gene in cardiovascular disease. However, transgenic animals are not available to all cardiovascular researchers, and most laboratories are unable to generate particular transgenic animal models when needed owing to technical difficulties. This book includes three chapters documenting updated techniques and useful protocols for the successful production of transgenic models for cardiac research. It is expected that these exemplary chapters will stimulate the generation of additional novel transgenic animal models for cardiac research.

Chapter 24 offers technical protocols necessary for the generation of mouse models that overexpress different sarcoplasmic reticulum Ca^{2+} ATPase (SERCA) isoforms and a SERCA2 knockout mouse model with decreased SERCA levels. Chapter 25 describes detailed methods for the maintenance and breeding of two diabetic animal models, OVE26 and agouti mice, for type 1 and type 2 diabetes, respectively. Protocols for producing cardiac-targeted transgenic mice are presented in this chapter. Transgenic rats overexpressing the AT_1 receptor in cardiomyocytes offer an excellent paradigm for studying a target gene in a specific type of cell or tissue (Chapter 26). The transgenic rat is more suitable than the mouse for studying the role of the AT_1 receptor in cardiac function and heart diseases. Thus, the generation of transgenic animals and the subsequent phenotypic characterization of these genetic manipulations in intact animals and isolated hearts have greatly enhanced our current knowledge of cardiac development, Ca^{2+} handling, excitation–contraction coupling, receptor-mediated signal transduction, and heart disease processes. Ultimately, these advances will help identify optimal therapeutic targets for heart diseases.

Thus, molecular cardiology has initiated new and exciting approaches to the study of cardiovascular diseases. These new approaches have challenged traditional cardiology in many ways, including disease pathogenesis, diagnosis, and treatment. Gene analysis and transgenic techniques have provided a new understanding of cardiovascular disease pathogenesis. Gene therapy and cell therapy have provided physicians and scientists with novel ideas for the treatment of heart diseases, although there is a lack of clinical success at this time. Therefore, there is an urgent demand for significant and rapid advances in molecular cardiology. These advances largely depend on the development of innovative technology in molecular and cellular biology.

References

1. Schneider, M. D. and French, B. A. (1993) The advent of adenovirus: gene therapy for cardiovascular disease. *Circulation* **88,** 1937–1942.
2. Svensson, E. C., Marshall, D. J., Woodard, K., et al. (1999) Efficient and stable transduction of cardiomyocytes after intramyocardial injection or intracoronary perfusion with recombinant adeno-associated virus vectors. *Circulation* **99,** 201–205.
3. Sakoda, T., Kasahara, N., Hamamori, Y., and Kedes, L. (1993) A high-titer lentiviral production system mediates efficient transduction of differentiated cells including beating cardiac myocytes. *J. Mol. Cell. Cardiol.* **31,** 2037–2047.
4. Stolberg, S. G. (1999) The biotech death of Jesse Gelsinger. *New York Times,* November 28.
5. Wang, W. and Sun, Z. (2004) eNOS gene delivery attenuates cold-induced hypertension (CIH). *FASEB J.* **18,** A1221, 823.4 (abstract).
6. Xia, H., Mao, Q., Paulson, H., and Davidson, B. L. (2002) siRNA- mediated gene silencing *in vitro* and *in vivo. Nature Biotechnol.* **20,** 1006–1010.
7. Huentelman, M. J., Teschemacher, A. G., Paton, J. F. R., Raizada, M. K., and Kasparov S. (2004) Evaluation of tetracycline response element (TRE)-based genetic switches for control of gene expression in adeno- and lentiviral vectors. *FASEB J.* **18,** A1221, 823.5 (abstract).

8. Pfeffer, J. M., Pfeffer, M. A., Fletcher, P. F., and Braunwarld, E. (1991) Progressive ventricular remodeling in rat with myocardium infarction. *Am. J. Physiol.* **260,** 1406–1414.

9. Fukuda, K. (2003) Application of mesenchymal stem cells for the regeneration of cardiomyocyte and its use for cell transplantation therapy. *Hum. Cell.* **16,** 83–94.

10. Kand, H. J., Kim, H. S., Zhang, S. Y., et al. (2004) Effects of intracoronary infusion of peripheral blood stem-cells mobilised with granulocyte-colony stimulating factor on left ventricular systolic function and restenosis after coronary stenting in myocardial infarction: the MAGIC cell randomised clinical trial. *Lancet* **6,** 751–756.

11. Ozbaran, M., Omay, S. B., Nalbantgil, S., et al. (2004) Autologous peripheral stem cell transplantation in patients with congestive heart failure due to ischemic heart disease. *Eur. J. Cardiothorac. Surg.* **25,** 342–350.

12. Ott, H. C., Bonaros, N., Marksteiner, R., et al. (2004) Combined transplantation of skeletal myoblasts and bone marrow stem cells for myocardial repair in rats. *Eur. J. Cardiothorac. Surg.* **25,** 627–634.

13. Menasche, P. (2004) Skeletal myoblast transplantation for cardiac repair. *Expert. Rev. Cardiovasc. Ther.* **2,** 21–28.

14. Murry, C. E., Soonpaa, M. H., Reinecke, H., et al. (2004) Haematopoietic stem cells do not transdifferentiate into cardiac myocytes in myocardial infarcts. *Nature* **428,** 664–668.

15. Basam, L. B., Wagers, A. J., Christensen, J. L., Kofidis, T., Weissman, I. L., and Robbins, R. C. (2004) Haematopoietic stem cells adopt mature haematopoietic fates in ischaemic myocardium. *Nature* **428,** 668–673.

16. Dowell, J. D., Rubart, M., Pasumarthi, K. B., Soonpaa, M. H., and Field, L. J. (2003) Myocyte and myogenic stem cell transplantation in the heart. *Cardiovasc. Res.* **58,** 336–350.

17. Mangi, A. A., Noiseux, N., Kong, D., et al. (2003) Mesenchymal stem cells modified with Akt prevent remodeling and restore performance of infracted hearts. *Nature Med.* **9,** 1195–1201.

18. Sun, Z., Cade, R., Fregly, M. J., and Rowland, N. E. (1997) Effect of chronic treatment with propranolol on the cardiovascular responses to chronic cold exposure. *Physiol. Behav.* **62,** 379–384.

19. Sun, Z., Zhang, Z., and Cade, R. (2003) Angiotensinogen gege knockout delays and attenuates cold-induced hypertension. *Hypertension* **41,** 322–327.

20. Hamawaki, M., Coffman, T. M., Lashus, A., et al. (1998) Pressure-overload hypertrophy is unabated in mice devoid of AT_{1A} receptor. *Am. J. Physiol.* **274,** H868–H873.

21. Sun, Z., Wang, X., and Cade, R. (2003) AT_{1A} receptors are essential to the development of cold-induced hypertension. *Circulation* **108,** 421.

22. Green, D. L., Malhotra, A., and Scheuer, J. (1993) Angiotensin II increases cardiac protein synthesis in adult rat heart. *Am. J. Phsiol.* **265,** H238–H243.

23. Waeber, B. and Brunner, H. R. (1996) Cardiovascular hypertrophy: role of angiotensin II and bradykinin. *J. Cardiovasc. Pharmacol.* **27,** S36–S40.

24. Ohtani, S., Fujiwara, H., Hasegawa, K., et al. (1997) Upregulated expression of angiotensin II type 1 receptor gene in human pathologic hearts. *J. Card. Fail.* **3,** 303–310.
25. Xiao, G., Mao S., Baumgarten, G., et al. (2001) Inducible activation of c-Myc in adult myocardium in vivo provokes cardiac myocyte hypertrophy and reactivation of DNA synthesis. *Circ. Res.* **89,** 1122–1129.
26. Kroumpouzou, E., Gomatos, I. P., Kataki, A., Karayannis, M., Dangas, G. D., and Toutouzas, P. (2003) Common pathways for primary hypertrophic and dilated cardiomyopathy. *Hybrid. Hybridomics.* **22,** 41–45.
27. Field, L. J. (1988) Atrial natriuretic factor-SV 40 Tantigen transgenes produce tumors and cardiac arrhythmias in mice. *Science* **239,** 1029–1033.

II

GENE TRANSFER AND GENE THERAPY FOR CARDIOVASCULAR DISEASE

2

Gene Therapy Approaches to Cardiovascular Disease

J. Mark Jones and Walter J. Koch

Summary

The potential of enhanced cardiovascular function via gene therapy has aroused extensive interest. Both viral and nonviral vectors have shown promise in the realm of cardiovascular gene therapy. Modification of vectors or addition of further transgenes to the expression cassette has permitted targeted and regulated gene expression. The many potential targets of cardiovascular gene therapy can be considered under the following headings: vascular, congenital heart disease, and myocardial. Cardiac gene delivery may be to either the endothelium of either native coronary vessels or coronary artery bypass grafts, or to the myocardium. Myocardial gene delivery is possible either via direct myocardial injection or via the coronary vasculature.

However, alteration of any cardiac cellular signaling pathway may have cardiotoxic effects. Thus, any genes that appear to cause enhanced cardiac function, must undergo extensive toxicity studies in animals before similar experiments are performed in human subjects. The techniques described may be utilized in the future to deliver various genes targeted to combat many different disease processes, in different animal models, and ultimately to provide feasible gene therapy approaches to human cardiovascular disease.

Key Words: Gene transfer; viral vector; nonviral vector; transcriptional targeting; translational targeting; regulatable transgene expression; intracoronary; coronary catheterization; cardiac surgery; cardiopulmonary bypass; cardiac-selective; adrenergic receptor; vascular; endothelial; myocardium.

From: *Methods in Molecular Medicine, vol. 112: Molecular Cardiology: Methods and Protocol.*
Edited by: Z. Sun © Humana Press Inc., Totowa, NJ

1. Introduction

The potential of enhanced cardiovascular function via gene therapy approaches has aroused extensive interest *(1–4)*, and in this chapter we review some of the major areas. First, the role of both viral and nonviral vectors in the realm of cardiovascular gene therapy is considered. Second, the methods of targeted and regulated gene expression by modification of the vector or addition of further transgenes to the expression cassette are explored. Third, an overview is given of some of the existing animal models whereby vector delivery can be achieved. Finally, we discuss the potential targets of cardiovascular gene therapy.

2. Vectors Available for Cardiac Gene Therapy

Many vectors have been advocated for gene transfer. These may be classified as either viral or nonviral *(5,6)*.

2.1. Viral Vectors

The viral genome contains the essential viral genes, genes required for replication and structural products, and a packaging domain. These regions are surrounded by regulatory sequences. After cell entry, replication and associated activity of the early genes occurs. This is followed by activity of the late genes and packaging of new viral particles prior to release of these new virions *(7)*.

Generation of a viral vector system involves the creation of vector DNA as well as helper DNA (**Fig. 1**). Vector DNA contains the regulatory sequences and a packaging domain, but a therapeutic expression cassette replaces the essential viral genes. This vector DNA is incapable of replication without the assistance of the helper DNA. The helper DNA contains the essential viral genes surrounded by regulatory sequences placed in a heterologous or unrelated DNA context. This may be a plasmid, a helper virus, or the host chromosomal DNA of the packaging cell. The helper DNA does not contain a packaging domain, and thus, in itself, is incapable of producing new virions *(6)*.

2.1.1. Adenovirus

Adenoviruses have a 36-kb double-stranded DNA genome that contains five early transcription units (E1A, E1B, E2, E3, and E4), two delayed early units (IX and IVa2), and one late unit (major late). This late unit is processed to generate five families of late mRNAs (L1–L5). Following cell entry, proteins in the viral particle are efficient at endosomal lysis. This allows the virus to escape, and subsequently the genome enters the nucleus. The E1 gene acts as a master transcriptional regulator originating the process of viral gene expression leading to viral replication. E1 in combination with the E2 and E4 genes is required for viral genome replication. E3 genes are dispensible for the viral life

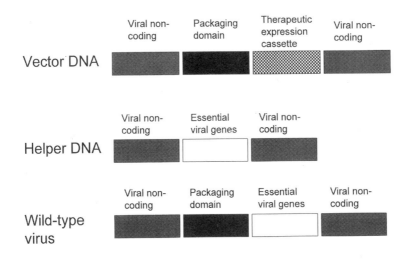

Fig. 1. Engineering virus into vector.

cycle. "Late" genes encode viral structural protein genes that are transcribed, allowing for encapsidation of the newly replicated genomes *(8)*.

First-generation adenoviral vectors have an E1 deletion. The E1 deleted viral genome containing the transgene is added to a cell line that contains a stable E1a expression cassette. This allows the added DNA to replicate and be packaged into E1 deleted vectors, which, in theory, are not capable of replication. However, even in the absence of E1 gene products, transcription occurs at a low rate, inducing an early inflammatory cytokine response. This is followed by an antigen-dependent immune response that includes the cell-mediated destruction of transduced cells *(9)*. The E3 gene may play a role in immune surveillance in infected hosts and deletion of it may offer protection against some of the immune-mediated responses directed against the vector or vector-transduced cells.

There are more than 50 different human adenoviral serotypes *(8)*. The possibility of using adenovirus as a vector was demonstrated following systemic intravenous delivery in neonatal mice *(10)*. This resulted in widespread β-galactosidase (β-gal) expression that persisted for almost 1 yr *(11)*. Adenoviral vectors can efficiently infect nondividing cells. The DNA remains episomal, rather than being incorporated into the host cell chromosome, although the period of persistence of the episomal genes is unknown. Current vectors are primarily derived from types 2 and 5, the most common serotypes to which adults have been exposed. It may be possible to use other serotypes or nonhuman adenovirus to avoid potential problems related to preexisting immunity.

Secondary vector delivery using a different serotyped capsid has also been demonstrated in animal models *(12)*. Adenoviral vectors have many favorable characteristics suggesting their utilization as vectors for gene transfer. They can infect a wide range of target cells including nondividing cells, and they can be produced in high titers with relative ease. Despite initial concerns over the possibility of germline gene insertion, it appears that adenoviruses cannot infect oocytes and so the risk of female germline transduction is low *(13)*. However, limitations include the generation of an inflammatory and immune response, which may be related to the relatively short duration of gene expression *(14–18)*. To avoid the immune response to the vector, it may be possible to use newer, improved adenoviral vectors. An adenoviral vector with deletion of E2b, in addition to E1 and E3, has diminished late adenoviral gene expression compared with the conventional vector *(19)*. This vector can also be produced with relative ease in large quantities and so may be suitable for large animal studies.

Recent interest has focused on high-capacity, "gutted" or "gutless" adenoviral vectors *(20,21)*. These vectors have two main advantages over earlier generation adenoviral vectors. First, all viral coding sequences are deleted from the vector genome, so that viral proteins are not expressed from the vector, thus reducing its toxicity. Second, with the absence of viral coding sequences, the capacity for incorporation of heterologous DNA is increased to 36 kb, allowing the simultaneous expression of several genes, large cDNAs, and regulatory elements. However, transgene expression with "gutted" adenoviral vectors has been shown to be lower than with earlier generation adenoviral vectors, although this was corrected by addition of the E4 region of the adenovirus genome *(20)*. It has been established that additional stuffer DNA has to be included in a "gutted" adenoviral vector genome if the gene or the expression cassette that is incorporated is less than 27 kb in size. This stuffer DNA may contain nuclear matrix attachment regions which can also influence gene expression *(21)*.

2.1.2. Adeno-Associated Virus

Adeno-associated virus (AAV) is a human parvovirus that is not able to replicate unless a helper virus, such as adenovirus or herpesvirus, is present in the same cell. There are six known human serotypes but AAV-2 has been the major focus of attention. AAV has not been linked to human disease and can infect a wide range of target cells, establishing latent infection by integration into the cell genome. The viral genome consists of two genes, the *rep* gene required for viral genome replication and the *cap* gene, which encodes structural proteins. These two genes are flanked by viral inverted terminal repeats (ITRs). AAV vectors can be produced by adding separate plasmids containing the ITRs flanking the therapeutic gene cassette, the *rep* and *cap* genes, and the addition of a helper adenovirus or another plasmid containing the essential adenoviral helper genes *(6)*. AAV efficiently transduces both dividing and non-dividing cells, through both episomal transgene expression and by random chromosomal integration. It has given stable β-gal expression 8 wk after vector delivery by intramuscular cardiac injection to mice and 6 mo expression after intracoronary delivery to the pig circumflex artery, with no evidence of cardiac inflammation or myocardial necrosis *(22,23)*. This may be owing to the absence of viral coding sequences from the AAV vector genome. However, the maximum transgene size is approx 5 kb, and production is currently very labor-intensive; this may improve with recent advances. Furthermore, it is not usually produced in as high a titer as recombinant adenovirus *(24)*. In vivo expression has a delayed onset with minimal expression until 1 mo *(25)*. This may be related to a requirement for generation of double-stranded (ds) DNA genomes by either vector single-stranded (ss) DNA annealing, or second-strand synthesis followed by vector genome linking. Moreover, vector genome linking has allowed effective doubling of the limited coding capacity by splitting an expression cassette into two vectors and administering them simultaneously *(6)*.

2.1.3. Retrovirus

Retroviruses encode RNA-dependent DNA polymerase, reverse transcriptase, which converts the viral ss RNA genome to ds DNA, which is then inserted into the host chromosome. For this integration to occur, the infected cell must undergo mitosis shortly after infection, thus limiting the delivery of DNA to replicating cells. Retroviral genomes have two long terminal repeat (LTR) sequences at their ends. These frame the *gag, pol,* and *env* genes encoding the structural proteins, nucleic acid polymerases/integrases, and surface glycoprotein, respectively. A transgene of up to 8 kb can be inserted and expressed in place of the viral genes, which are expressed by heterologous transcriptional signals from two separate constructs lacking most viral *cis*-acting sequences and stably incorporated in packaging cell lines. This split construct design improves vector safety by increasing the number of recombination events required to reconstruct a replication-competent genome.

Lentiviruses have a more complex genome, which encodes two additional regulatory genes, *tat* and *rev*, essential for expression of the genome, and a variable set of accessory genes. Unlike retroviruses, they rely on active transport of the preintegration complex into the nucleus of the target cell, which allows integration into the host genome in the absence of replication. In addition, they do not trigger an inflammatory response. Safety concerns remain regarding the use of these members of the human immunodeficiency virus (HIV) family, including potential mutation into its pathogenic phenotype. New generations of vectors that contain only the essential packaging genes may increase vector biosafety. Moreover, self-inactivating transfer vectors contain a deletion in the downstream LTR that, when transduced into target cells, results in the transcriptional inactivation of the upstream LTR and reduces the risk of vector recombination *(6,26)*. A lentivirus-based vector system has been developed that can transduce nondividing cardiac myocytes and integrate the transgene into the genome of target cells *(27)*. However, generation of lentiviral vectors is also labor-intensive. Moreover, the issue of attenuation of gene expression owing to vector silencing remains unresolved. It has been suggested that multiple integration events may need to be achieved for long-term expression, since probably only a proportion of the integrated vectors remain transcriptionally active *(26)*. Restraints are placed on the viral genome by the obligatory RNA step in the retroviral life cycle such that the transgene expression cassette must be of limited size and without introns or internal polyadenylation signals *(6)*.

A summary of some characteristics of these viral vectors is shown in **Table 1**.

2.2. Nonviral Vectors

Cationic liposomes rely on receptor-mediated endocytosis or fusion of cell membranes. Negatively charged DNA is contained within a positively charged lipid vesicle. Plasmid DNA is released in the cytoplasm, but only a small proportion of it enters the nucleus. There it remains separate from the host genome and is associated with transient transgene expression. Liposomes have a favorable safety profile. They contain no viral sequences, and, unlike viral vectors, they have no cDNA size constraints in vector construction. Efficiency of transfection is enhanced in proliferating cells, although cell division is not required *(5,27)*. The role of nonviral vectors has been thought to be limited owing to their markedly reduced efficiency of myocardial gene transfer *(5,28–30)*. However, in a functional heterotopic rabbit heart transplant model, despite lower efficiency of liposome-mediated gene transfer, the efficacy of liposome-mediated interleukin-10 gene transfer was much higher than that mediated by adenovirus. Significant negative inotropic and arrhythmogenic adverse effects on transplanted hearts were observed owing to viral cytotoxic and immune responses, which attenuated the therapeutic efficacy of the first-generation adenovirus-mediated gene therapy *(31)*. A carrier system incorporating low-density lipoprotein (LDL), lipids, and plasmid DNA has demonstrated enhanced myocardial transfection, which may be related to LDL receptor-mediated endocytosis *(32)*.

Plasmid DNA and RNA can be directly injected into skeletal and cardiac muscle. Antisense oligonucleotides are short DNA sequences complementary to the RNA message of interest. These are chemically modified to resist nuclease degradation. After direct injection, much of it is degraded in the intra-

Table 1
Properties of Different Viral Vectors for Cardiovascular Gene Therapy

	Adenovirus	Adeno-associated virus (AAV)	Retrovirus
Ease of production	Produced in high titers with ease	Moderately high titers but labor-intensive	Low titers
Onset of expression	Early	Delayed	Delayed
Duration of expression	Short term	Prolonged	Prolonged but vector silencing may occur
Infect nondividing cells	Yes	Yes	No, except lentivirus
Inflammatory/immune response	Marked, but reduced with "gutted" adenovirus	Relatively nonimmuno-genic	Relatively nonimmuno-genic
Integration into host genome	No, episomal	Both episomal and chromosomal insertion	Chromosomal insertion, potential for mutagenesis

cellular lysosomal compartment. Only a fraction, therefore, escapes intracellular or extracellular degradation. Transfection efficiency is lower than with liposome complexes and adenoviral vectors *(28,29)*. The nucleotide sequence hybridizes to target RNA, which prevents translation of RNA. However, antisense oligonucleotides bind to other mRNAs showing partial similarity to the complementary target RNA, and even to various proteins, which can cause altered functional characteristics *(5,30)*.

3. Regulation of Gene Expression

Expression levels of an introduced gene depend mostly on the transduction efficiency of the vector and on the strength of the transcriptional regulatory elements. Typically, strong and ubiquitously active viral promoters such as human cytomegalovirus (CMV) have been used to drive transgene expression *(33)*. A complication of protracted, unrestricted gene expression, which could be offered by many of the newer viral vectors, is the potential for deleterious side effects *(34)*. Thus, it has been suggested that regulatable promoters and vectors are required *(35)*. Several systems for controlling exogenous transgene expression have been used including steroid hormones such as glucocorticoids *(36)*. A limitation of using steroids is the interference of endogenous gene expression. The tetracycline-controllable expression system enables tight on/off regulation, high inducibility, fast response times, no pleitropic effect owing to the use of the tetracycline operon derived from bacteria, and a well-characterized inducer, namely, tetracycline or doxycycline *(37)*. Two types of system, tet-off and tet-on, have been used to regulate transgene expression. In the tet-off system, the tetracycline-responsive transcriptional activator (tTA) induces the transcription of a gene containing the tet-responsive element, and transcription is turned off in the presence of tetracycline. In the tet-on system, the reverse tetracycline-responsive transcriptional activator (rtTA), binds to the tet-responsive element and turns on the transcription in the presence of tetracycline. In an adenovirus-mediated tetracycline-controllable expression system, the tet-off system was demonstrated to be functionally superior, in terms of tightly regulatable transgene expression *(38)*.

The acetylation state of histones is correlated with gene expression, in that deacetylated histones are associated with repressed gene expression. A single vector system that contained a chimeric tetracycline repressor, which interacts with histone deacetylases, and a tetracycline-sensitive promoter was created. In vitro experiments showed tight control of gene expression in a doxycycline dose- and time-dependent fashion *(39)*. Tetracycline regulation has been combined with glucocorticoid regulation in chimeric promoters *(40)*. Tetracycline-dependent lentiviral vectors have also been developed, resulting in efficient regulation of transgene expression *(41)*. A hypoxia-regulatory element, which is activated by transactivating hypoxia-inducible factor (HIF)-1 in response to a reduction in oxygen has been combined with a cardiac-specific promoter in an AAV vector. This "vigilant vector" has been tested to give proof of principle that therapeutic genes could be switched on in the heart during times of ischemic stress *(42)*.

4. Transductional and Transcriptional Targeting

Gene expression following systemic adenoviral vector delivery is affected by the natural tropism of the virus for the coxsackie/adenoviral receptor (CAR). CAR is expressed to high levels in the liver, which consequently has a high capacity for nonspecific vector uptake. Transductional targeting alters the natural infection pathway and can be performed by pseudotyping, whereby modulation of the viral envelope allows manipulation of viral vector cell targeting specificity. This has been performed in a range of vectors including adenovirus, AAV, and lentivirus *(43)*. It has been possible to perform transductional targeting to, for example, the pulmonary endothelium *(44)*.

Transcriptional targeting via tissue-specific promoters has also been investigated. A suitable cardiac-specific promoter is the myosin light chain *(42,45)*. An additional benefit of tissue-specific promoters is the reduction of gene expression in antigen-presenting cells, thus reducing the host immune response *(46)*. However, a limiting factor in the use of tissue-specific promoters is the lower level of expression compared with their viral counterparts, such as the CMV promoter. This can be overcome by constructing synthetic promoter libraries or by exploiting endogenous genomic sequences that enhance tissue-specific expression *(47)*. A further problem with such tissue-specific promoters is that the selectivity of some promoters is altered or lost when they are placed in the context of an adenoviral genome. It has been demonstrated that enhancer elements or transcription start sites within the adenoviral sequences surrounding the transgene expression cassette interact with the promoter elements, which can activate transcription in nontarget cells *(48,49)*.

5. Animal Models

Cardiac gene delivery can be performed with targeting of genes to the endothelium of either native coronary vessels or coronary artery bypass grafts, or to the myocardium. Myocardial gene delivery can be performed either via direct myocardial injection or via the coronary vasculature. Direct myocardial injection requires multiple injections causing high levels of gene expression within a 1.5-cm radius of the site of injection *(50–52)*.

Intracoronary delivery of vector in a Langendorff perfused heart model has shown that prolonged contact time with the virus improves gene transfer *(53)*. Adenoviral-mediated gene transfer has been achieved during transplantation of rat and rabbit hearts, but this technique is limited to viral exposure of the donor heart prior to transplantation *(54–56)*. Intracoronary delivery in rats and rabbits has been performed during thoracotomy, with the aorta cross-clamped and the virus introduced by injection into the left ventricle (LV) cavity *(57–60)*. Owing to the occluded aorta, LV ejection forces the virus down the coronary arteries. However, the acute pressure overload of the LV limits the period of cross-clamping to a matter of seconds. A more clinically applicable method of gene delivery is direct catheterization of the right or left coronary artery. Here too, exposure of the heart to the virus is limited. Present systems require high infusion pressure to inject the virus, which could result in endothelial or myocardial injury *(61,62)*. Following these methods of gene delivery, the adenovirus was also distributed systemically, and noncardiac tissues have shown evidence of transgene expression *(57,58,63)*. We have therefore developed a cardiac-selective method of vector delivery in which the vector is delivered to the cardioplegic arrested heart following application of an aortic cross-clamp during standard cardiopulmonary bypass (CPB) *(64,65; see* Chapter 4).

Continuous circulation of an adenoviral vector solution through the heart has been suggested as another potential method of gene delivery during CPB, although this requires the use of two separate circuits and oxygenators, unlike the standard approach *(66)*. Gene transfer has been documented using retrograde delivery of vector through the coronary sinus in a porcine beating heart model *(67)*. This is another method that could also be utilized for vector delivery during cardiac surgery. Additional work in the Langendorff perfused rabbit heart suggested that agents that increase endothelial permeability can greatly enhance the efficiency of gene transfer *(68)*. Further experiments have demonstrated that vascular endothelial growth factor (VEGF), which is known to produce a transient increase in microvascular permeability within the coronary circulation, can also enhance escape of virus particles from the vasculature *(69,70)*. Increased myocardial transcapillary gradient and high-pressure infusion of adenoviral vectors are some of the physical methods that have been demonstrated to optimize myocardial gene transfer *(69,71)*. Utilization of these principles has been used to deliver a deficient structural protein, δ-sarcoglycan, to cardiomyopathic hamsters, resulting in a slowing of the progression of LV dysfunction compared with controls. The method of vector delivery involved deep hypothermia to 18–25°C, followed by the delivery of cold crystalloid cardioplegia containing histamine. This allowed homogenous transgene expression in more than 75% of LV myocytes *(72)*.

Of particular pertinence in this setting is the fact that cardioplegia has detrimental effects on endothelial structure and function *(73,74)*. Contact with cardioplegia and the associated relative ischemia may increase endothelial permeability, thus overcoming one of the barriers to adenoviral infection of cardiac myocytes. It is interesting to note that in a transplant heart model adenovirus-mediated gene transfer was enhanced when the vector had a prolonged dwell time during warm ischemia *(75)*. Furthermore, if delivery of a gene that could enhance postoperative cardiac function was possible during CPB, as we have shown with adenoviral-mediated gene transfer of the human β_2-adrenergic receptor (β_2AR), this might be especially desirable toward the end of a prolonged cross-clamp period when impaired cardiac function may be more likely *(76–76b)*.

6. Targets for Cardiac Gene Transfer

6.1. Vascular

A range of targets for vascular gene therapy exists *(5)*. Therapeutic angiogenesis in ischemic myocardium has been attempted in canine and porcine models using VEGF *(51,77)*. In a pacing model of congestive heart failure, adenovirus-mediated VEGF gene transfer improved cardiac function *(78)*. Moreover, a preliminary placebo-controlled, double-blind trial of naked plasmid-mediated VEGF gene transfer in patients with chronic myocardial ischemia demonstrated a statistically significant reduction in anginal class and a trend towards improved exercise duration *(79)*. Fibroblast growth factor (FGF) also stimulates many cell types including endothelial cells *(80)*.

Restenosis following coronary angioplasty is a significant clinical problem. Gene transfer of an inhibitor of β-adrenergic receptor kinase (βARKct) can alter vascular smooth muscle proliferation via G protein-coupled signal transduction and so reduce the severity of restenosis *(81)*. Following peripheral arterial grafting and coronary artery bypass grafting (CABG), venous graft occlusion is linked to neointimal hyperplasia *(82)*. Ex vivo gene transfer of EGF decoy oligonucleotides to saphenous vein grafts has been performed with encouraging results *(83)*. Similar treatment of venous grafts during CABG could be performed *(83a)*. Alternatively, the present model of gene transfer could be utilized during CABG, thus allowing treatment of disease in tissues downstream to the location of the graft, via overexpression of a secreted therapeutic protein from the transduced graft *(84)*.

The etiology of atherosclerosis is multifactorial, and thus many potential targets exist. It may be possible to have cardiac-selective delivery of genes encoding compounds, such as the LDL, very low-density lipoproteins, high-density lipoproteins, or apolipoprotein E, which may alter the progress of atherosclerosis *(24,85)*.

6.2. Congenital Heart Disease

In many congenital cardiac disorders the development of cardiac chambers is abnormal. For example, the arterial switch operation performed for transposition of the great arteries requires that the morphological LV be able to take on the workload of the systemic ventricle postoperatively *(86)*. The βAR system is known to influence myocardial remodeling *(87)*. Delivery of such genes during congenital cardiac surgery may permit "genetic remodeling" and so allow surgery to be performed in infants with a suboptimally prepared LV.

6.3. Myocardial Targets

In vitro gene transfer of the human $β_2AR$ or βARKct to cardiomyocytes isolated from various animal models has confirmed enhanced contraction at the cellular level *(58–60,88)*. Another protein whose expression is altered in heart failure is SERCA2a, which is involved in mobilization of intracellular calcium stores *(89)*. Improved survival and cardiac metabolism after adenoviral-mediated gene transfer of SERCA2a has been shown in a rat model of heart failure *(90)*. Infection of cardiomyocytes, isolated from failing human LV at the time of transplantation, with adenoviral vector containing the SERCA2a gene has documented improved myocyte contraction compared with infection with empty vector *(91)*. Similar experiments have also confirmed that adenoviral gene transfer of antisense phospholamban likewise improves contractile function in failing human cardiomyocytes *(92)*. Proof of benefit of β_2AR and $\beta ARKct$ gene transfer in human tissue has been obtained *(92a)*. Although such in vitro studies have limitations, it will be of interest to document the effects of transfer of the β_2AR and $\beta ARKct$ transgenes in these models prior to undertaking in vivo human clinical studies of gene transfer.

Cardiac-specific overexpression of β_2AR and $\beta ARKct$ is associated with enhanced LV function in transgenic murine models. Moreover, cross-breeding transgenic heart failure models with a $\beta ARKct$-overexpressing strain has confirmed rescue of the failure phenotype *(93–95)*. These beneficial effects have been confirmed in an adenoviral-mediated gene transfer model to rabbits with chronic heart failure subsequent to myocardial infarction *(60)*. Evidence suggests that $\beta ARK1$ inhibition is beneficial in many models of heart failure, perhaps by dampening sympathetic overdrive *(96)*. Moreover, the combination of $\beta ARKct$ expression and chronic βAR antagonism by metoprolol has been shown to increase survival and improve cardiac function in the calsequestrin-overexpressing mouse model of heart failure *(95)*. In a neonatal porcine model we have confirmed that cardioplegic arrest and CPB induces downregulation of the βAR system, with associated impairment of LV function, which can, however, be ameliorated with β_2AR gene transfer *(76b)*. A Langendorff perfused rabbit heart model demonstrated elevation of $\beta ARK1$ following cardioplegic arrest. Interestingly, pretreatment with an adenoviral vector encoding the $\beta ARKct$ transgene restored LV function to normal *(97)*. It would be of further interest to develop an adult porcine model of heart failure and assess whether gene transfer of β_2AR or $\beta ARKct$ has beneficial effects. A suitable model may be rapid pacing, which has already been documented to induce heart failure in pigs *(78,98)*.

β_2AR gene transfer is associated with acute enhancement of cardiac function in a rabbit heterotopic heart transplant model *(99)*. This raises the possibility of using genetic manipulation of β_2AR signaling as an adjunct to mechanical assist devices to facilitate functional myocardial recovery. Polymorphisms of the human β_2AR exist *(100–102)*. In addition, a reengineered β_2AR that responds to synthetic agonists has been described *(103)*. Such targets for gene transfer may allow treatment to be tailored for individuals with particular genetic abnormalities. Alternatively, genes could be overexpressed, but manipulation of the desired effect could be achieved by administration of synthetic pharmacological agents.

A novel cell signaling mechanism has been induced in cardiomyocytes in which a vector encoding the V2 vasopressin receptor was delivered to the heart *(104)*. Cardiomyocytes do not normally express this receptor, but it did couple satisfactorily to the cellular second messenger systems, resulting in enhanced LV function.

Other targets for myocardial gene transfer abound. Myocardial apoptosis involves complex regulated cell suicide machinery, in which two main signaling pathways lead to activation of the caspase family of cysteine proteases. These pathways involve, first, death receptor signaling, via substances such as tumor necrosis factor or Fas, and second, release of cytochrome c from mitochondria and subsequent *trans*-activation of procaspase 9 by apoptosis protease-activating factor. In vitro studies showed that caspase 3 induced sarcomeric disruption and reduced myocyte contractility, whereas adenovirus-mediated gene delivery of a caspase 3 inhibitor enhanced LV function in a rapid pacing model of cardiac failure *(105)*.

Ischemia and oxidative stress are major mechanisms of tissue injury. According to the duration and severity, myocardial ischemia and reperfusion may lead to cell injury and death. Superoxide dismutase (SOD) catalyzes the dismutation of superoxide anion to oxygen and hydrogen peroxide. Ischemic preconditioning is associated with an increase in the activity of manganese SOD, an isoform found in the mitochondrial matrix. In a rat model of ischemia–reperfusion, adenoviral-mediated transfer of manganese SOD reduced infarct size *(106)*. The catalytic byproducts of hemoxygenase (HO-1) exert wide-ranging antioxidant and cytoprotective effects. AAV-mediated transfer of the HO-1 gene before myocardial injury conferred long-term myocardial protection from ischemia-reperfusion injury, which may be beneficial as preventive therapy for patients with or at risk of developing coronary ischemic events *(107)*.

7. Perspectives

An exciting prospect for translating much work from animal models to human studies has been opened up by the recent demonstration of quantitative imaging of transgene expression in living animals *(108)*. The development of micro-positron emission tomography has allowed improved resolution to approx 2 mm^3. Such technology has been utilized to correlate expression of therapeutic and reporter genes in a time-dependent fashion using inducible promoters *(109)*. However, it must be remembered that alteration of any cardiac cellular signaling pathway may ultimately turn out to have cardiotoxic effects, including arrhythmias. Thus, any genes that appear to cause enhanced cardiac function must undergo extensive toxicity studies in animals prior to similar experiments being performed in human subjects *(1,2,34,110)*. Although many issues still remain unresolved, the techniques described in this chapter may be utilized in the future to deliver various genes, targeted to combat many different disease processes, in different animal models, and ultimately to provide feasible gene therapy approaches to human cardiovascular disease.

References

1. Barry, W. H. (1999) Molecular inotropy: A future approach to the treatment of heart failure. *Circulation* **100,** 2303, 2304.
2. Hajjar, R. J., del Monte, F., Matsui, T., Rosenzweig, A. (2000) Prospects for gene therapy for heart failure. *Circ. Res.* **86,** 616–621.
3. Lefkowitz, R. J., Rockman, H. A., and Koch, W. J. (2000) Catecholamines, cardiac β-adrenergic receptors, and heart failure. *Circulation* **101,** 1634–1637.
4. Liggett, S. B. (2001) β-adrenergic receptors in the failing heart: the good, the bad, and the unknown. *J. Clin. Invest.* **107,** 947, 948.
5. Ylä-Herttuala, S., and Martin, J. F. (2000) Cardiovascular gene therapy. *Lancet* **355,** 213–222.
6. Kay, M. A., Glorioso, J. C., and Naldini, L. (2001) Viral vectors for gene therapy: the art of turning infectious agents into vehicles of therapeutics. *Nature Med.* **7,** 33–40.
7. Roizman, B. and Palese, P. (1996) Multiplication of viruses: an overview. In: *Fields Virology* (Fields, B. N., Knipe, D. M., Howley, P. M., and Chanock, R. M., eds.), Lippincott-Raven, Philadelphia, PA, pp. 101–111.
8. Shenk, T. (1996) Adenoviridae: the viruses and their replication. In: *Fields Virology* (Fields, B. N., Knipe, D. M., Howley, P. M., and Chanock, R. M., eds.), Lippincott-Raven, Philadelphia, PA, pp. 2149–2171.
9. Searle, P. F. and Mautner, V. (1998) Adenoviral vectors: not to be sneezed at. *Gene Ther.* **5,** 725–727.
10. Stratford-Perricaudet, L. D., Levrero, M., Chasse, J. F., Perricaudet, M., and Briand, P. (1990) Evaluation of the transfer and expression in mice of an enzyme-encoding gene using a human adenovirus vector. *Hum. Gene Ther.* **1,** 241–256.
11. Stratford-Perricaudet, L. D., Makeh, I., Perricaudet, M., and Briand, P. (1992) Widespread long-term gene transfer to mouse skeletal muscles and heart. *J. Clin. Invest.* **90,** 626–630.
12. Kass-Eisler, A., Leinwand, L. A., Gall, J., Bloom, B., and Falck-Pederson, E. (1996) Circumventing the immune response to adenovirus-mediated gene therapy. *Gene Ther.* **3,** 154–162.
13. Gordon, J. W. (2001) Direct exposure of mouse ovaries and oocytes to high doses of an adenovirus gene therapy vector fails to lead to germ cell transduction. *Mol. Ther.* **3,** 557–564.
14. Yang, Y., Nunes, F. A., Berencsi, K., Furth, E. E., Gönczöl, E., and Wilson, J. M. (1994) Cellular immunity to viral antigens limits E1-deleted adenoviruses for gene therapy. *Proc. Natl. Acad. Sci. USA* **91,** 4407–4411.
15. Yang, Y., Jooss, K. U., Su, Q., Ertl, H. C. J., and Wilson, J. M. (1996) Immune response to viral antigens versus transgene product in the elimination of recombinant adenovirus-infected hepatocytes in vivo. *Gene Ther.* **3,** 137–144.
16. Muruve, D. A., Barnes, M. J., Stillman, I. E., Libermann, T. A. (1999) Adenoviral gene therapy leads to rapid induction of multiple chemokines and acute neutrophil-dependent hepatic injury in vivo. *Hum. Gene Ther.* **10,** 965–976.

17. Nunes, F. A., Furth, E. E., Wilson, J. M., and Raper, S. E. (1999) Gene transfer into the liver of nonhuman primates with E1-deleted recombinant adenoviral vector: safety of readministration. *Hum. Gene Ther.* **10,** 2515, 2526.
18. Thomas, C. E., Birkett, D., Anozie, I., Castro, M. G., Lowenstein, P. R. (2001) Acute direct adenoviral vector cytotoxicity and chronic, but not acute, inflammatory responses correlate with decreased vector-mediated transgene expression in the brain. *Mol. Ther.* **3,** 36–46.
19. Amalfitano, A., Hauser, M. A., Hu, H., Serra, D., Begy, C. R., and Chamberlain, J. S. (1998) Production and characterization of improved adenovirus vectors with the E1, E2b, and E3 genes deleted. *J. Virol.* **72,** 926–933.
20. Gilbert, R., Nalbantoglu, J., Howell, J. M., et al. (2001) Dystrophin expression in muscle following gene transfer with a fully deleted ("gutted") adenovirus is markedly improved by trans-acting adenoviral gene products. *Hum. Gene Ther.* **12,** 1741–1755.
21. Schiedner, G., Hertel, S., Johnston, M., Biermann, V., Dries, V., and Kochanek, S. (2002) Variables affecting in vivo performance of high-capacity adenovirus vectors. *J. Virol.* **76,** 1600–1609.
22. Kaplitt, M. G., Xiao, X., Samulski, R. J., et al. (1996) Long-term gene transfer in porcine myocardium after coronary infusion of an adeno-associated virus vector. *Ann. Thorac. Surg.* **62,** 1669–1676.
23. Svensson, E. C., Marshall, D. J., Woodard, K., Lin, H., Jiang, F., Chu, L., and Leiden, J. M. (1999) Efficient and stable transduction of cardiomyocytes after intramyocardial injection or intracoronary perfusion with recombinant adeno-associated virus vectors. *Circulation* **99,** 201–205.
24. Kozarsky, K. F. (2001) Gene therapy for cardiovascular disease. *Curr. Opin. Pharmacol.* **1,** 197–202.
25. Chu, D., Sullivan, C. C., Weitzman, M. D., Du, L., Wolf, P. L., Jamieson, S. W., and Thistlethwaite, P. A. (2003) Direct comparison of efficiency and stability of gene transfer into the mammalian heart using adeno-associated virus versus adenovirus vectors. *J. Thorac. Cardiovasc. Surg.* **126,** 671–679.
26. Lever, A. M. L. (2000) Lentiviral vectors: progress and potential. *Curr. Opin. Mol. Ther.* **2,** 488–496.
27. Sakoda, T., Kasahara, N., Hamamori, Y., and Kedes, L. (1999) A high-titer lentiviral production system mediates efficient transduction of differentiated cells including beating cardiac myocytes. *J. Mol. Cell. Cardiol.* **31,** 2037–2047.
28. Guzman, R. J., Lemarchand, P., Crystal, R. G., Epstein, S. E., and Finkel, T. (1993) Efficient gene transfer into myocardium by direct injection of adenovirus vectors. *Circ. Res.* **73,** 1202–1207.
29. Kass-Eisler, A., Falck-Pederson, E., Alvira, M., et al. (1993) Quantitative determination of adenovirus-mediated gene delivery to rat cardiac myocytes in vitro and in vivo. *Proc. Natl. Acad. Sci. USA* **90,** 11,498–11,502.
30. Duckers, H. J. and Nabel, E. G. (2000) Prospects for genetic therapy of cardiovascular disease. *Med. Clin. N. Am.* **84,** 199–213.
31. Sen, L., Hong, Y. S., Luo, H., Cui, G., and Laks, H. (2001) Efficiency, efficacy, and adverse effects of adenovirus vs. liposome-mediated gene therapy in cardiac allografts. *Am. J. Physiol.* **281,** H1433–1441.

32. Affleck, D. G., Yu, L., Bull, D. A., Bailey, S. H., and Kim, S. W. (2001) Augmentation of myocardial transfection using TerplexDNA: a novel gene delivery system. *Gene Ther.* **8,** 349–353.

33. Xu, Z. L., Mizuguchi, H., Ishii-Watabe, A., Uchida, E., Mayumi, T., and Hayakawa, T. (2001) Optimization of transcriptional regulatory elements for constructing plasmid vectors. *Gene* **272,** 149–156.

34. Isner, J. M. (2002) Myocardial gene therapy. *Nature* **415,** 234–239.

35. Blau, H. M. and Banfi, A. (2001) The well-tempered vessel. *Nature Med.* **7,** 532–534.

36. Inazawa, T., Tanabe, T., Yamada, H., et al. (2001) Glucocorticoid-regulated expression of exogenous human growth hormone gene in rats. *Mol. Ther.* **4,** 267–272.

37. Gould, D. J., Berenstein, M., Dreja, H., Ledda, F., Podhajcer, O. L., and Chernajovsky, Y. (2000) A novel doxycycline inducible autoregulatory plasmid which displays "on"/"off" regulation suited to gene therapy applications. *Gene Ther.* **7,** 2061–2070.

38. Mizuguchi, H. and Hayakawa, T. (2001) Characteristics of adenovirus-mediated teracycline-controllable expression system. *Biochim. Biophys. Acta.* **1568,** 21–29.

39. Jiang, W., Zhou, L., Breyer, B., et al. (2001) Tetracycline-regulated gene expression mediated by a novel chimeric repressor that recruits histone deacetylases in mammalian cells. *J. Biol. Chem.* **276,** 45,168–45,174.

40. Bohner, S. and Gatz, C. (2001) Characterisation of novel target promoters for the dexamethasone-inducible/tetracycline-repressible regulator TGV using luciferase and isopentenyl transferase as sensitive reporter genes. *Mol. Gen. Genet.* **264,** 860–870.

41. Vigna, E., Cavalieri, S., Ailles, L., Geuna, M., Loew, R., Bujard, H., and Naldini, L. (2002) Robust and efficient regulation of transgene expression in vivo by improved tetracycline-dependent lentiviral vectors. *Mol. Ther.* **5,** 252–261.

42. Phillips, M. I., Tang, Y., Schmidt-Ott, K., Qian, K., and Kagiyama, S. (2002) Vigilant vector: heart-specific promoter in an adeno-associated virus vector for cardioprotection. *Hypertension* **39,** 651–655.

43. Auricchio, A., Kobinger, G., Anand, V., et al. (2001) Exchange of surface proteins impacts on viral vector cellular specificity and transduction characteristics: the retina as a model. *Hum. Mol. Genet.* **10,** 3075–3081.

44. Reynolds, P. N., Nicklin, S. A., Kaliberova, L., et al. (2001) Combined transductional and transcriptional targeting improves the specificity of transgene expression in vivo. *Nat. Biotechnol.* **19,** 838–842.

45. Franz, W. M., Rothman, T., Frey, N., and Katus, H. A. (1997) Analysis of tissue-specific gene delivery by recombinant adenoviruses containing cardiac-specific promoters. *Cardiovasc. Res.* **35,** 560–566.

46. Weeratna, R. D., Wu, T., Efler, S. M., Zhang, L., and Davis, H. L. (2001) Designing gene therapy vectors: avoiding immune responses by using tissue-specific promoters. *Gene Ther.* **8,** 1872–1878.

47. Ribault, S., Neuville, P., Mechine-Neuville, A., et al. (2001) Chimeric smooth muscle-specific enhancer/promoters: valuable tools for adenovirus-mediated cardiovascular gene therapy. *Circ. Res.* **88,** 468–475.

48. Rubinchik, S., Lowe, S., Jia, Z., Norris, J., and Dong, J. (2001) Creation of a new transgene cloning site near the right ITR of Ad5 results in reduced enhancer interference with tissue-specific and regulatable promoters. *Gene Ther.* **8,** 247–253.

49. Buvoli, M., Langer, S. J., Bialik, S., and Leinwand, L. A. (2002) Potential limitations of transcription terminators used as transgene insulators in adenoviral vectors. *Gene Ther.* **9,** 227–231.

50. French, B. A., Mazur, W., Geske, R. S., and Bolli, R. (1994) Direct in vivo gene transfer into porcine myocardium using replication deficient adenoviral vectors. *Circulation* **90,** 2414–2424.

51. Magovern, C. J., Mack, C. A., Zhang, J., et al. (1996) Direct in vivo gene transfer to canine myocardium using a replication-deficient adenovirus vector. *Ann. Thorac. Surg.* **62,** 425–434.

52. Mühlhauser, J., Jones, M., Yamada, I., et al. (1996) Safety and efficacy of in vivo gene transfer into the porcine heart with replication-deficient, recombinant adenovirus vectors. *Gene Ther.* **3,** 145–153.

53. Donahue, J. K., Kikkawa, K., Johns, D. C., Marban, E., and Lawrence, J. H. (1997) Ultrarapid, highly efficient viral gene transfer to the heart. *Proc. Natl. Acad. Sci. USA* **94,** 4664–4668.

54. Kypson, A. P., Peppel, K., Akhter, S. A., Lilly, R. E., Glower, D. D., Lefkowitz, R. J., and Koch, W. J. (1998) Ex vivo adenovirus-mediated gene transfer to the adult rat heart. *J. Thorac. Cardiovasc. Surg.* **115,** 623–630.

55. Kypson, A. P., Hendrickson, S. C., Akhter, S. A., et al. (1999) Adenoviral-mediated gene transfer of the β_2-adrenergic receptor to donor hearts enhances cardiac function. *Gene Ther.* **6,** 1298–1304.

56. Shah, A. S., White, D. C., Tai, O., et al. (2000) Adenovirus-mediated genetic manipulation of the myocardial β-adrenergic signalling system in transplanted hearts. *J. Thorac. Cardiovasc. Surg.* **120,** 581–588.

57. Hajjar, R. J., Schmidt, U., Matsui, T., et al. (1998) Modulation of ventricular function through gene transfer in vivo. *Proc. Natl. Acad. Sci. USA* **95,** 5251–5256.

58. Maurice, J. P., Hata, J. A., Shah, A. S., et al. (1999) Enhancement of cardiac function after adenoviral-mediated in vivo intracoronary β_2-adrenergic receptor gene delivery. *J. Clin. Invest.* **104,** 21–29.

59. White, D. C., Hata, J. A., Shah, A. S., Glower, D. D., Lefkowitz, R. J., and Koch, W. J. (2000) Preservation of myocardial of β-adrenergic receptor signalling delays the development of heart failure after myocardial infarction. *Proc. Natl. Acad. Sci. USA* **97,** 5428–5433.

60. Shah, A. S., White, D. C., Emani, S., et al. (2001) In vivo ventricular gene delivery of a β-adrenergic receptor kinase inhibitor to the failing heart reverses cardiac dysfunction. *Circulation* **103,** 1311–1316.

61. Shah, A. S., Lilly, E., Kypson, A. P., et al. (2000) Intracoronary adenovirus-mediated delivery and overexpression of the β_2-adrenergic receptor in the heart: prospects for molecular ventricular assistance. *Circulation* **101,** 408–414.

62. Emani, S. M., Shah, A. S., Bowman, M. K., Emani, S., Wilson, K., Glower, D. D., and Koch, W. J. (2003) Catheter-based intracoronary myocardial adenoviral

gene delivery: importance of intraluminal seal and infusion flow rate. *Mol. Ther.* **8,** 306–313.

63. Barr, E., Carroll, J., Kalynych, A. M., Tripathy, S. K., Kozarsky, K., Wilson, J. M., and Leiden, J. M. (1994) Efficient catheter-mediated gene transfer into the heart using replication-defective adenovirus. *Gene Ther.* **1,** 51–58.

64. Davidson, M. J., Jones, J. M., Emani, S., Wilson, K. H., Jaggers, J., Koch, W. J., and Milano, C. A. (2001) Cardiac gene delivery with cardiopulmonary bypass. *Circulation* **104,** 131–133.

65. Jones, J. M., Wilson, K. H., Koch, W. J., and Milano, C. A. (2002) Adenoviral gene transfer to the heart during cardiopulmonary bypass: effect of myocardial protection technique on transgene expression. *Eur. J. Cardiothorac. Surg.* **21,** 847–852.

66. Bridges, C. R., Burkman, J. M., Malekan, R., et al. (2002) Global cardiac-specific transgene expression using of cardiopulmonary bypass with cardiac isolation. *Ann. Thorac. Surg.* **73,** 1939–1946.

67. Boekstegers, P., von Degenfeld, G., Giehrl, W., et al. (2000) Myocardial gene transfer by selective pressure-regulated retroinfusion of coronary veins. *Gene Ther.* **7,** 232–240.

68. Donahue, J. K., Kikkawa, K., Thomas, A. D., Marban, E., and Lawrence, J. H. (1998) Acceleration of widespread adenoviral gene transfer to intact rabbit hearts by coronary perfusion with low calcium and serotonin. *Gene Ther.* **5,** 630–634.

69. Logeart, D., Hatem, S. N., Heimburger, M., Le Roux, A., Michel, J. B., Mercadier, J. J. (2001) How to optimize in vivo gene transfer to cardiac myocytes: mechanical or pharmacological procedures? *Hum. Gene Ther.* **12,** 1601–1610.

70. Nagata, K., Marban, E., Lawrence, J. H., and Donahue, J. K. (2001) Phosphodiesterase inhibitor-mediated potentiation of adenovirus delivery to myocardium. *J. Mol. Cell. Cardiol.* **33,** 575–580.

71. Wright, M. J., Wightman, L. M., Latchman, D. S., and Marber, M. S. (2001) In vivo myocardial gene transfer: optimization and evaluation of intracoronary gene delivery in vivo. *Gene Ther.* **8,** 1833–1839.

72. Ikeda, Y., Gu, Y., Iwanaga, Y., et al. (2002) Restoration of deficient membrane proteins in the cardiomyopathic hamster by in vivo cardiac gene transfer. *Circulation* **105,** 502–508.

73. He, G.-W. (1999) Myocardial protection during cardiac surgery from the viewpoint of coronary endothelial function. *Clin. Exp. Pharmacol. Physiol.* **26,** 810–814.

74. Sellke, F. W. (1999) Vascular changes after cardiopulmonary bypass and ischemic cardiac arrest: roles of nitric oxide synthase and cyclooxygenase. *Braz. J. Med. Biol. Res.* **32,** 1345–1352.

75. Yap, J., Pellegrini, C., O'Brien, T., Tazelaar, H. D., and McGregor, C. G. (2001) Conditions of vector delivery improve efficiency of adenoviral-mediated gene transfer to the transplanted heart. *Eur. J. Cardiothorac. Surg.* **19,** 702–707.

76. Jones, J. M., O'Kane, H., Gladstone, D. J., et al. (2001) Repeat heart valve surgery: risk factors for operative mortality. *J. Thorac. Cardiovasc. Surg.* **122,** 913–918.

76a. Jones, J. M., Wilson, K. H., Steenbergen, C., Koch, W. J., and Milano, C. A. Dose dependent effects of cardiac β_2 adrenoceptor gene therapy. *J. Surg. Res.*, in press.

76b. Jones, J. M., Petrofski, J. A., Wilson, K. H., Steenbergen, C., Koch, W. J., and Milano, C. A. β_2 adrenoreceptor gene therapy ameliorates left ventricular dysfunction following cardiac surgery. *Eur. J. Cardiothorac. Surg.*, in press.

77. Mack, C. A., Patel, S. R., Schwarz, E. A., et al. (1998) Biologic bypass with the use of adenovirus-mediated gene transfer of the complementary deoxyribonucleic acid for vascular endothelial growth factor 121 improves myocardial perfusion and function in the ischemic porcine heart. *J. Thorac. Cardiovasc. Surg.* **115,** 168–177.

78. Leotta, E., Patejunas, G., Murphy, G., et al. (2002) Gene therapy with adenovirus-mediated myocardial transfer of vascular endothelial growth factor 121 improves cardiac performance in a pacing model of congestive heart failure. *J. Thorac. Cardiovasc. Surg.* **123,** 1101–1113.

79. Losordo, D. W., Vale, P. R., Hendel, R. C., et al. (2002) Phase 1/2 placebo-controlled, double-blind, dose-escalating trial of myocardial vascular endothelial growth factor 2 gene transfer by catheter delivery in patients with chronic myocardial ischemia. *Circulation* **105,** 2012–2018.

80. Giordano, F. J., Ping, P., McKirnan, M. D., et al. (1996) Intracoronary gene transfer of fibroblast growth factor-5 increases blood flow and contractile function in an ischemic region of the heart. *Nature Med.* **2,** 534–539.

81. Iaccarino, G., Smithwick, L. A., Lefkowitz, R. J., and Koch, W. J. (1999) Targetting $G_{\beta\gamma}$ signalling in arterial vascular smooth muscle proliferation: a novel strategy to limit restenosis. *Proc. Natl. Acad. Sci. USA* **96,** 3945–3950.

82. Akowuah, E. F., Sheridan, P. J., Cooper, G. J., and Newman, C. (2003) Preventing saphenous vein graft failure: does gene therapy have a role? *Ann. Thorac. Surg.* **76,** 959–966.

83. Mann, M. J., Whittemore, A. D., Donaldson, M. C., et al. (1999) Ex-vivo gene therapy of human vascular bypass grafts with E2F decoy: the PREVENT single-centre, randomised, controlled trial. *Lancet* **354,** 1493–1498.

83a. Petrofski, J. A., Hata, J. A., Gehrig, T. R., et al. (2004) Gene delivery to aortocoronary saphenous vein grafts in a large animal model of intimal hyperplasia. *J. Thorac. Cardiovasc. Surg.* **127,** 27–33.

84. Dzau, V. J., Mann, M. J., Ehsan, A., and Griese, D. P. (2001) Gene therapy and genomic strategies for cardiovascular surgery: The emerging field of surgiomics. *J. Thorac. Cardiovasc. Surg.* **121,** 206–216.

85. Hasty, A. H., Linton, M. F., Brandt, S. J., Babaev, V. R., Gleaves, L. A., and Fazio, S. (1999) Retroviral gene therapy in ApoE-deficient mice: ApoE expression in the artery wall reduces early foam cell lesion formation. *Circulation* **99,** 2571–2576.

86. Di Donato, R. M. and Castaneda, A. R. (1995) Anatomic correction of transposition of the great arteries at the arterial level. In: *Surgery of the Chest* (Sabiston, D. C. and Spencer, F. C., eds.), WB Saunders, Philadelphia, PA, pp. 1592–1602.

87. Dzimiri, N. (1999) Regulation of β-adrenoceptor signalling in cardiac function and disease. *Pharmacological Reviews* **51,** 465–501.
88. Drazner, M. H., Peppel, K. C., Dyer, S., Grant, A. O., Koch, W. J., and Lefkowitz, R. J. (1997) Potentiation of β-adrenergic signalling by adenoviral-mediated gene transfer in adult rabbit ventricular myocytes. *J. Clin. Invest.* **99,** 288–296.
89. Houser, S. R., Piacentino, V. III, and Weisser, J. (2000) Abnormalities of calcium cycling in the hypertrophied and failing heart. *J. Mol. Cell. Cardiol.* **32,** 1595–1607.
90. del Monte, F., Williams, E., Lebeche, D., et al. (2001) Improvement in survival and cardiac metabolism after gene transfer of sarcoplasmic reticulum Ca^{2+}-ATPase in a rat model of heart failure. *Circulation* **104,** 1424–1429.
91. del Monte, F., Harding, S. E., Schmidt, U., et al. (1999) Restoration of contractile function in isolated cardiomyocytes from failing human hearts by gene transfer of SERCA2a. *Circulation* **100,** 2308–2311.
92. del Monte, F., Harding, S. E., Dec, G. W., Gwathmey, J. K., and Hajjar, R. J. (2002) Targeting phospholamban by gene transfer in human heart failure. *Circulation* **105,** 904–907.
92a. Williams, M. L., Hata, J. A., Schroder, J., et al. (2004) Targeted β-adrenergic receptor kinase (βARK1) inhibition by gene transfer in failing human hearts. *Circulation* **109,** 1590–1593.
93. Rockman, H. A., Chien, K. R., Choi, D.-J., et al. (1998) Expression of a β-adrenergic receptor kinase 1 inhibitor prevents the development of myocardial failure in gene-targeted mice. *Proc. Natl. Acad. Sci. USA* **95,** 7000–7005.
94. Freeman, K., Lerman, I., Kranias, E. G., et al. (2001) Alterations in cardiac adrenergic signalling and calcium cycling differentially affect the progression of cardiomyopathy. *J. Clin. Invest.* **107,** 967–974.
95. Harding, V. B., Jones, L. R., Lefkowitz, R. J., Koch, W. J., and Rockman, H. A. (2001) Cardiac βARK1 inhibition prolongs survival and augments β blocker therapy in a mouse model of severe heart failure. *Proc Natl Acad Sci USA* **98,** 5809–5814.
96. Rockman, H. A., Koch, W. J., and Lefkowitz, R. J. (2002) Seven-transmembrane-spanning receptors and heart function. *Nature* **415,** 206–212.
97. Tevaearai, H. T., Eckhart, A. D., Shotwell, K. F., Wilson, K. H., and Koch, W. J. (2001) Ventricular dysfunction after cardioplegic arrest is improved after myocardial gene transfer of a β-adrenergic receptor kinase inhibitor. *Circulation* **104,** 2069–2074.
98. Helmer, G. A., McKirnan, M. D., Shabetai, R., Boss, G. R., Ross, J., and Hammond, H. K. (1996) Regional deficits of myocardial blood flow and function in left ventricular pacing–induced heart failure. *Circulation* **94,** 2260–2267.
99. Tevaearai, H. T., Eckhart, A. D., Walton, G. B., Keys, J. R., Wilson, K., and Koch, W. J. (2002) Myocardial gene transfer and overexpression of β$_2$-adrenergic receptors potentiates the functional recovery of unloaded failing hearts. *Circulation* **106,** 124–129.

100. Green, S. A., Cole, G., Jacinto, M., Innis, M., and Liggett, S. B. (1993) A polymorphism of the human β_2-adrenergic receptor within the fourth transmembrane domain alters ligand binding and functional properties of the receptor. *J. Biol. Chem.* **268**, 23,116–23,121.

101. Turki, J., Lorenz, J. N., Green, S. A., Donnelly, E. T., Jacinto, M., and Liggett, S. B. (1996) Myocardial signalling defects and impaired cardiac function of a human β2-adrenergic receptor polymorphism expressed in transgenic mice. *Proc. Natl. Acad. Sci. USA* **93**, 10,483–10,488.

102. Liggett, S. B., Wagoner, L. E., Craft, L. L., Hornung, R. W., Hoit, B. D., McIntosh, T. C., and Walsh, R. A. (1998) The Ile164 β_2-adrenergic receptor polymorphism adversely affects the outcome of congestive heart failure. *J. Clin. Invest.* **102**, 534–539.

103. Small, K. M., Brown, K. M., Forbes, S. L., and Liggett, S. B. (2001) Modification of the β_2-adrenergic receptor to engineer a receptor-effector complex for gene therapy. *J. Biol. Chem.* **276**, 31,596–31,601.

104. Weig, H.-J., Laugwitz, K.-L., Moretti, A., et al. (2000) Enhanced cardiac contractility after gene transfer of V2 vasopressin receptors in vivo by ultrasound-guided injection or transcoronary injection. *Circulation* **101**, 1578–1585.

105. Laugwitz, K.-L., Moretti, A., Weig, H.-J., et al. (2001) Blocking caspase-activated apoptosis improves contractility in failing myocardium. *Hum. Gene Ther.* **12**, 2051–2063.

106. Abunasra, H. J., Smolenski, R. T., Morrison, K., et al. (2001) Efficacy of adenoviral gene transfer with manganese superoxide dismutase and endothelial nitric oxide synthase in reducing ischemia and reperfusion injury. *Eur. J. Cardiothorac. Surg.* **20**, 153–158.

107. Melo, L. G., Agrawal, R., Zhang, L., et al. (2002) Gene therapy strategy for long-term myocardial protection using adeno-associated virus-mediated delivery of heme oxygenase gene. *Circulation* **105**, 602-607.

108. Wu, J. C., Inubushi, M., Sundaresan, G., Schelbert, H. R., and Gambhir, S. S. (2002) Positron emission tomograpgy imaging of cardiac reporter gene expression in living rats. *Circulation* **106**, 180–183.

109. Sun, X., Annala, A. J., Yaghoubi, S. S., et al. (2001) Quantitative imaging of gene induction in living animals. *Gene Ther.* **8**, 1572–1579.

110. Marban, E. (2000) Gene therapy for common acquired diseases of the heart: the Sirens' song. *Circulation* **101**, 1498–1500.

3

Gene Therapy for Myocardial Ischemia Using the Hypoxia-Inducible Double Plasmid System

Yi Tang

Summary

There are repeated ischemic events and nonischemic intervals in the heart affected by coronary artery disease. In the current study, we designed a hypoxia-inducible double plasmid system. By using a hypoxia response element, this system can be switched on by low oxygen but turned off by normal oxygen tension. Furthermore, the design of the double plasmid system, which contains a transactivator plasmid and a reporter plasmid, dramatically amplified the gene expression. This system could be used to carry cardioprotective genes for effective and regulated gene therapy for the ischemic heart.

Key Words: Hypoxia response element; myocardial ischemia; chimeric transcriptional factor; gene therapy; gene amplification.

1. Introduction

Coronary artery disease frequently involves repeated bouts of myocardial ischemia and nonischemic intervals. Therefore, we want to design a gene therapy strategy for the ischemic heart, which expresses cardioprotective genes on hypoxic ischemic attacks but keeps silent during nonischemic intervals, since constitutive overexpression of transgenes may lead to deleterious side effects. In the current study, we utilized hypoxia response element to regulate transgene expression in response to hypoxia.

How to increase the expression level of transgenes to reach the optimal therapeutic level is another problem facing gene therapy. Here, we adopted a novel double plasmid system, which can amplify the gene expression by several hundred fold.

From: *Methods in Molecular Medicine, vol. 112: Molecular Cardiology: Methods and Protocols*
Edited by: Z. Sun © Humana Press Inc., Totowa, NJ

2. Materials

1. Plasmids: pGL-SV40 (pGL2-promoter), pRL-TK (Promega, Madison, WI), pGene/V5-His/*lacZ* (Invitrogen, Carlsbad, CA).
2. H9c2 cell line (cat. no. CRL1446, ATCC, Manassas, VA).
3. Cell culture reagents (Mediatech, Herndon, VA), including Dulbecco's modified Eagle's medium (DMEM), sodium pyruvate (store at 4°C), and heat-inactivated fetal bovine serum (FBS; store at –20°C).
4. Transfection reagents (Invitrogen, Carlsbad, CA), including lipofectamine (store at 4°C) and Opti-MEM (store at 4°C).
5. Endofree Plasmid Max Prep kit (Qiagen, Valencia, CA).
6. The hypoxia chamber system (Oxygen Sensors).
7. Dual luciferase assay system (Promega).
8. Monolight 3010 luminometer (PharMingen, San Diego, CA).

3. Methods

3.1. Amplification Method: The Double Plasmid System

We developed an amplification method that we called the double plasmid system (**Fig. 1**). It consists of two plasmids, the transactivator plasmid and the reporter plasmid. It can amplify the power of promoters based on the strong transcription activity of GAL4/p65 fusion protein, which is expressed by the transactivator plasmid. The transactivator (GAL4/p65) consists of the yeast GAL4 DNA binding domain and the p65 activation domain. It binds to the GAL4 upstream activating sequence (UAS) in the reporter plasmid and activates transcription.

3.1.1. The Cardiomyocyte-Specific Transactivator Plasmid (pGS-MLC)

The pGS-MLC (**Fig. 2**) is based on the pGS-CMV, a generous gift from Dr. Sean M. Sullivan (University of Florida, Gainesville). pGS-CMV contains cytomegalovirus (CMV) enhancer/promoter and a coding sequence for a chimeric transcription factor (GAL4/p65) consisting of the yeast GAL4 DNA binding domain (amino acids 1–93) (2) and the human p65 activation domain (amino acids 283–551) (3) from nuclear factor κB (NF-κB). A 281-bp myosin light chain 2v promoter fragment was amplified by polymerase chain reaction (PCR) from pMLC-Luc (4) with primer pairs designed with 5' *Sbf*I or 3' *Sac*I sites on the ends. The PCR products were digested by *Sbf*I and *Sac*I and ligated to *Sbf*I/*Sac*I-digested pGS-CMV plasmid to replace the CMV enhancer/promoter. For an alternative way to obtain the fragment coding the GAL4 binding domain and the p65 activation domain, *see* **Note 1**.

3.1.2 The Hypoxic Inducible Transactivator Plasmid (pGS-HRE/SV40)

In pGS-HRE/SV40 (**Fig. 3**), a 68-bp human enolase (ENO) 1 hypoxia response element (HRE) sequence (–416 to –349, Genebank, X16287) was

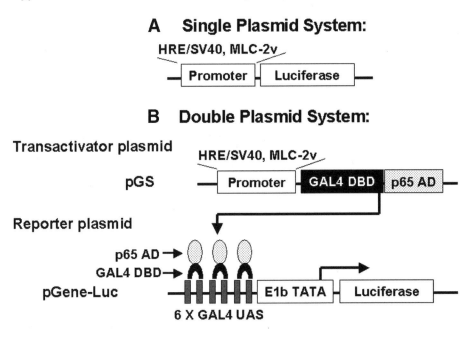

Fig. 1. Diagram of the amplification system. (**A**) The single plasmid system is the traditional way to express transgene; in which a promoter drives a transgene (luciferase) directly in one plasmid. The promoter could be MLC-2v, the HRE/SV40 promoter, or other promoters. (**B**) The double plasmid system can amplify the power of promoters based on the strong transcription activity of the GAL4/p65 fusion protein. The promoter in the transactivator plasmid (pGS) could be replaced with the SV40, HRE/SV40, CMV, and MLC-2v promoter. The reporter plasmid contains GAL4 upstream activation sequence (UAS) in front of an adenovirus E1b TATA box and the firefly luciferase reporter gene. (Reprinted from **ref.** *1*, with permission from Elsevier.)

incorporated upstream of the SV40 promoter in pGS-SV40. The HRE served as a gene switch. It turned on the SV40 promoter under hypoxia and switched it off under normoxia. Therefore, the expression level of the GAL4/p65 transcriptional factor also fluctuated with the change in oxygen tension. The ENO1 HRE fragment was amplified by PCR from pGL-HRE/SV40 (**Fig. 4**; a kind gift of Dr. Semenza *[5]*, Johns Hopkins University, Baltimore, MD), and then inserted in front of the SV40 promoter in pGS-SV40.

3.1.3 The Reporter Plasmid (pGene-Luc)

The pGene-Luc (**Fig. 5**) was derived from pGene/V5-His/*lac*Z. The promoter of pGene/V5-His/*lac*Z has six copies of a 17-bp GAL4 UAS (*6*), an

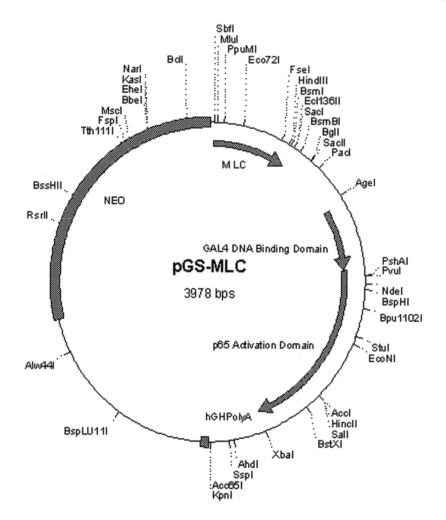

Fig. 2. Map of pGS-MLC. The MLC-2v promoter drives the expression of a chimeric transcription factor consisting of the GAL4 DNA binding domain and the p65 activation domain. The plasmid has human growth hormone polyA signal (hGH polyA) and the neomycin resistance gene.

adenovirus E1b TATA box *(7)*, and the coding sequence of *lac*Z. We replaced the coding sequence of lacZ with the coding sequence of luciferase (*see* **Note 2**). The coding sequence of luciferase was amplified from pGL-SV40 by PCR with 5′ *Hind*III and 3′ blunt-end. The pGene/V5-His/*lac*Z was digested with

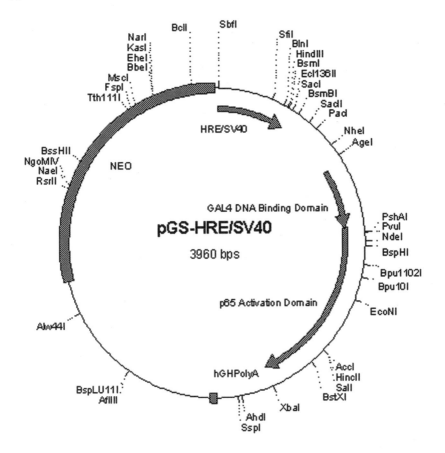

Fig. 3. Map of pGS-HRE/SV40. HRE is a hypoxia response element, which can activate the SV40 promoter under hypoxia. The HRE/SV40 enhancer/promoter drives the expression of GAL4/p65 protein. The plasmid has human growth hormone polyA signal (hGH polyA) and the neomycin resistance gene.

*Hind*III and *Pme*I. Then the fragment of luciferase cDNA was ligated with the backbone of pGene/V5-His/*lac*Z. The GAL4 UAS plus the E1b TATA box itself has very little activity. Since it contains GAL4 binding sites (GAL4 UAS), it can be recognized and activated by the chimeric transcription factor GAL4/p65. The identity of clones was confirmed by nucleotide sequence analysis.

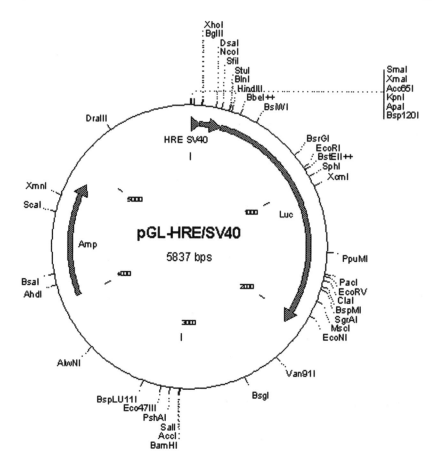

Fig. 4. Map of pGL-HRE/SV40. HRE/SV40 enhancer/promoter drives the reporter gene luciferase. The plasmid has the ampicillin resistance gene.

3.1.4. Single Plasmid System (**Fig. 1**)

The single plasmid system is defined as one plasmid in which the promoter (e.g., the MLC-2v promoter) drives the expression of a reporter gene (e.g., luciferase). The single plasmid system was used for comparison with the double plasmid system. In pMLC-Luc *(3)*, the MLC-2v promoter drives luciferase. pGL-HRE/SV40 (**Fig. 4**) is based on pGL-SV40, with the 68-bp ENO1 HRE in the 5' primer of SV40 promoter.

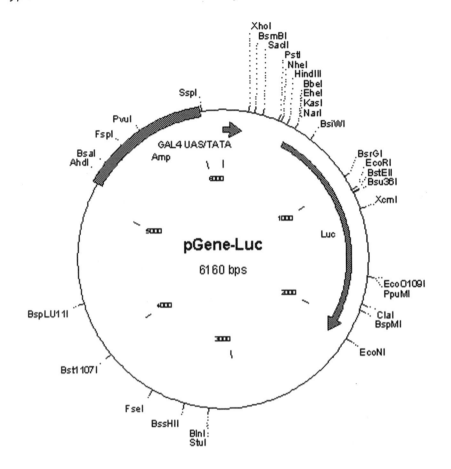

Fig. 5. Map of pGene-Luc. This is the reporter plasmid in the double plasmid system. It contains GAL4 upstream activation sequence (UAS) in front of an adenovirus E1b TATA box and the firefly luciferase reporter gene. The plasmid has the ampicillin resistance gene.

3.2. Cell Culture

A rat embryonic cardiac myoblast cell line, H9c2 (ATCC, cat. no. CRL1446) was used to test the expression of our plasmids in vitro (*see* **Note 3**). H9c2 cells were maintained in DMEM supplemented with 1 mM sodium pyruvate and 10% FBS under normoxic conditions (5% CO_2, 20% O_2, 75% N_2) in a humidified incubator at 37°C. The cells were passaged before they reached 80% confluence and at a 1:3 ratio. For transfection, the passage of cells is less than 50.

MPV, an endothelial cell line, was cultured in DMEM supplemented with sodium pyruvate and 10% FBS.

3.3. Transient Transfection

1. H9c2 cells were seeded within 24 h before transfection. At the time of transfection, the confluence of cells was at 70–80%.
2. The plasmid for transfection was purified with the Endofree Plasmid Max Prep kit (*see* **Note 4**).
3. Transfection was performed with lipofectamine according to the manufacture's protocol. A typical transfection involves the addition of 2–4 mg plasmid and 10 µL of lipofectamine diluted with 1 mL Opti-MEM (Invitrogen) into a 60-mm diameter dish.
4. Five hours after transfection, fresh growth media with 20% FBS was added to the dish without descanting the transfection mixture.
5. Twenty-four hours after transfection, the old media was replaced with fresh growth media (*see* **Note 5**). The cells were then put into the hypoxia chamber.

3.4. Hypoxic Treatment

The hypoxia chamber is an airtight chamber with the inlet connecting to a gas tank and the outlet connecting to a vacuum. The gas tank has premixed hypoxic gas, for example, 1% O_2, 5% CO_2, and 94% N_2. The chambers were evacuated and gassed six times, and then the tightly sealed chambers were incubated at 37°C for the desired hypoxic treating time.

3.5. Reporter Gene Assays

The pRL-TK plasmid, which expresses *Renillan* luciferase, was used to control transfection efficiency between different dishes and batches of transfection. All the plasmids in double and single systems express firefly luciferase. Luciferase assays were performed with a dual luciferase assay system. Results were quantified with a Monolight 3010 luminometer and expressed as a ratio of firefly luciferase activity over *Renilla* luciferase activity.

3.6. Results

3.6.1. The Cardiomyocyte Specific Amplification System

The MLC double plasmid system dramatically increased reporter gene expression compared with the MLC single plasmid (**Fig. 6**). Luciferase expression in the MLC double plasmid system was elevated in a dose-dependent manner with increasing amounts of transfected transactivator plasmid (pGS-MLC). The maximal level was 346.08 ± 22.50-fold higher than that of the single plasmid system (pMLC-Luc). Furthermore, this amplification did not compromise the cardiac specificity of the MLC-2v promoter. The MLC double plasmid

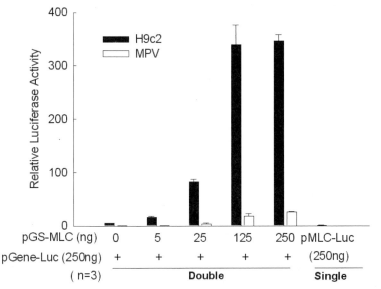

Fig. 6. Double plasmid systems amplified the power of the MLV-2v promoter and still maintained its cardiac specificity. For double plasmid system transfection, H9c2 cells seeded in 6-well plates received 125 ng/well control plasmid (pRL-TK), 250 ng/well reporter plasmid (pGene-Luc), 0–250 ng/well transactivator plasmid (pGS-MLV), and various amounts of empty vector such that all cells received a total of 625 ng plasmid per well. The transfection of 250 ng/well pMLC-Luc served as the single plasmid system. The relative luciferase activity from double plasmid transfection was normalized to that obtained from the single plasmid system (x-fold). (mean ± SD; $n = 3$ independent samples).

system still maintained the expression profile more in cardiac (H9c2) but less in noncardiac (MPV) cells, although at the high dose of transactivator plasmid there was a slight increase in expression of MPV.

3.6.2. The Hypoxia-Inducible Double Plasmid System

The absolute expression levels of the HRE/SV40 double plasmid system under both low and normal oxygen conditions were greatly increased compared with that of the single plasmid system (pGL-HRE/SV40) (**Fig. 7**). pGS-HRE/SV40 at 10 ng/well increased reporter expression by 58.78 ± 21.65-fold under hypoxia and 8.83 ± 2.23-fold under normal oxygen relative to the expression of the single plasmid system (pGL-HRE/SV40) at 20% O_2. The reporter expression can be further increased up to 412.79 ± 185.27-fold at 1% O_2 and 205.35 ± 65.44-fold at 20% O_2 by a higher dose (100 ng/well) of pGS-HRE/SV40 compared with the expression of the single plasmid system (pGL-HRE/SV40) at 20% O_2.

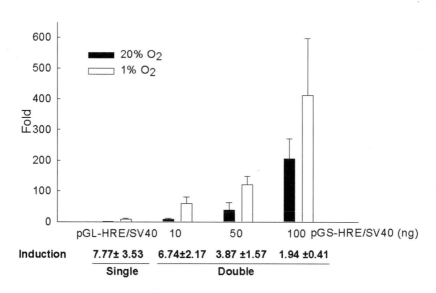

Fig. 7. Hypoxia-responsive ability of the HRE/SV40 double plasmid system. H9c2 cells seeded in 60-mm dishes were cotransfected with 1 µg/well pRL-TK, 2 µg/well reporter plasmid (pGene-Luc), 10–100 ng/well transactivator plasmid (pGS-HRE/SV40), and the various amount of empty vector such that all cells received a total of 3.5 µg plasmids. As single plasmid control, 1 µg/well pRL-TK, 2 µg/well pGL-HRE/SV40, and 0.5 µg/well empty vector were cotransfected into H9c2 cells. At 24 h after transfection, duplicate plates were incubated in 1 or 20% O_2 for 24 h prior to preparation of cell lysates. The ratio of firefly luciferase/*Renilla* luciferase activity was normalized to the result obtained from cells transfected with pGL-HRE/SV40 and exposed to 20% O_2 (*relative luciferase activity*). Expression at 1% relative to 20% O_2 was calculated (*Induction*), and mean ± SD is shown (*n* = three independent experiments). (Adapted from **ref. 8**, with permission from Lippincott Williams & Wilkins.)

4. Notes

1. The fragments that code the GAL4 binding domain and the p65 activation domain can also be obtained from plasmid pSwitch in the Gene Switch Kit (Invitrogen).
2. The reason to replace the *lacZ* with luciferase is that it is easier to quantitate the expression level of luciferase. The luciferase assay has very low background. The linear order for luciferase assay is from 10^3 to 10^8. However, the quantitative *lacZ* assay has a higher background and a narrow range of linear order. Therefore, luciferase is a better reporter gene to be used for comparing expression levels of different plasmids. Luciferase reacts with its substrate and emits light instantly. The whole reaction takes only several seconds. However, the *lacZ* assay requires 20–50 min of incubation time and has multiple steps. Therefore, the results of the luciferase assay are more repeatable, and the whole assay is time-saving.

3. H9c2 cells have the basic characteristics of cardiac myocytes, such as expression of myosin light chain, and stimulation by acetylcholine. It can be expanded in vitro. It is a more convenient resource to test our plasmid than the primary culture of adult cardiomyocytes, which is hard to prepare and culture. After we obtained positive results from these embryonic cardiac myoblast cells, we further confirmed the results in the primary culture of adult rat cardiomyocytes.
4. It is important to keep the transfection plasmid from being contaminated by endotoxin. Endotoxin will severely damage H9c2 cells during transfection.
5. For better gas exchange between the cell culture media and air, use a minimal volume of media to just cover the cells. For a 60-mm diameter dish, 2 mL media was usually added.

Acknowledgments

This work was supported by NIH MERIT award HL 27334 and a Predoctoral Fellowship from the American Heart Association Florida/Puerto Rico Affiliate (0110140B).

Reference

1. Tang, Y., Schmitt-Ott, K., Qian, K., Kagiyama, S., and Phillips, M. I. (2002) Vigilant vectors: adeno-associated virus with a biosensor to switch on amplified therapeutic genes in specific tissues in life-threatening diseases. *Methods* **28,** 259–266.
2. Keegan, L., Gill, G., and Ptashne, M. (1986) Separation of DNA binding from the transcription-activating function of a eukaryotic regulatory protein. *Science* **231,** 699–704.
3. Schmitz, M. L. and Baeuerle, P. A. (1991) The p65 subunit is responsible for the strong transcription activating potential of NF-kappa B. *EMBO J.* **10,** 3805–3817.
4. Phillips, M. I., Tang, Y., Schmidt-Ott, K., Qian, K., and Kagiyama, S. (2002) Vigilant vector: heart-specific promoter in an adeno-associated virus vector for cardioprotection. *Hypertension* **39,** 651–655.
5. Semenza, G. L., Jiang, B. H., Leung, S. W., Passantino, R., Concordet, J. P., Maire, P., and Giallongo, A. (1996) Hypoxia response elements in the aldolase A, enolase 1, and lactate dehydrogenase A gene promoters contain essential binding sites for hypoxia-inducible factor 1. *J. Biol. Chem.* **271,** 32,529–32,537.
6. Giniger, E., Varnum, S. M., and Ptashne, M. (1985) Specific DNA binding of GAL4, a positive regulatory protein of yeast. *Cell* **40,** 767–774.
7. Lillie, J. W. and Green, M. R. (1989) Transcription activation by the adenovirus E1a protein. *Nature* **338,** 39–44.
8. Tang, Y., Jackson, M., Qian, K., and Phillips, M. I. (2002) Hypoxia inducible double plasmid system for myocardial ischemia gene therapy. *Hypertension* **39,** 695–698.

4

Cardiac Gene Delivery Using DNA–Adenoviral Constructs

J. Mark Jones and Walter J. Koch

Summary

In view of the limitations of current cardiac gene transfer techniques by direct myocardial injection, or via the coronary vasculature, we have been attempting to develop potentially clinically applicable methods. Selective catheterization of the coronary arteries has been performed, but the duration of exposure of the heart to the virus is limited. Present systems require high infusion pressure to inject the virus, which could result in endothelial or myocardial injury, and extracardiac transgene expression occurs.

An alternative method has been developed in which the adenoviral vector is administered following cardioplegic arrest of the heart during cardiopulmonary bypass (CPB), which allows prolonged myocardial contact with the adenoviral vector. This may be advantageous since intracoronary delivery of vector in a Langendorff perfused heart model has shown that prolonged contact time with the virus improves gene transfer. Despite the detrimental effect of cold temperatures and contact with blood on transgene expression in the in vitro and ex vivo studies, we have demonstrated that these factors are unimportant in this in vivo model. Exposure of extracardiac tissues to the vector is limited. Moreover, administration of the β_2AR transgene has resulted in amelioration of impaired cardiac function following CPB and cardioplegic arrest.

Key Words: Gene transfer; intracoronary; adenoviral vector; coronary catheterization; cardiac surgery; cardiopulmonary bypass; cardiac-selective.

From: *Methods in Molecular Medicine, vol. 112: Molecular Cardiology: Methods and Protocols*
Edited by: Z. Sun © Humana Press Inc., Totowa, NJ

1. Introduction

Transgenic murine models have suggested potential molecular therapeutic targets in the cardiovascular system *(1)*. Against this background there has been interest in the potential of gene therapy to improve cardiac function *(2)*. However, it must be acknowledged that gene transfer models differ significantly from transgenic models. In order to achieve overexpression of transgenes by gene transfer, appropriate vectors and delivery methods are required.

Cardiac gene delivery can be performed with targeting of genes to the endothelium of either native coronary vessels or coronary artery bypass grafts, or to the myocardium. Myocardial gene delivery is possible, either via direct myocardial injection or via the coronary vasculature. Direct myocardial injection requires multiple injections causing high levels of gene expression within a 1.5-cm radius of the site of injection *(3)*.

Our laboratory has been investigating the genetic modulation of the myocardial β-adrenergic receptor (βAR) system using adenoviral-mediated gene transfer. Myocardial gene delivery of the potentially therapeutic β_2AR and β-adrenergic receptor kinase C-terminal (βARKct) transgenes has been performed. In addition, we have used the marker genes β-galactosidase and green fluorescent protein, which do not influence βAR density or signaling but do provide an indication of the distribution of the transgene. Several experimental methods of intracoronary gene transfer have been used. Gene transfer has been achieved during transplantation of rat and rabbit hearts, but this technique is limited to viral exposure of the donor heart prior to transplantation *(4)*. Intracoronary delivery in rabbits has been performed during thoracotomy, with the aorta cross-clamped, and the virus introduced by injection into the left venticular (LV) cavity *(5)*. Owing to the occluded aorta, LV ejection forces the virus down the coronary arteries. However, the acute pressure overload of the LV limits the period of cross-clamping to a matter of seconds.

We have thus been attempting to develop methods that could be more clinically applicable, given the limitations of existing experimental methods of myocardial gene delivery. In this chapter we describe two alternative potentially clinically applicable methods of intracoronary adenoviral-mediated myocardial gene transfer.

Selective catheterization of the right or left coronary artery has been performed in both rabbits and piglets, but the duration of exposure of the heart to the virus is limited *(6)*. Present systems require high infusion pressure to inject the virus, which could result in endothelial or myocardial injury. Following these methods of intracoronary gene delivery, the adenovirus was also distributed systemically, and noncardiac tissues have shown evidence of transgene expression *(5,7,8)*.

An alternative method for global myocardial gene transfer in piglets has been developed in which the adenoviral vector is administered following cardioplegic arrest of the heart during cardiopulmonary bypass (CPB). The neonatal piglet model of CPB was chosen since it was well established, although the existing studies did not require survival of the animal following surgery *(9)*. Furthermore, in view of the fact that vector quantity may be a limiting factor, a relatively small animal was deemed desirable. Such a method of delivery allows prolonged myocardial contact with the adenoviral vector. This may be advantageous since intracoronary delivery of vector in a Langendorff perfused heart model has shown that prolonged contact time with the virus improves gene transfer *(10)*. Despite the detrimental effect of cold temperatures and contact with blood on transgene expression in the in vitro and ex vivo studies, we have demonstrated that these factors are unimportant in this in vivo model *(11,12)*. In particular, the presence of cold cardioplegic solutions or blood in the coronary circulation prior to administration of the vector did not impair gene transfer *(12)*. We have also confirmed that exposure of noncardiac tissues to the vector is limited, although not prevented, by this technique *(13)*. Unlike a recently described experimental method of gene delivery that involves two separate CPB circuits, this model of gene delivery could be easily utilized in routine clinical cardiac surgical practice *(14)*. Moreover, administration of the β_2AR transgene has resulted in amelioration of impaired cardiac function following CPB and cardioplegic arrest *(15)*.

These two clinically applicable methods of gene delivery may prove to be useful techniques. Obviously, the former cardiac catheterization method is less invasive but carries with it the risk of endothelial or myocardial injury, as well as extracardiac transgene expression. In contrast, gene transfer during CPB is controlled and cardiac selective. The beneficial functional effects of cardiac transgene expression counter the detrimental effects of CPB on cardiac function. Moreover, this technique could be combined with cardiac-specific or regulatable promoters to reduce the toxicity of uncontrolled transgene expression further *(16,17)*.

2. Materials

2.1. Technique 1: Selective Coronary Gene Delivery

1. 100 mg/mL Ketamine (Abbott Laboratories, North Chicago, IL).
2. Lidocaine HCl (Abbot Laboratories).
3. Contrast liquid (Renografin®-60, Bracco Diagnostics, Princeton NJ).
4. Heparin (Elkins-Sinn, Cherry Hill, NJ).
5. Phosphate buffered saline (PBS; Dulbecco's phosphate-buffered saline, Gibco-BRL, Life Technologies, Grand Island, NY).

6. Surgical instruments: surgical blade no. 15 (Becton Dickinson), scissors, pickups, right-angle forceps, atraumatic bulldog clamp.
7. Sutures: 2/0 silk, 3/0 vicryl (Ethicon, Somerville, NJ).
8. 24-Gage cannula (Quik-Cath®, Baxter Healthcare Corporation).
9. Fluoroscopy system: 4-Fr Introducer and 3-Fr Angled tip access catheter (Cook, Bloomington, IN).
10. Infusion pump with 3-mL tubing (Universal administration set, Baxter fluven 0153/C; 26 in. contains 3 mL) and two three-way connectors with male Luer slip adapters (Baxter).

2.2. Technique 2: Gene Delivery During Cardiopulmonary Bypass

1. 100 mg/mL Ketamine (Abbott Laboratories).
2. Isoflurane (Abbott Laboratories).
3. Dexamethasone (American Regent Laboratories, Shirley, NY).
4. Heparin (Elkins-Sinn, Cherry Hill, NJ).
5. Furosemide (American Regent Laboratories).
6. Lidocaine (Abbott Laboratories).
7. Sodium bicarbonate (Abbott Laboratories).
8. Protamine sulfate (American Pharmaceutical Partners, Los Angeles, CA).
9. Bupivicaine (Abbott Laboratories).
10. 10 mg/ml Butorphenol tartrate (Fort Dodge Animal Health, Fort Dodge, IA).
11. Cold crystalloid cardioplegia composed of lactated Ringer's solution containing 40 mM/L KCl (Abbott Laboratories, North Chicago, IL).
12. PBS (Gibco-BRL).
13. Saline slush.
14. Surgical instruments: sternal retractor, aortic cross-clamp, haemostats, dissecting scissors, Mayo scissors, pickups, no. 11 and 15 surgical blades, right-angle forceps, atraumatic bulldog vascular clamp.
15. Sutures: 5/0 prolene, 2/0 polydioxanone, 2/0 and 3/0 vicryl, 2/0 silk (Ethicon).
16. Cannulae: 18- and 24-gage Teflon cannula (Quik-Cath®, Baxter Healthcare Corporation), 19-gage butterfly cannulae (Abbott Laboratories).
17. 3-mm Orotracheal tube (Intermediate Hi-Lo Cuffed Tracheal Tube®, Mallinckrodt Medical Inc., MO).
18. Positive pressure Sechrist Infant Ventilator (model IV-100B, Sechrist Industries, Anaheim, CA).
19. Blood gas analyzer (GEM Premier Plus, Instrumentation Laboratory, Lexington, MA).
20. Electrocardiograph (ECG) electrodes.
21. Pressure transducer (Gould Disposable Transducer model TDN) and signal amplifier (model 450, Mennen Medical).
22. Rectal temperature probe (probe YSI402, model 431D, Yellow Springs, OH).
23. Water mattress (K-20, American Pharmaseal).
24. Diathermy plate and machine (Valleylab).
25. Pediatric membrane oxygenator (Medtronic Minimax, Medtronic Cardiopulmonary, Anaheim, CA).

26. Integral heat exchanger in the oxygenator reservoir and water bath system (BIO-CAL 370, Biomedicus).
27. Two nonpulsatile roller pumps (Stöckert-Shiley, Irvine, CA).
28. Gas mixer (Sechrist) to control gas flow through the membrane oxygenator.
29. Life Pak 6S Cardiac Monitor (Hewlett Packard).
30. 8-Fr Infant arterial cannula (DLP, Grand Rapids, MI) and 18-Fr venous cannula (CR Bard, Tewksbury, MA).
31. 8-Fr Chest drain.

3. Methods

3.1. Technique 1: Selective Coronary Gene Delivery

3.1.1. Catheterization Technique

1. Anesthetize the piglet with ketamine (60 mg/kg im). Cannulate the ear vein, and inject 300 IU heparin. Position the animal supine, and stabilize with cord, thus exposing the anterior neck.
2. Scrub and drape.
3. Prepare the infusion system: fill a 30-mL syringe with saline containing 20 IU/mL heparin, and connect successively to a three-way connector, the 3-mL tubing, a second three-way connector, and then the coronary catheter. Expel all air bubbles. Prepare the introducer, and also flush it with heparinized saline solution. Fill a 10-mL syringe with contrast (8.0 mL) mixed with heparin (2.0 mL). Connect the contrast syringe to the distal three-way connector.
4. Infiltrate the proposed area of incision with 2 mL 1% lidocaine. Incise along the anterior border of the sternocleidomastoid muscle. Retract the muscle laterally to expose the common carotid artery.
5. Ligate the carotid artery distally with a 2/0 silk suture, and place a 2/0 silk suture loop around the artery proximally.
6. Clamp the artery proximally before performing a small arteriotomy. Insert the introducer, and remove the inner guide.
7. Insert the coronary catheter into the introducer, and conduct its tip under fluoroscopic assistance and intermittent delivery of contrast until it enters the right or left coronary ostium as required.

3.1.2. Gene Delivery

1. Thaw the adenoviral vector solution, and mix with PBS at room temperature to a final volume of 3 mL.
2. Slowly infuse the solution into the 3-mL tubing via the proximal stopcock to ensure that the solution remains in the tubing prior to controlled infusion via the pump.
3. Advance the coronary catheter until resistance is felt, and confirm the wedged position of the catheter by injecting 1 mL contrast. The coronary artery should be easily visualized, but there should be no backflow into the aorta.
4. Drive the pump at 80 mL/min for a total volume of 3 mL.

5. Slowly remove the coronary catheter (*see* **Note 1**).
6. Remove the introducer, and ligate the carotid artery using the loop suture.
7. Close the skin with a continuous 3/0 vicryl suture.

3.2. Technique 2: Gene Delivery During Cardiopulmonary Bypass

3.2.1. Anesthetic and Surgical Preparation

1. Anesthetize with 10 mg ketamine followed by isoflurane administered by face mask, initially at a concentration of 5%. Place an intravascular cannula in a marginal ear vein (*see* **Note 2**). Intubate under direct vision, using a laryngoscope with the piglet lying prone, and inflate the cuff with 2 mL of room air. Turn the piglet supine, and place it on a water heating mattress on the operating table. Secure its legs with cord, to increase stability.
2. Mechanically ventilate the piglet with 1–2% isoflurane (*see* **Note 3**).
3. Place three ECG electrodes on shaved skin to monitor the ECG and heart rate. Insert the rectal temperature probe, and maintain the temperature at 36–38°C by means of the water mattress. Ensure that a diathermy plate is placed underneath the animal, and connect to the diathermy machine.
4. Scrub the anterior chest and abdomen with chlorhexidine followed by ethanol.
5. Surgically expose the left femoral artery, and introduce an 18-gage cannula into the distal aorta. This arterial catheter is used to facilitate continuous blood pressure monitoring and arterial blood gas sampling. Connect the catheter to a pressure transducer and signal amplifier.
6. Perform a skin incision from the sternal notch to just below the xiphoid process. Perform a median sternotomy using Mayo scissors, and achieve hemostasis from subcutaneous and bone edges. Insert a sternal retractor, and open gradually.
7. Partially remove the thymus gland by blunt and sharp dissection, taking care not to damage the phrenic nerves. Open the pericardium in the midline, and use 2/0 silk stay sutures to improve access.
8. Develop plane between the aorta and the pulmonary trunk by sharp and blunt dissection, and pass a 2/0 silk suture around the aorta.
9. Administer 300 IU/kg heparin IV.
10. The CPB circuit should already be primed with fresh heparinized blood (450 mL) from an adult donor pig (*see* **Note 4**). The temperature of the perfusate is controlled by an integral heat exchanger in the oxygenator reservoir together with a water bath system. The water temperature is set to 40°C initially, and the perfusate is continuously circulated thereafter with a nonpulsatile roller pump at 100 mL/kg/min. A Sechrist Gas Mixer is used to control gas flow through the membrane oxygenator (*see* **Note 5**).
11. Insert an 8-Fr infant arterial cannula into the ascending aorta, through a 5/0 prolene purse-string suture with teflon pledgets. Insert a single 18-Fr venous cannula into the right atrial appendage through a 5/0 prolene purse-string suture with teflon pledgets.

12. Establish nonpulsatile CPB at 100 ml/kg/min. A collapsed right ventricle and absent LV ejection confirms satisfactory venous drainage. Return shed blood to the venous reservoir by a second roller pump.
13. Vent the LV through the left atrium using a 19-gage butterfly cannula connected to the pump suction.
14. After establishment of CPB, apply a cross-clamp to the aorta just proximal to the aortic cannula.
15. Inject 30 ml/Kg cold crystalloid cardioplegia at a rate of approx 50 mL/min, through a 21-gage butterfly cannula inserted into the proximal aorta (*see* **Note 6**). Judge satisfactory delivery by observing blanching of the coronary circulation and cardiac arrest.
16. Place saline slush within the pericardial cavity to provide topical cooling and aid myocardial protection.

3.2.2. Gene Delivery

1. Simultaneously, thaw the adenoviral vector from –80°C and reconstitute it in 8 mL of PBS at room temperature.
2. Immediately following delivery of cardioplegia, inject the adenoviral vector through the cardioplegia cannula. Flush the catheter and proximal aorta with a further 2 mL of PBS.
3. Attach the end of the butterfly cannula to the barrel of a 50-mL syringe to vent the aortic root passively.

3.2.3. Weaning From CPB and Recovery

1. Add 5 mg furosemide and 10 mg lidocaine to the venous reservoir, 5 min and 2 min, respectively, before releasing the aortic cross-clamp.
2. Defribrillate the heart as necessary with a 5-J shock.
3. Allow the heart to stabilize for 10 min prior to weaning from CPB.
4. Administer sodium bicarbonate as required according to arterial blood gas analysis.
5. Wean from CPB by partially and then totally occluding the venous cannula. Visually assess preload (right atrial filling) and cardiac contractility. Monitor arterial blood pressure. Guided by these parameters, additional transfusion via the aortic or femoral cannulae may be given.
6. Remove the venous and arterial cannulae, and tie the purse-string sutures. Additional 5/0 prolene sutures may be required to achieve hemostasis.
7. Reverse heparin with 10 mg protamine sulfate.
8. Insert an 8-Fr anterior mediastinal chest drain through the subxiphoid region.
9. Perform routine hemostasis prior to sternal closure with 2/0 polydioxanone. Close the subcutaneous tissues and skin in two layers with 2/0 and 3/0 vicryl.
10. After hemodynamic and metabolic stability are confirmed, remove the femoral arterial cannula, and ligate the femoral artery. Also close the groin wound in two layers. Inflitrate both the sternal and groin wounds with 10 mL 0.25% bupivicaine.

11. Following the cessation of isoflurane anesthesia, disconnect the piglet from the ventilator, and administer oxygen via a face mask when it is breathing satisfactorily. Continue ECG monitoring until the piglet makes attempts to gain sternal recumbency. At this stage, remove the chest drain and peripheral venous cannula.

12. Transfer the piglet to an infant incubator. Remove the endotracheal tube when the piglet is deemed able to maintain a patent airway. After sternal recumbency is achieved, the piglet may be transferred to the vivarium, and postoperative opioid analgesia is administered as required (0.5 mg im Butorphenol every 4 h).

4. Notes

1. After coronary gene delivery, wait approx 30 min for a hypotensive reaction, which is common after this technique of gene delivery. An easy way to record arterial pressure continuously is to insert a catheter connected to a pressure transducer into the carotid introducer instead of the coronary catheter. If hypotension develops, elevate the animal's legs, thus placing it in a Trendelenbug position to enhance venous return to the heart. Additional volume replacement by infusion of saline solution is only occasionally necessary.

2. To reduce postoperative pulmonary edema, an im injection of dexamethasone (12.5 mg) is administered 12 h preoperatively, as well as an intravenous bolus of dexamethasone (25 mg) on induction of anesthesia. Prophylactic antibiotics are also administered on induction of anesthesia.

3. Initial ventilator settings are as follows: inspired oxygen fraction 0.6, ventilation rate 24 breaths/min, inspiratory/expiratory ratio 1:1.2, peak inspiratory pressure 12 mmHg, positive end-expiratory pressure 0 mmHg, but adjust according to blood gas analysis.

4. Adult donor preparation: an adult pig weighing approx 30 kg is anesthetized with 15 mg/kg sodium penthol (Abbott Laboratories) im. A standard dose of 10,000 IU heparin is administered iv. The carotid artery is cannulated, and the blood drained into a fresh empty saline bag containing 3000 IU heparin. It is advisable to discard the last 200 mL of blood owing to activation of inflammatory mediators.

5. The initial settings on the gas mixer are as follows: total gas flow rate 3 L/min, oxygen fraction 60%, carbon dioxide fraction 2%.

6. Preliminary studies demonstrated an aortic root pressure of 80 mmHg under this infusion rate, which is within physiological limits and thus should minimize endothelial and myocardial damage.

References

1. Koch, W. J., Lefkowitz, R. J., and Rockman, H. A. (2000) Functional consequences of altering myocardial adrenergic receptor signalling. *Annu. Rev. Physiol.* **62,** 237–260.
2. Lefkowitz, R. J., Rockman, H. A., and Koch, W. J. (2000) Catecholamines, cardiac β-adrenergic receptors, and heart failure. *Circulation* **101,** 1634–1637.

3. French, B. A., Mazur, W., Geske, R. S., and Bolli, R. (1994) Direct in vivo gene transfer into porcine myocardium using replication deficient adenoviral vectors. *Circulation* **90,** 2414–2424.
4. Kypson, A. P., Hendrickson, S. C., Akhter, S. A., et al. (1999) Adenoviral-mediated gene transfer of the β_2-adrenergic receptor to donor hearts enhances cardiac function. *Gene Ther.* **6,** 1298–1304.
5. Maurice, J. P., Hata, J. A., Shah, A. S., et al. (1999) Enhancement of cardiac function after adenoviral-mediated in vivo intracoronary β_2-adrenergic receptor gene delivery. *J. Clin. Invest.* **104,** 21–29.
6. Shah, A. S., Lilly, E., Kypson, A. P., et al. (2000) Intracoronary adenovirus-mediated delivery and overexpression of the β_2-adrenergic receptor in the heart - prospects for molecular ventricular assistance. *Circulation* **101,** 408–414.
7. Barr, E., Carroll, J., Kalynych, A. M., Tripathy, S. K., Kozarsky, K., Wilson, J. M., and Leiden, J. M. (1994) Efficient catheter-mediated gene transfer into the heart using replication-defective adenovirus. *Gene Ther.* **1,** 51–58.
8. Hajjar, R. J., Schmidt, U., Matsui, T., et al. (1998) Modulation of ventricular function through gene transfer in vivo. *Proc. Natl. Acad. Sci. USA* **95,** 5251–5256.
9. Lodge, A. J., Chai, P. J., Daggett, C. W., Ungerleider, R. M., and Jaggers, J. (1999) Methylprednisolone reduces the inflammatory response to cardiopulmonary bypass in neonatal piglets: timing of dose is important. *J. Thorac. Cardiovasc. Surg.* **117,** 515–522.
10. Donahue, J. K., Kikkawa, K., Johns, D. C., Marban, E., Lawrence, and J. H. (1997) Ultrarapid, highly efficient viral gene transfer to the heart. *Proc. Natl. Acad. Sci. USA* **94,** 4664–4668.
11. Jones, J. M., Wilson, K. H., Koch, W. J., and Milano, C. A. (2002) Adenoviral gene transfer to the heart during cardiopulmonary bypass: effect of myocardial protection technique on transgene expression. *Eur. J. Cardiothorac. Surg.* **21,** 847–852.
12. Davidson, M. J., Jones, J. M., Emani, S., Wilson, K. H., Jaggers, J., Koch, W. J., and Milano, C. A. (2001) Cardiac gene delivery with cardiopulmonary bypass. *Circulation* **104,** 131–133.
13. Jones, J. M., Wilson, K. M., Steenbergen, C., Koch, W. J., and Milano, C. A. Dose dependent effects of cardiac β_2 adrenoceptor gene therapy. *J. Surg. Res.,* in press.
14. Bridges, C. R., Burkman, J. M., Malekan, R., et al. (2002) Global cardiac-specific transgene expression using of cardiopulmonary bypass with cardiac isolation. *Ann. Thorac. Surg.* **73,** 1939–1946.
15. Jones, J. M., Petrofski, J. A., Wilson, K. H., Steenbergen, C., Koch, W. J., and Milano, C. A. β_2 adrenoreceptor gene therapy ameliorates left ventricular dysfunction following cardiac surgery. *Eur. J. Cardiothorac. Surg.,* in press.
16. Franz, W. M., Rothman, T., Frey, N., and Katus, H. A. (1997) Analysis of tissue-specific gene delivery by recombinant adenoviruses containing cardiac-specific promoters. *Cardiovasc. Res.* **35,** 560–566.
17. Phillips, M. I., Tang, Y., Schmidt-Ott, K., Qian, K., and Kagiyama, S. (2002) Vigilant vector: heart-specific promoter in an adeno-associated virus vector for cardioprotection. *Hypertension* **39,** 651–655.

5

Manipulation of Neuronal Nitric Oxide Synthase Within the Paraventricular Nucleus Using Adenovirus and Antisense Technology

Yi-Fan Li, Yu Wang, Keith M. Channon, Harold D. Schultz, Irving H. Zucker, and Kaushik P. Patel

Summary

Congestive heart failure (CHF) is characterized by impaired cardiovascular reflexes and increased neurohumoral drive. The long-term sympatho-excitation increases the progression and risk of mortality during CHF. The paraventricular nucleus (PVN) of the hypothalamus is a very important central site for integration of sympathetic outflow and cardiovascular function. Within the PVN, nitric oxide (NO), mainly generated by neuronal nitric oxide synthase (nNOS), functions in inhibitory regulation of sympathetic outflow. Our previous study has indicated that in rats with experimental heart failure, the NO mechanism within the PVN is attenuated. We hypothesize that this alteration may contribute to the sympatho-excitation commonly observed in CHF. To investigate the role of NO within the PVN in sympathetic dysfunction in CHF, we have manipulated nNOS expression using adenoviral gene transfer of nNOS or nNOS antisense. These techniques have allowed us to observe the effects of alterations in nNOS on sympathetic outflow and cardiovascular function. In this chapter, we describe the methods for delivering nNOS adenoviral vector or nNOS antisense into the PVN using microinjection, as well as the protocols for detecting nNOS expression after these manipulations, using Western blot, NADPH-diaphorase staining, and immunofluorescent staining.

Key Words: Paraventricular nucleus of the hypothalamus; nitric oxide; neuronal nitric oxide synthase; sympatho-excitation; congestive heart failure; adenoviral gene transfer; antisense; microinjection; Western blot; NADPH-diaphorase staining; immunofluorescence.

From: *Methods in Molecular Medicine, vol. 112: Molecular Cardiology: Methods and Protocols*
Edited by: Z. Sun © Humana Press Inc., Totowa, NJ

1. Introduction

1.1. NO Within the PVN is Involved in Sympatho-Excitation in CHF

Sympatho-excitation is one of the major complications of congestive heart failure (CHF) *(1)*. The elevated sympathetic action causes an increase in cardiac afterload owing to vasoconstriction *(2,3)*, as well as an increase in cardiac preload owing to venoconstriction and water/sodium retention *(4)*. Long-term sympathetic excitation and high concentrations of plasma noradrenaline directly induce myocardial damage and apoptosis, which decrease myocardial contractility *(5)*. Overall, the elevated sympathetic action aggravates CHF. Although there has been significant progress in elucidating the peripheral mechanisms involved in this abnormality, the central mechanisms of the sympathetic abnormality in CHF are poorly understood *(6)*.

The paraventricular nucleus (PVN) of the hypothalamus is a key area that integrates sympathetic outflow *(6–8)*. Nitric oxide (NO) has been identified as an important modulator in the central nervous system (CNS) *(9)*. Neuronal NO synthase (nNOS) is a major resource of NO generation in the CNS. nNOS is densely localized in the PVN of the hypothalamus *(10–12)*, suggesting that NO may serve as a physiological modulator in that region. Previous studies have indicated that NO within the PVN exerts an inhibitory effect on sympathetic outflow and cardiovascular function *(13,14)*. We observed that microinjection into the PVN of an inhibitor of NO synthase, N^G-monomethyl-L-arginine (L-NMMA), increased renal sympathetic nerve discharge (RSND), arterial blood pressure, and heart rate in rats *(14)*. These data indicate that the endogenous NO system within the PVN is involved in mediating sympathetic outflow.

Our further studies have indicated that NO function within the PVN is altered in rats with experimental HF. First, we observed that the genetic message for nNOS is decreased in the hypothalamus of rats with HF *(15)*. We subsequently observed that the number of nNOS-positive neurons detected using the NADPH-diaphorase staining method was significantly decreased in the PVN of rats with HF compared with sham-operated control rats *(16)*. In a recent study, using microdissection of the PVN combined with reverse transcriptase-polymerase chain reaction (RT-PCR) and Western blot techniques, we confirmed that nNOS expression within the PVN was downregulated in HF compared with sham-operated rats *(17)*. Furthermore, our functional studies indicated that the response of sympathetic activity to blockade of NO within the PVN was attenuated in rats with HF compared with sham-operated control rats, suggesting that the endogenous NO-mediated inhibitory effect within the PVN on sympathetic outflow is less potent in HF rats compared with control rats *(18)*. These data support the concept that the reduced NO production within the PVN owing to the downregulation of nNOS causes an attenuated inhibition of sympathetic outflow. This may contribute to the elevated sympatho-excitation commonly observed during HF.

To investigate the role of NO within the PVN in the integration of sympathetic and cardiovascular function, we have used multiple approaches. Pharmacological stimulation or inhibition of NOS within the PVN are very powerful approaches. However, most of the selective NO synthase inhibitors currently used are only relatively selective, which sometimes makes it difficult to determine further the roles of specific NOS subtypes within the PVN in the regulation of sympathetic outflow. In addition, the relatively short-term effect of the injected compounds limits the efforts to determine long-term effects of NO in the PVN on sympathetic outflow.

Adenoviral vectors have been widely used to induce localized overexpression of a transferred gene in a target tissue *(19)*. Gene transfer of neuronal NOS, using an adenoviral vector (Ad.nNOS) generates high levels of recombinant nNOS protein and augments agonist-stimulated NO production in cultured vascular smooth muscle and endothelial cells and in vascular tissues in vivo *(20,21)*. Recently, we have used Ad.nNOS for transferring the nNOS gene into the PVN to test the role of NO production in the regulation of sympathetic outflow in rats *(22)*. The results indicated that Ad.nNOS gene transfer induced the local overexpression of nNOS within the PVN and an increased tonic suppression of sympathetic outflow.

Antisense technology is a widely used method of inhibition for many genes of interest *(23,24)*. This technique has been used to study cardiovascular regulation in both physiological and pathophysiological conditions *(25,26)*. Antisense to nNOS in the nucleus tractus solitarii has been shown to influence the regulation of blood pressure *(27)*. In our studies, we used nNOS antisense to inhibit nNOS expression specifically within the PVN and determine the role of NO in the regulation of sympathetic outflow.

In this chapter, we summarize the protocols using the Ad.nNOS vector to overexpress nNOS and using antisense to nNOS to block the effects of endogenous nNOS in order to study the role of NO within the PVN in the regulation of sympathetic outflow.

1.2. Overexpression of nNOS by the Adenovirus Vector

Adenoviral vectors encoding rat nNOS (Ad.nNOS) or β-galactosidase (Ad.β-gal) were constructed by Channon et al. (20). They recombined an adenoviral vector system derived from the 340 mutant strain of adenovirus type 5, inserted a nuclear localizing β-galactosidase expression cassette in the E1 cloning region, and induced unique restriction sites at the 3' end of the E1 cloning site. The resulting viral vector (Ad.β-gal) served as a control virus. The Ad.nNOS vector was created by replacing the β-galactosidase cassette with one containing an nNOS cDNA. The rat nNOS cDNA was cloned into a pGEM CMV plasmid. This plasmid was modified and digested into a linearized fragment containing the left Ad5 inverted terminal repeat (ITR), cytomegalovirus (CMV) promotor, nNOS cDNA, and simian virus 40 (SV40) pA. The vector "backbone" DNA was a fragment with an ITR and the viral packaging signal at the extreme 5' end, which was prepared from the parent vector Ad.β-gal. These two fragments were ligated for 1 h at room temperature using T4 DNA ligase. The ligated DNA was transfected into 293 cells using the calcium phosphate method. Following the observation of a cytopathic effect, the recombinant Ad.nNOS was isolated and purified by double cesium chloride density centrifugation, as previously described *(20,21)*. This recombinant Ad.nNOS vector contains a rat nNOS cDNA under the control of the CMV immediate-early promoter. The vector expresses functional nNOS protein in human vascular smooth muscle cells and human umbilical vein endothelial cells *(20)*. The construct also expressed functional nNOS protein when infused in the carotid arteries of rabbits *(21)*.

1.3. Inhibition of nNOS by Antisense

The general concept of antisense inhibition of gene expression is that a short DNA sequence in the antisense direction binds to its complementary site of the specific mRNA of the protein of interest in the cytoplasm and prevents ribosomal assembly and reading through the message, or induces mRNA degradation by RNase H. Consequently, the synthesis of the target protein is inhibited. There are many potential target sequences of antisense oligonucleotides (AS-ODNs). However, three regions are considered the most promising target sites for designing effective AS-ODNs: the 5' cap region, the AUG translation initiation codon, and the 3'-untranslated region of the mRNA. The common length of an AS-ODN is 15–20 bp.

In our study, we used nNOS antisense to inhibit nNOS expression within the PVN. The antisense sequence was 5'-ACGTGTTCTCTTCCATG, which is designed according to the neuronal NOS mRNA sequence (GenBank accession number NM 052799). The target site chosen for AS-ODN is the AUG translation initiation codon and some nearby downstream bases of the mRNA sequence of nNOS. To avoid nonspecific binding with mRNA of other genes, the chosen antisense sequence should not have significant homology with other genes. We checked the specificity of our antisense sequence of nNOS with a BLAST search of GenBank. The result of the BLAST search indicated that the chosen sequence had no significant overlap with other rat mRNAs. A mismatched ODN consisting of the same number of bases in random order was used as a control. The ODNs were modified with phosphorothiate oligodeoxynucleotides to improve their stability.

1.4. Determination of nNOS Expression Within the PVN

We focused on the role of nNOS within the PVN in the regulation of cardiovascular function and autonomic activities. It is always necessary to determine the changes in nNOS gene expression to confirm the correlation between the functional change and the change in nNOS gene expression. AS-ODNs may inhibit target gene function in several ways, including the induction of mRNA degradation or the disruption of protein translation. Consequently, in some cases, both mRNA and protein levels are decreased after antisense treatment. In other cases, however, a decrease in protein level can occur without a decrease in mRNA level. Regarding function, the protein level is the most important, although measuring both mRNA and protein levels simultaneously may provide more information.

The nNOS expression within the PVN can be determined by many methods. NADPH-diaphorase staining is an easily and widely used method to determine NOS activity. Immunohistochemistry with anti-nNOS antibody offers a very specific method to measure nNOS protein. Western blot combined with the PVN punch technique *(29)*, allows for a specific and quantitative measurement of nNOS protein levels within the PVN.

1.5. Functional Study: Effect of Manipulation of nNOS Within the PVN on Sympathetic Nerve Activity, Blood Pressure, and Heart Rate

The combination of molecular approaches for manipulation of nNOS with functional studies is critical to determine the effect of NO on sympathetic outflow and cardiovascular function within the PVN. To test the effects of manipulation of nNOS within the PVN on cardiovascular function and sympathetic outflow, we observed the responses in RSND, blood pressure (BP), and heart rate (HR) in anesthetized and conscious rats subjected to Ad.nNOS transfection or to the microinjection of antisense to nNOS into the PVN (*see* **Note 1**).

2. Materials

2.1. Delivery of the Ad.nNOS Vector or ODNs Into the PVN by Microinjection

1. Male Sprague-Dawley rats, 250–300 g.
2. Sodium pentobarbital.
3. Hamilton microsyringe, model 7000.5 (*see* **Note 2**).
4. Stereotaxic apparatus (Davis Kopf Instruments, Tujanga, CA).
5. Artificial cerebrospinal fluid (aCSF), composition: 3.0 mM KCl, 0.65 mM MgCl$_2$, 1.5 mM CaCl$_2$, 132 mM NaCl. Before use, add 24.6 mM NaHCO$_3$, and 3.3 mM glucose. Adjust pH to 7.4, Sterilize the solution with a 0.22-μm filter (*see* **Note 3**).

6. Dilute Ad.nNOS or Ad.β-gal vectors with sterilized aCSF to the working concentration of 10^8 pfu/mL (*see* **Note 4**).
7. Dissolve ODNs in aCSF to a concentration of 10 μg/μL. Sterilize with a 0.22-μm filter. Aliquot and store at −70°C.

2.2. NADPH-Diaphorase Staining

1. Perfusion machine.
2. Cryostat (Leica).
3. Sodium pentobarbital.
4. Heparinized saline (200 U/mL).
5. 4% Paraformaldehyde in 0.1 M phosphate-buffered saline (PBS) (500 mL): Add 7 g sodium phosphate dibasic in 400 mL ddH$_2$O. Dissolve using a stirbar and stirplate. Add 20 g paraformaldehyde, and immediately cover with foil. Leave the foil-covered container on the stirplate, and allow the solution to heat and mix until it becomes transparent. Do not allow the solution to boil. Cool it to room temperature. Adjust the pH to 7.4. Add ddH$_2$O to adjust the solution to 500 mL. Filter the solution with filter paper, and keep at 4°C.
6. 20% sucrose: add 20 g sucrose to 100 mL ddH$_2$O. Dissolve using a stirbar and stirplate. Store solution at 4°C.
7. 24-Well cell culture plates. These can be reused, but the inside of the well must be clear. It is not necessary to sterilize them.
8. NADPH-diaphorase solution: in 20 mL of 0.1 M PBS, pH 7.4, add 0.3% Triton X-100, 4 mg nitroblue tetrazolium (0.2 mg/mL). Dissolve using a stirrer to mix. Add 20 mg β-NADPH (1.0 mg/mL), and allow the solution to mix on the stirrer for 10 min.

2.3. nNOS Immunofluorescent Staining

1. Materials for transcardial perfusion and fixation are as mentioned previously in **Subheading 2.2.**
2. Monoclonal anti-nNOS antibody (Transduction Lab, Lexington, KY).
3. Donkey anti-mouse IgG secondary antibody conjugated with fluorescence Cy2 (Jackson).
4. Normal donkey serum (Jackson).
5. 0.1 M PBS.
6. 0.1 M PBS plus 0.1 % Triton X-100.
7. Blocking solution: 10 % of normal donkey serum in 0.1 M PBS.
8. Humidified chamber.

2.4. nNOS Western Blot

1. Cryostat (Leica).
2. 15-gage Luer Stub Adaptor (Becton Dickinson) for punching tissues.
3. Lysing buffer: 10 mM PBS, 1% Nonidet P-40, 0.5% sodium deoxycholate, 1% sodium dodecyl sulfate (SDS).
4. Protease inhibitor cocktail (Sigma).

5. Extraction buffer: add protease inhibitor cocktail to lysing buffer (100 μL/mL) just prior to extracting the samples.
6. 30% Acrylamide: dissolve 146 g of acrylamide and 4 g of *N,N'*-methylene-bis-acrylamide in 100 mL of Milli Q water. Filter and store at 4°C in the dark.
7. 10% SDS: dissolve 10 g of SDS into 100 mL Milli Q water. Store at room temperature.
8. Lower Tris buffer (4X): dissolve 18.17 g of Tris base in 90 mL Milli Q water. Add 4 mL of 10% SDS. Adjust the pH to 8.8. Make up solution to 100 mL. Store at 4°C.
9. Upper Tris buffer (4X): dissolve 6.06 g of Tris base in 90 mL Milli Q water. Add 4 mL of 10% SDS. Adjust the pH to 6.8. Make up solution to 100 mL. Store at 4°C.
10. 15% Ammonium persulfate (APS): dissolve 1.5 g in 10 mL of double-distilled water. Aliquot and store at –20°C.
11. TEMED (Sigma).
12. Reservoir buffer (10X): dissolve 30 g of Tris base and 144 g of glycine in 900 mL Milli Q water. Adjust the pH to 8.3. Make up to 1000 mL.
13. Tank buffer: take 100 mL of reservoir buffer and 10 mL of 10% SDS, and add Milli Q water to 1000 mL.
14. Transfer buffer: take 100 mL of reservoir buffer and 200 mL of methanol, and add Milli Q water to 1000 mL (*see* **Note 5**).
15. Loading buffer (2X): mix 0.5 mL of β-mercaptoethanol, 3 mL of 10% SDS, 1.25 mL of upper Tris buffer, 1 mg of pyronin Y, 4 mg of bromophenol blue, 5 mL of glycerol. Add Milli Q water to 10 mL. Alloquot and store at –20°C.
16. TBS buffer (10X): dissolve 80 g of NaCl, 2 g of KCl, and 30 g of Tris base in 800 mL of Milli Q water. Adjust the pH to 7.4. Add Milli Q water to 1000 mL.
17. TBST buffer: mix 100 mL of TBS buffer, 0.5 mL of Tween-20 in 800 mL of Milli Q water. Adjust the pH to 7.0. Add Milli Q water to 1000 mL.
18. Polyvinylidene difluoride (PVDF) membrane (Millipore) (*see* **Note 6**).
19. Bio-Rad Mini-protean system.

2.5. Functional Studies

1. General surgery instruments.
2. Grass amplifier (P55).
3. Grass bridge amplifier (S72).
4. Statham pressure transducer.
5. PowerLab data recording and analysis system.
6. UA-10 telemetry system (Data Sciences International): consists of a radiofrequency transducer, receiver panel, consolidation matrix, and computer with a PowerLab System.

3. Methods

3.1. Delivery of the Ad.nNOS Vector or ODNs Into the PVN by Microinjection (see Note 1)

1. Anesthetize the rat with 40 mg/kg pentobarbital ip.

2. Place the rat in a stereotaxic apparatus. Make a small burr hole on the skull using a dental drill. The coordinates for the right PVN are determined from the Paxinos and Watsons rat atlas *(29)*, i.e., 1.8 mm posterior, 0.4 mm lateral to the Bregma, and 7.8 mm ventral to the dura.
3. Advance a cannula (outer diameter 0.5 mm and inner diameter 0.1 mm) of the microsyringe that contains application agents into the right PVN (*see* **Note 2**).
4. Inject 100–300 nL of adenoviral vector (*see* **Note 4**), or 200 nL (2 µg) of ODN (*see* **Note 7**), slowly into the PVN over 20 min.
5. Following the injection, leave the microsyringe in place for 5 min, and then slowly withdraw the microsyringe cannula from the PVN.
6. After the injection, suture the wound. Allow the rats to recover in a cage. The analgesics (1 mL/kg Nubain-Stadol sc) are administered on each of the next 2 d (*see* **Note 8**).

3.2. NADPH-Diaphorase Staining

3.2.1. Transcardial Perfusion

1. Deeply anesthetize the rats with 70 mg/kg pentobarbital ip.
2. Open the rat up to the chest cavity. Hold the base of the heart with forceps, and puncture the left ventricle with a dulled needle that is connected to the perfusion machine.
3. Turn on the perfusion machine to perfuse the rat with heparinized saline. Clip a lobe of the liver so as to allow for the exit of the excess fluid.
4. When the paws and nose of the rat turn white, switch the machine to the 4% paraformaldehyde solution. When this solution enters the system, the body of the rat should begin to twitch noticeably and will eventually become stiff (*see* **Note 9**).
5. Remove the brain and put it into the 4% paraformaldehyde solution for further fixation at 4°C overnight.
6. Put the brain into 20% sucrose for 24 h for cryostat protection.

3.2.2. Staining Procedure

1. Just prior to sectioning the brain, add 0.5 mL of NADPH-diaphorase solution into the wells of a 24-well culture plate.
2. Block the brain in the coronal plane, and section it at 30-µm thickness in a cryostat (*see* **Note 10**).
3. Collect the sections of the PVN area, and place the sections into the NADPH-diaphorase solution in the wells of a 24-well culture plate.
4. Place the plate in an oven at 37°C for 60 min (*see* **Note 11**).
5. Following the reaction, rinse the sections in phosphate buffer, pH 7.4.
6. Mount the sections onto chrome-alum-coated slides (*see* **Note 12**). Air-dry the slides overnight. Rinse the slides in distilled water, and dry them again. Mount cover slips onto the slides.
7. Observe the slides with a light microscope, and record their images with a digital camera.

Examples of the NADPH-diaphorase staining of the PVN in transfected rats are shown in **Fig. 1**. There is an increase in the positively stained cells in the Ad.nNOS-transfected side of the PVN compared with the contralateral uninfected PVN (**Fig. 1A**). In contrast, in the Ad.β-gal-treated side of the PVN, there is no significant change in NADPH-diaphorase staining compared with the noninjected contralateral PVN (**Fig. 1B**).

3.3. nNOS Immunofluorescent Staining

The limitation of NADPH-diaphorase is its nonselective staining of all NOS isoforms. Immunohistochemistry is a very specific method to determine different NOS isoforms by using specific antibodies. In our study, we use immunofluorescent staining to determine the alterations in nNOS expression following the manipulations with adenoviral gene transfection or antisense inhibition.

1. Prepare the rats and fix the brains (*see* **Note 13**) as mentioned previously in **Subheading 3.2.1.**
2. Section the brains at 20-μm thickness in the coronal plane in a cryostat at –18°C (*see* **Note 14**). Mount the sections containing the PVN area on a glass slide.
3. Incubate the slides for 5 min in 0.1 *M* PBS + 0.1% Triton X-100 to increase the permeability of the cells.
4. Incubate the slides with blocking solution for 1 h at room temperature to prevent non-specific binding (*see* **Note 15**).
5. Incubate the slides with the primary antibody in blocking solution (1:100) for 1 h at room temperature or overnight at 4°C (*see* **Note 16**).
6. Following 3 washes with PBS, incubate the sections with a secondary antibody (1:500) (*see* **Note 17**) for 30 min at room temperature. After three washes, air-dry and mount the sections with Fluoromount (BDH Laboratory Supplies, England) and cover slips. Observe the slides under a Leica microscope with appropriate excitation/emission filters. Capture the pictures using a digital camera system (*see* **Note 15**).

Figure 2 shows an example of immunofluorescent staining of antisense inhibition of nNOS. In the antisense-injected side of the PVN, nNOS-positive neurons are significantly reduced. Conversely, within the noninjected contralateral PVN, a number of nNOS-positive neurons are stained with bright green fluorescence.

3.4. nNOS Western Blot

NADPH-diaphorase and immunofluorescent staining provides valuable *in situ* information on nNOS expression. The limitation is that histological data are difficult to analyze aquantitatively. In our study, we punched the PVN tissues for protein extraction and performed immunoblot studies (Western) with

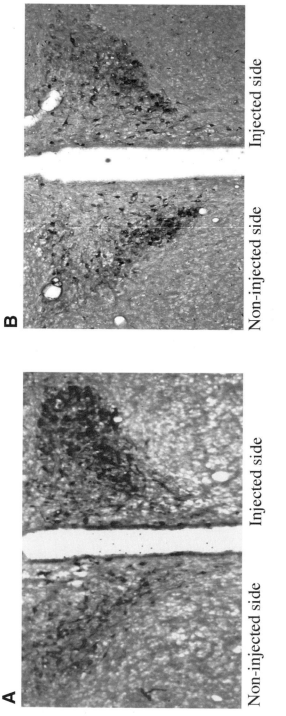

Fig. 1. NADPH-diaphorase staining of nNOS in the PVN infected with adenoviral vectors. (**A**) The injected side of the PVN infected with control adenovirus vector (Ad.β-gal) did not induce a significant increase in nNOS expression compared with the non-injected side. (**B**) The injected side of the PVN infected with Ad.nNOS induced a significant increase in nNOS expression compared with the noninjected side.

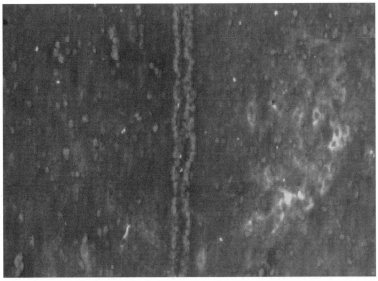

Antisense-injected side   Non-injected side

Fig. 2. Immunofluorescence staining of nNOS in the PVN injected with ODNs. The nNOS-positive neurons show bright green flourescence (Cy2 staining) in the noninjected side of the PVN. Conversely, in the antisense-injected side, the nNOS-positive neurons are significantly reduced.

anti-nNOS antibody to determine nNOS expression quantitatively within the PVN.

3.4.1. Sample Preparations

1. Deeply anesthetize the rats with 70 mg/kg pentobarbital ip and immediately remove and freeze the brains on dry ice.
2. Block the brains in the coronal plane, and section them at 300-μm thickness in a cryostat.
3. Collect and flatten the sections. Precool a Luer Stub Adapter needle on dry ice. According to the method of Palkovits and Brownstein *(28)*, punch the PVN area using the precooled needle from the injected side or the contralateral control side. Rinse the punched tissue in a labeled tube containing 100 μL of extract buffer.
4. Using a sonicator (GraLab 545), homogenize the punches on ice for 15 s.
5. Leave the samples at room temperature for 10 min.
6. Centrifuge the samples at 13,400g for 20 min. Pour the supernatants into new microcentrifuge tubes.
7. Determine protein contents in the supernatants using a BCA protein assay kit (Pierce).

8. Adjust the protein concentration in the samples to 0.5 μg/μL. Mix the protein sample with loading buffer at a ratio of 1:1.

3.4.2. SDS-PAGE and Immunoblotting

1. Prepare the 7.5% running gel by mixing 5.02 mL of 30% acrylamide stock with 4.98 mL of lower Tris buffer and 11.66 mL of Milli Q water. Add 99.74 μL of 10% APS and 10 μL of TEMED to polymerize the gel. Pour the gel into the space between the glass plates of the gel apparatus, leaving about 2 cm clear at the top. Layer water onto the top of the gel. Allow the gel to polymerize for 40 min.
2. Prepare the stacking gel by mixing 1 mL of 30% acrylamide stock with 2 mL of upper Tris buffer and 4 mL of Milli Q water. Add 27 μL of 10% APS and 7 μL of TEMED to polymerize the gel. Remove the top water and pour the stacking gel on top. Insert the comb of choice. Allow to polymerize for 30 min. Remove the comb.
3. Prior to loading, boil the prepared samples for 5 min. Load 20–30 μL of the samples (10–15 μg protein) into the wells of the stacking gel (*see* **Note 18**).
4. Electrophorese the samples in the tank buffer at 40 mA until the blue dyes have reached the bottom of the gel.
5. Wet the PVDF membrane (*see* **Note 16**) with methanol, and soak in transfer buffer. Wet several pieces of filter paper and two pieces of sponge with transfer buffer. Make the sandwich in the following order: one piece of sponge, two pieces of filter paper, the gel, the membrane, two pieces of filter paper, and one piece of sponge.
6. Electrotransfer for 90 min at 300 mA (*see* **Note 6**).
7. Block membrane by incubating in 5% fat-free milk powder in TBST for 30 min at room temperature.
8. Incubate membrane with monoclonal anti-nNOS antibody (Transduction Lab) in the 5% fat-free milk in TBST (1:1000) overnight at 4°C (*see* **Notes 19** and **20**).
9. Following three washes with TBST, incubate the membrane with a peroxidase-conjugated goat antimouse IgG secondary antibody (Pierce Chemical, Rockford, IL) in the 5 % fat-free milk in TBST (1:5000) for 1–2 h at room temperature (*see* **Note 20**).
10. Following three washes with TBST, visualize the signals on the membrane using enhanced chemiluminescence substrate (Pierce Chemical) (*see* **Note 21**) and Renaissance X-ray film (NEN/DuPont).
11. Capture the bands on the film using a Kodak digital camera, and analyze the net intensity of the bands using Kodak 1D Image Analysis Software (*see* **Note 20**).

Figure 3 shows examples of the Western blot detection of nNOS protein levels in the punched PVN samples. **Figure 3A** shows that nNOS gene transfection with Ad.nNOS induces an increase in nNOS protein level compared with the noninfected side and the side infected with Ad.β-gal. **Figure 3B** shows that injection into the PVN of the AS-ODN to nNOS induces a decrease in nNOS protein.

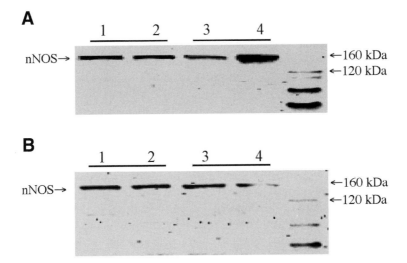

Fig. 3. Western blotting for nNOS in the punched PVN tissues. (**A**) Western blotting of nNOS protein in the samples of the PVN infected with adenoviral vectors. The samples of the noninjected side (lane 1) and injected side (lane 2) of the PVN in the rat infected with the control adenovirus vector (Ad.β–gal) did not exhibit in a significant increase in nNOS protein levels. The sample of the injected side (lane 4) of the PVN infected with Ad.nNOS exhibited in a significant increase in nNOS protein levels compared with the non-injected side (lane 3). (**B**) Western blotting for nNOS in punched PVN tissues injected with antisense to nNOS or missense. The samples of the noninjected side (lane 1) and injected side (lane 2) of the PVN injected with missense did not exhibit significantly increased nNOS protein levels. Conversely, the sample of the side (lane 4) of the PVN injected with nNOS antisense exhibited significantly reduced nNOS protein levels compared with the noninjected side (lane 3).

3.5. Functional Studies: Measuring Sympathetic and Cardiovascular Activities

3.5.1. Radiotelemetry Monitoring of Blood Pressure and Heart Rate in Conscious Rats

1. Calibrate the transducer to an accuracy of within ±3 mmHg.
2. Anesthetize the rats with 55 mg/kg ketamine and 10 mg/kg xylazine, ip (*see* **Note 22**).
3. Make a central abdominal incision. Place a radiotelemetry device (model TA11PA-C40) in the intraperitoneal space. Insert a flexible catheter attached to the transducer into the left femoral artery pointing upstream (against the blood flow).
4. For ODN administration, make a small burr hole in the skull. Place a guide cannula (0.7 mm OD and 0.2 mm ID) into the PVN, and fix it with dental acrylic.

5. Suture the incision, and allow the rats to recover for 3–5 d. House the rats in individual cages. Place the cages over a receiver panel connected to the computer for data acquisition.
6. Inject AS-ODN or missense ODN (2 µg in 200 nL) into the PVN through the guide cannula. The rats are unrestrained and free to move in their cages during the injection.
7. After administration of antisense or missense ODN, record the BP and HR signals continuously over the next 24 h.

3.5.2. Acute Recording of RSND

1. Three days after the Ad.nNOS or Ad.β-gal transfection of the PVN as described previously in this chapter, anesthetize the rat with 0.75 g/kg urethane ip and 70 mg/kg α-chloralose ip (*see* **Note 22**).
2. Catheterize the left femoral artery with polyethylene tubing (PE-50, filled with saline) connected to a Statham pressure transducer. Input the pressure signal from the transducer to a Grass bridge amplifier (S72), and then record the amplified signal with a PowerLab data acquisition system.
3. Place the rat in a stereotaxic apparatus, and insert a microinjection syringe cannula into the right PVN as described previously in **Subheading 3.1.**
4. Expose the left kidney through a left retroperitoneal flank incision. You can see the renal nerve track go between the artery and vein. Carefully isolate a branch of the renal nerve from the adipose and connective tissues and place the nerve on a thin bipolar steel electrode (*see* **Note 23**). Drop a mixture of Wacker Silgel 604A and 604B on the nerve–electrode junction to insulate it electrically from the surrounding tissues (*see* **Notes 24** and **25**).
5. Connect the electrode to a Grass amplifier (P55). Set the high- and low-frequency cutoffs at 1000 and 100 Hz, respectively. Direct the electrical signal output from the Grass amplifier to a Grass Integrator, which rectifies the signal and integrates the raw nerve discharge. The output of the Grass Integrator is recorded and stored for later analysis in a computer-based data acquisition system, PowerLab.
6. Following a 30–40-min stabilization period, record baseline RSND. All RSND recordings are corrected by subtraction of background noise, defined as the signal remaining after administration of 20 mg/kg hexamethonium iv or postmortem.
7. Inject an inhibitor of NO synthase, L-NMMA, in doses of 50, 100, and 200 pM in 50, 100, and 200 nL, respectively, into the PVN with intervals of 30 min between each dose. Record the responses in BP, HR, and RSND after each dose of L-NMMA. The response of RSND to the administration of drugs into the PVN during the experiment is subsequently expressed as a percentage change from the basal value.
8. At the end of the experiments, inject monastral blue dye into the brain for histological verification of injection sites. Remove and fix the brain in 4% formaldehyde for at least 24 h. Section the brain (30 µm) using a cryostat at −18°C. Mount the sections on microscope slides, and stain the slides with 1% aqueous neutral red. Verify the presence of the blue dye within the PVN microscopically.

Injection of ODN

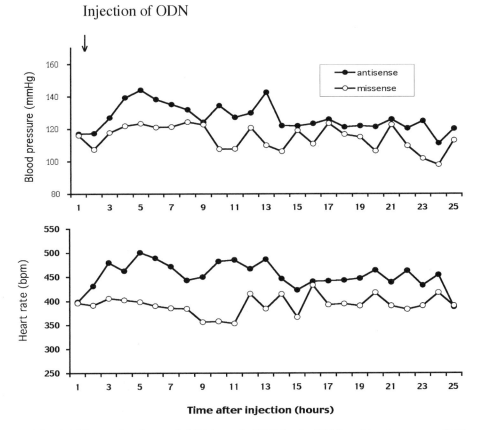

Fig. 4. Effects of antisense inhibition of nNOS in the PVN on blood pressure (BP) and heart rate (HR) in one conscious rat treated with antisense (closed circles) and one rat treated with missense (open circles). Following ODN injection in the PVN, the BP and HR increased over the next 5 h in the rat treated with antisense to nNOS. There was no significant change in BP and HR in the rat treated with missense ODN.

As shown in **Fig. 4**, in the conscious rat, BP and HR were markedly increased during an 8-h period following the administration of nNOS antisense. Conversely, there were no significant changes in BP and HR in the rat treated with missense control ODN.

Figure 5 shows the responses to the NO blocker L-NMMA in Ad.nNOS- or Ad.β-gal–transfected rats. Microinjection of L-NMMA induces a significantly greater response in RSND in the Ad.nNOS rat compared with that of the control Ad.β-gal rat, suggesting an increased inhibitory action of NO on sympathetic outflow in the PVN.

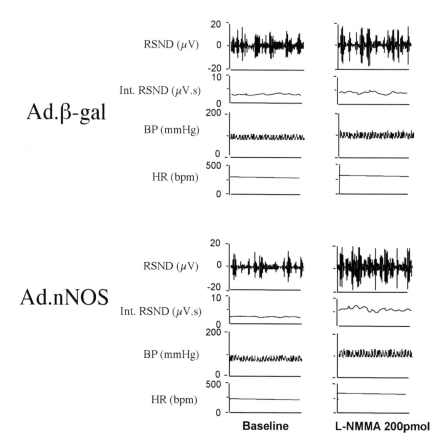

Fig. 5. Recordings of RSND, BP, and HR in anesthetized rats whose PVNs were transfected with either Ad.β-gal (top panel) or Ad.nNOS (bottom panel). The response in RSND to L-NMMA was greater in the Ad.nNOS-transfected rat (right bottom) than in the Ad.β-gal-transfected rat (right top).

4. Notes

1. The entire procedure must be performed under bacteria-free conditions.
2. The cannula of the microsyringe can be sterilized using 75% ethanol followed by several washes with sterile aCSF.
3. Appropriate preparation of aCSF is very important for the success of the gene transfection. NaHCO$_3$ and glucose must be added freshly. The pH value must be corrected before use.
4. The appropriate concentrations of Ad.nNOS used for injection need to be optimized. NADPH-diaphorase staining can be used to evaluate the efficiencies of the different doses. In our previous study, a 200-nL solution (final conc. 1×10^8 pfu/mL) of Ad.nNOS or Ad.β-gal was injected into the PVN. Initially, we

observed that higher Ad.nNOS concentrations of 1×10^{10}–1×10^{12} PFU/mL resulted in the destruction of neurons at the site of injection. With a concentration of 1×10^{8} PFU/mL, no damage to the neurons within the PVN was observed from light microscopic evaluation.

5. The transfer buffer can be reused several times. However, an additional 5% of methanol needs to be added into the transfer buffer when it is reused.

6. The other kind of membrane commonly used for Western blot is a nitrocellulose membrane. A nitrocellulose membrane has a lower binding affinity for proteins than a PVDF membrane. Thus, when a nitrocellulose membrane is used, the transfer time may be reduced to 1 h.

7. The appropriate amount of ODN administered into the PVN may vary owing to the differences in length, sequence, modification, and purity of the ODN. The optimization should always be performed. A common range for the amounts of ODN applied via brain microinjection is 1–10 μg.

8. The periods for transfection also need to be evaluated and chosen according to the objectives of the experiment. In our previous study, we observed that after 3 d of injections, the injected sites showed significant increases in nNOS expression.

9. A good perfusion is very important for the success of the staining. Once the chest cavity is open, the puncture procedure should be done quickly and the perfusion of saline should be started before the heartbeat stops so as to wash the blood out of the body completely. The 4% paraformaldehyde in $0.1\ M$ PBS should be made freshly and prechilled on ice.

10. Make a small cut at the edge of the brain block as a marker to indicate the different sides. Once the sections are put into the staining solution, the sides of the section will be difficult to identify. The section can be mounted correctly according to the marker.

11. The period of incubation for the sections with the NADPH-diaphorase solution is 30–60 min at 37°C. After 30 min of incubation, check the color of the section. Once the color of the section becomes bright blue, stop the incubation. If the blue is dim and faint, prolong the time of incubation. If the color is still faint after a 60-min incubation, prolonging the incubation is not helpful. Check whether errors were made in the previous steps.

12. Mounting the section on the slide is tricky. Fill a large culture dish with PBS. Float the section in the PBS. Put a slide into the PBS under the section. Using a fine painting brush, carefully move the section in the solution onto the slide and get the slide slowly out of the solution. Great care should be taken to avoid getting the section twisted, stretched, or wrinkled.

13. Fresh tissue without perfusion fixation can also be used for immunoflourescent staining of nNOS. In this case, some post-fixations may be used. The sectioned tissues can be incubated with prechilled 100% acetone, or 50% ethanol + 50% methanol, or 100% methanol for 10–30 min at –20°C. The sections can also be incubated with prechilled 4% paraformaldehyde solution for 30 min at 4°C. Following the fixation, the sections are rinsed with $0.1\ M$ PBS + 0.1% Triton X-100 followed by the regular blocking procedure.

14. High quality of the tissue section is important. Do not use a blunt blade. Avoid folding of the section.

15. The background is a common problem in immunofluorescent staining. If a monoclonal antibody of nNOS (for example, the product of Transduction Lab) is used, the background is unlikely due to the concentration of the primary antibody; it is probably caused by to the nonspecific reaction of the secondary antibody. The appropriate blocking procedure is crucial. Always use a suitable serum from the species in which the secondary antibody has been developed. A longer (up to overnight at 4°C) blocking incubation may be helpful. The concentrations of the secondary antibody should be optimized. Finally, the complete washes following the incubation with the primary and secondary antibodies are always important. Prolong the wash time, and use additional washes if the background is still high.

16. The alternative is to incubate with the primary antibody for 1–2 h at room temperature. This is a time-saving procedure. However, incubation with the primary antibody for a longer time (24–48 h) at 4°C is likely to give a better signal-to-noise ratio.

17. In our experience, for rat tissues, the secondary antibody developed in donkey (Jackson) gives a better signal-to-noise ratio compared with that from rabbit and goat.

18. In our experiments, a detectable band of nNOS can be obtained when loading as little as 1 μg of total protein of the PVN sample. However, a common range of loading amount is 5–15 μg of total proteins per lane.

19. An alternative incubation time for the primary antibody is 1–2 h at room temperature followed by the same wash procedure. This is a time-saving method, and it always works well with our samples. However, if the signal appears faint or the background noise appears high, incubation with the primary antibody overnight at 4°C is recommended.

20. A high background signal is a common problem in Western blotting. Several alternatives may be used to reduce the noise signal. For example, prolong the time of blocking incubation with 5% milk to 1–2 h, or use 10% milk instead of 5%. The wash is very important to prevent noise signal. To reduce the background, it is helpful to try a longer time or larger volume of wash following the primary and secondary antibody incubations. If both the background and expected signal are high, reducing the amount of secondary antibody or shortening the incubation time may be considered.

21. Different grades of chemiluminescent agents have different sensitivities. We usually use Piece SuperSignal West Pico Chemiluminescent Substrate, which produces a good signal with our experimental condition. Its lower detection limit is in the low-picogram (10^{-12}) range. If lower concentrations or lesser amounts of samples have to be used, owing to the limited sample resource, for example, a more sensitive chemiluminescent agent may be used. For example, Piece SuperSignal West Femto Chemiluminescent Substrate provides a lower detection limit in the low-femtogram (10^{-15}) range.

22. Anesthesia significantly affects the nerve discharge and blood pressure. Be sure to use the same kind of anesthesia and the same ratio of anesthesia to body weight in the rats for the same experiments. For long-term (more than 4 h) recording, additional anesthesia may be needed. Give the additional anesthesia intraperitoneally instead of intravenously to maintain a constant level.

23. To isolate an intact, well-functioning branch of the renal nerve track, great care needs to be taken. Use a glass bar to separate the nerve from the connective tissue. Never stretch the nerve too tight. Start the isolation at the far peripheral end of the branch so as to leave some spare part of the branch. In case the first part is damaged, you can move forward centrally to the spare part to try again.

24. Once the nerve is isolated, bath it in mineral oil or normal saline immediately to avoid drying out.

25. The most common method used to insulate the electrode–nerve junction from tissues and fluid involves the use of mineral oil. However, for long-term recording (more than 1 h), this method is not very good. We used the approach of insulating the junction from the surrounding tissues with a mixture of Wacker silgel 604A and 604B. The ratio of gel A and B is 5:1. Incubate the mixed gels at 60°C for 3 min to promote solidifying. When the mixture cools down to about 37°C and becomes as thick as a semiliquid, pour the gel onto the electrode–nerve junction. After about 20 min, the gel mixture becomes solid. This solid cover serves multiple roles including insulating, bathing, and fixing the junction so as to stabilize the signal recording for a long time (up to 8 h).

References

1. Cohn, J. N., Levine, T. B., Olivari, M. T., et al. (1984) Plasma norepinephrine as a guide to prognosis in patients with chronic congestive heart failure. *N. Engl. J. Med.* **311**, 819–823.

2. Eisenhofer, G., Friberg, P., Rundqvist, B., et al. (1996) Cardiac sympathetic nerve function in congestive heart failure. *Circulation* **93**, 1667–1676.

3. Patel, K. P., Zhang, K., and Carmines, P. K. (2000) Norepinephrine turnover in peripheral tissues of rats with heart failure. *Am. J. Physiol. Regul. Integr. Comp. Physiol.* **278**, R556–R562.

4. Hillege, H. L., Girbes, A. R. J., De Kam, P. J., et al. (2000) Renal function, neurohormonal activation, and survival in patients with chronic heart failure. *Circulation* **102**, 203–210.

5. Singh, K., Communal, C., Sawyer, D. B., and Colucci, W. S. (2000) Adrenergic regulation of myocardial apoptosis. *Cardiovasc. Res.* **45**, 713–719.

6. Patel, K. P. and Zhang, K. (1996) Neurohumoral activation in heart failure: role of paraventricular nucleus. *Clin. Exp. Pharmacol. Physiol.* **23**, 722–726.

7. Kannan, H., Hayashida, Y., and Yamashita, H. (1989) Increase in sympathetic outflow by paraventricular nucleus stimulation in awake rats. *Am. J. Physiol. Regul. Integr. Comp. Physiol.* **256**, R1325–R1330.

8. Swanson, L. W. and Sawchenko, P. E. (1980) Paraventricular nucleus: a site for

the integration of neuroendocrine and autonomic mechanisms. *Neuroendocrinology* **31,** 410–417.

9. Garthwaite, J. and Boulton, C. L. (1995) Nitric oxide signaling in the central nervous system. *Annu. Rev. Physiol.* **57,** 683–706.

10. Vincent, S. R. and Kimura, H. (1992) Histochemical mapping of nitric oxide synthase in the rat brain. *Neuroscience* **46,** 755–784.

11. Bredt, D. S., Hwang, P. M., and Snyder, S. H. (1990) Localization of nitric oxide synthase indicating a neural role for nitric oxide. *Nature* **347,** 768–770.

12. Sanchez, F., Alonso, J. R., Arevalo, R., Blanco, E., Aijon, J., and Vanzquez, R. (1994) Coexistence of NADPH-diaphorase with vasopressin and oxytocin in the hypothalamic magnocellular neurosecretory nuclei of the rat. *Cell Tissue Res.* **276,** 31–34.

13. Horn, T., Smith, P. M., McLaughlin, B. E., Bauce, L., Marks, G. S., Pittman, Q. J., and Ferguson, A. V. (1994) Nitric oxide actions in paraventricular nucleus: Cardiovascular and neurochemical implications. *Am. J. Physiol. Regul. Integr. Comp. Physiol.* **266,** R306–R313.

14. Zhang, K., Mayhan, W. G., and Patel, K. P. (1997) Nitric oxide within the paraventricular nucleus mediates changes in renal sympathetic nerve activity. *Am. J. Physiol.* **273,** R864–R872.

15. Patel, K. P., Zhang, K., Zucker, I. H., and Krukoff, T. L. (1996) Decreased gene expression of neuronal nitric oxide synthase in hypothalamus and brainstem of rats in heart failure. *Brain Res.* **734,** 109–115.

16. Zhang, K., Zucker, I. H., and Patel, K. P. (1998) Altered number of diaphorase (NOS) positive neurons in the hypothalamus of rats with heart failure. *Brain Res.* **786,** 219–225.

17. Li, Y.-F. and Patel, K. P. (2003) Paraventricular nucleus of the hypothalamus and elevated sympathetic activity in heart failure: altered inhibtory mechanisms. *Acta Physiol.Scand.* **177,** 17–26.

18. Zhang, K., Li, Y. F., and Patel, K. P. (2001) Blunted nitric oxide-mediated inhibition of renal nerve discharge within PVN of rats with heart failure. *Am. J. Physiol. Heart Circ. Physiol.* **281,** H995–H1004.

19. Davidson, B. L. and Breakefield, X. O. (2003) Viral vectors for gene delivery to the nervous system. *Nat. Rev. Neurosci.* **4,** 353–364.

20. Channon, K. M., Blazing, M. A., Shetty, G. A., Potts, K. E., and George, S. E. (1996) Adenoviral gene tranfer of nitric oxide synthase: high level expression in human vascular cells. *Cardiovasc. Res.* **32,** 962–972.

21. Channon, K. M., Qian, H., Neplioueva, V., et al. (1998) In vivo gene tranfer of nitric oxide synthase enhances vasomotor function in carotid arteries from normal and cholesterol-fed rabbits. *Circulation* **98,** 1905–1911.

22. Li, Y. F., Roy, S. K., Channon, K. M., Zucker, I. H., and Patel, K. P. (2002) Effect of in vivo gene transfer of nNOS in the PVN on renal nerve discharge in rats. *Am. J. Physiol. Heart Circ. Physiol.* **282,** H594–H601.

23. Meyers, K. J. and Dean, N. M. (2000) Sensible use of antisense: how to use oligonucleotides as reasearch tools. *Trends Pharmacol. Sci.* **21,** 19–23.

24. Leslie, R. A., Hunter, J., and Robertson, H. A. (2000) Antisense technology in the central nervous system. *Trends Neurosci.* **23,** 447.

25. Phillips, M. I., Wielbo, D., and Gyurko, R. (1994) Antisense inhibition of hypertension: a new strategy for renin-angiotensin candidate genes. *Kidney Int.* **46,** 1554–1556.

26. Diz, D. I., Westwood, B., and Averill, D. B. (2001) AT_1 antisense distinguishes receptors mediating angiotensin II actions in solitary tract nucleus. *Hypertension* **37,** 1292–1297.

27. Maeda, M., Hirano, H., Kudo, H., Doi, Y., Higashi, K., and Fujimoto, S. (1999) Injection of antisense oligos to nNOS into nucleus tractus solitarii increases blood pressure. *Neuroreport* **10,** 1957–1960.

28. Palkovits, M. and Brownstein, M. (1988) *Maps and Guide to Microdissection of the Rat Brain.* Elsevier, New York.

29. Paxinos, G. and Watson, C. (1986) *The Rat Brain in Stereotaxic Coordinates.* Academic Press, Orlando, FL.

6

TAT-Mediated Protein Transduction

Delivering Biologically Active Proteins to the Heart

Åsa B. Gustafsson, Roberta A. Gottlieb, and David J. Granville

Summary

TAT protein transduction is a novel method of delivering biologically active proteins into cells and tissues through the fusion of a protein transduction domain to the protein of interest. The present chapter outlines the methodology pertaining to the preparation of TAT-fusion proteins and how to efficiently transduce these proteins into cultured cells or isolated rat hearts perfused in Langendorff mode.

Key Words: TAT protein transduction; heart; cardiac myocytes; apoptosis; cell culture; protein expression; Langendorff perfusion; ischemia and reperfusion; necrosis; cardiovascular injury and repair; novel protein-based therapeutics.

1. Introduction

Biological manipulation of mammalian cell protein expression has traditionally been achieved by transfection of expression vectors or microinjection. Although these approaches have been fairly successful, the efficiency is relatively low in many cell types, and cell viability is often greatly compromised *(1–3)*. Furthermore, it is often impractical, especially when using isolated tissue or organ models in which viability is limited, to utilize standard adenoviral approaches because of the time required to synthesize the protein of interest. The ability to introduce proteins into the heart rapidly would greatly enhance our ability to study the function of various proteins in isolated, perfused heart models.

From: *Methods in Molecular Medicine, vol. 112: Molecular Cardiology: Methods and Protocols*
Edited by: Z. Sun © Humana Press Inc., Totowa, NJ

One recent method to circumvent these problems has been through the use of human immunodeficiency virus (HIV) TAT-mediated protein transduction. The technology requires the synthesis of a fusion protein, linking an arginine-rich, 11-amino acid TAT (amino acids 47–57) PTD (YGRKKRRQRRR [single letter amino acid code]) to the protein of interest using a bacterial expression vector followed by purification of this fusion protein under soluble or denaturing conditions. The protein can then be added directly to cells in culture, perfused into isolated tissues, or injected in vivo into mice. Protein transduction occurs in a concentration-dependent manner, achieving maximum intracellular levels within 15 min, with nearly equivalent concentrations among all cells in the transduced population (**Fig. 1**) *(1–3)*. However, this method does have drawbacks compared with that of other methods of transfection, as the protein is subject to degradation. Therefore, for long-term studies in which viability is not limited, an adenoviral approach may be preferable. Conversely, a combination of both TAT and adenoviral approaches in tandem may be required to achieve optimum results. One such example is transplantation, whereby infusion of an antiapoptotic TAT fusion protein into the donor heart may provide protection against early peritransplant/ischemic injury until sufficient levels of the adenovirus-mediated antiapoptotic protein can be achieved.

The precise mechanism by which the TAT PTD enters cells is poorly understood, but it seems to involve a charge–charge interaction between the basic PTD and acidic membrane motifs *(2)*. Furthermore, internalization does not appear to involve transporters, endocytosis, or receptors *(2)*. Once the TAT PTD is inside the cells, refolding of denatured proteins is believed to be mediated by chaperone proteins such as heat shock proteins *(2)*.

TAT-mediated transduction offers several advantages over standard DNA transfection methods for inducing protein expression: (1) all eukaryotic cell types are susceptible to transduction, (2) transduction is very rapid (<15 min) and highly efficient (>95% cells), (3) equivalent amounts of the protein are introduced into each cell and can be controlled by simply adjusting the amount injected into the animal or added to the medium, and (4) TAT fusion proteins can be injected intraperitoneally and are detected and functional in all tissues in the body *(1–4)*. In particular, Schwarze et al. *(4)* were able to demonstrate that intraperitoneal injection of a 120-kDa TAT-β-galactosidase protein into mice was not only detectable, but functional, in all tissues, including the heart, brain, and bone marrow. Since then, owing to the ability of these proteins to cross the blood–brain barrier, numerous experiments have been published dem-

Fig. 1. Overview of TAT protein transduction methodology. The cDNA of interest is cloned into the pTAT-HA plasmid (courtesy of Dr. Steven Dowdy, UCSD). *E. coli* (BL-21[DE]) are then transformed with the plasmid, bacteria are plated, and colonies

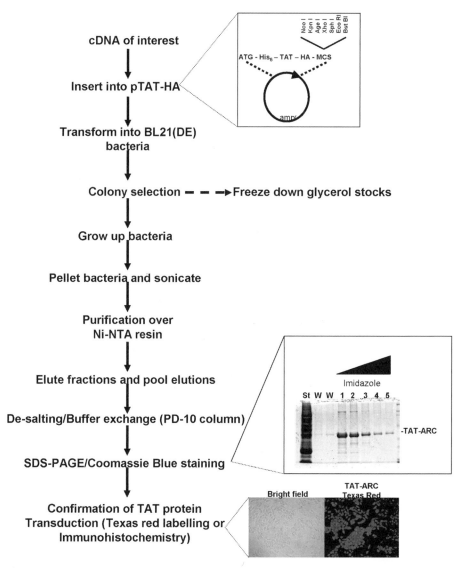

Fig. 1. *(continued)* are selected. Glycerol stocks are prepared for colonies expressing high levels of the TAT fusion protein (as determined by lysing 200 μL bacteria and Western blot analysis). High "TAT"-expressing bacteria are then grown up, pelleted, sonicated, and purified over an Ni-NTA column. Fractions are eluted with increasing concentrations of imidazole. Fractions expressing the protein of interest are then pooled and desalted using a PD-10 buffer exchange column. SDS-PAGE followed by Coomassie Blue staining or Western blotting for the protein of interest is performed to confirm that the protein of interest is present. TAT protein transduction can be confirmed by labeling the TAT–fusion protein with Texas Red or though immunostaining for the protein of interest. Functional assessment to confirm that the TAT protein is biologically active is also recommended when possible.

onstrating the utilization of this technology to introduce various types of proteins to the brain *(5–8)*. Furthermore, in our experience using Langendorff perfused rat hearts, infusion of the antiapoptotic TAT–ARC fusion protein for as little as 15 min was able to produce even dispersal of the protein in all cell types in the heart and provided significant protection against ischemia/reperfusion injury *(9)*.

In addition to TAT protein transduction, several other means have been used to transduce proteins into cells such as the *Drosophila* antennapedia transcription factor and the herpes simplex virus-1 DNA binding protein VP22 *(10)*. More recently, short oligomers of arginine have been utilized to facilitate uptake of agents into cells *(11)*. The latter polyarginine transporter system was shown to reduce ischemic heart injury significantly when conjugated to a cardioprotective εprotein kinase C agonist peptide *(11)*. However, in the current review, we will focus on the TAT protein transduction methodology.

2. Materials

1. 6xHis-TAT-HA cloning vector.
2. *Escherichia coli* strains DH5a and BL21(DE3) (Invitrogen, Carlsbad, CA).
3. Ampicillin (Sigma Chemical, St. Louis, MO).
4. IPTG (isopropyl-β-D-thio-galactopyranoside; Sigma).
5. Buffer Z: 8 M urea, 100 mM NaCl, 20 mM HEPES, pH 8.0.
6. Imidazole (Sigma).
7. Ni-NTA resin (Qiagen, Valencia, CA).
8. PD-10 desalting columns (Amersham Pharmacia, Piscataway, NJ).
9. Krebs-Ringer buffer: 118 mM NaCl, 4.75 mM KCl, 1.18 mM KH$_2$PO$_4$, 1.18 mM MgSO$_4$, 2.5 mM CaCl$_2$, 25 mM NaHCO$_3$, and 11 mM glucose.
10. Texas Red X succinimidyl ester (Molecular Probes, Eugene, OR).
11. Lysis buffer: 1% Nonidet NP-40, 20 mM Tris-HCl, pH 8.0, 137 mM NaCl, 10% glycerol supplemented with 1 mM phenylmethylsulfonyl fluoride (PMSF) and 0.15 U/mL aprotinin (Sigma).

3. Methods

The methods describe the expression and purification of TAT proteins, as well as the use of the TAT protein in Langendorff perfused hearts.

3.1. TAT Protein Expression and Purification

The method used to express and purify large quantities of transducible TAT proteins is described in **Subheadings 3.1.1.** and **3.1.2.** and, an overview is shown in **Fig. 1.** The TAT-HA-cDNA plasmid is transformed into BL21(DE) bacteria (Invitrogen), which has been optimized for recombinant protein expression. The BL21(DE) strain contains the T7 RNA polymerase gene, which can be induced by IPTG (*see* **Note 1**).

3.1.1. E. coli *Transformation and Selection*

1. Transform BL21(DE) bacteria by adding 10 ng of the pTAT-HA-cDNA plasmid to one vial of bacteria.
2. Mix by gently tapping the tube and incubate on ice for 30 min.
3. Heat-shock cells by incubating the vial in a 42°C waterbath for exactly 30 s, and then place back on ice.
4. Add 250 µL of prewarmed SOC, and incubate at 37°C for 1 h at 225 rpm.
5. Plate 20–200 µL of cells on LB plates containing 50 µg/mL ampicillin and incubate overnight at 37°C. Plate several different volumes to ensure well-spaced colonies on at least one plate.
6. Select six to eight colonies, and grow overnight in 4 mL LB media plus 50 µg/mL ampicillin and 100 µ*M* IPTG.
7. Screen for maximal protein production by first pelleting and lysing 200 µL of the cells with 50 µL 1X sample buffer. The sample buffer lysate is then boiled for 5 min, and proteins are separated by sodium dodecyl sulfate-polyacrylamide gel electrophoresis (SDS-PAGE) and analyzed by Western blotting.
8. Make glycerol stocks of the highest producing cultures by adding 500 µL culture to 500 µL sterile glycerol.
9. Store glycerol stocks at –80°C.

3.1.2. Protein Purification

1. Inoculate the highest expressing clone into a 1-L culture of LB plus 50 µg/mL ampicillin and 100 µ*M* IPTG overnight at 225 rpm and 37°C (*see* **Note 2**).
2. Recover the cells by centrifugation at 5000*g* for 15 min
3. Wash the cell pellets with 25 mL PBS, and combine pellets into one tube.
4. Resuspend bacterial pellet in 10 mL of buffer Z plus 20 m*M* imidazole.
5. Sonicate the bacteria on ice with three pulses of 15 s each with 30 s on ice in between pulses. Sonicate in biological safety cabinet (*see* **Note 3**).
6. Clarify the sonicate by centrifugation at 20,000*g* for 20 min at 4°C.
7. Pack 5 mL Ni-NTA resin into a column, and wash with 10 vol of buffer Z + 20 m*M* imidazole.
8. Apply the supernatant to the column with pre-equilibrated Ni-NTA resin at room temperature.
9. Allow binding to the resin by gravity flow, or a slight air pressure via syringe can be applied if needed.
10. Wash the column with 10 bed volumes of buffer Z plus 20 mM imidazole (*see* **Note 4**).
11. Elute the TAT fusion protein by stepwise adding 1 bed vol of buffer Z containing 100 m*M*, 250 m*M*, 500 m*M*, and 1 *M* imidazole.
12. Analyze each fraction by Coomassie Blue staining of an SDS-PAGE and immunoblot analysis.
13. Once the elution fraction has been identified, the stepwise elution can be replaced by one elution step with 2 vol of buffer Z + the concentration of imidazole in

which the protein elutes in. TAT–ARC and TAT–β-gal are eluted with buffer Z plus 250 mM imidazole.

14. Pool the appropriate fractions.
15. Apply onto PD-10 columns pre-equilibrated in PBS.
16. Determine the protein concentration by SDS-PAGE relative to a bovine serum albumin (BSA) standard, or by Bradford assay if the protein appears pure by Coomassie Blue staining.
17. Store the TAT protein at 4°C, and use within a week or freeze at –70°C for long-term storage (*see* **Note 5**).

3.2. TAT–Protein Transduction

3.2.1. TAT–Protein Transduction into Langendorff Perfused Hearts

1. Excise the heart from the anesthetized rat, and quickly cannulate onto the Langendorff perfusion apparatus.
2. Perfuse the heart at a constant pressure of 60 mmHg with Krebs-Ringer buffer, and bubble the perfusate with a mixture of 95% O_2 and 5% CO_2 at 37°C.
3. Equilibrate the heart for 5 min in Krebs-Ringer buffer.
4. Add the TAT–protein (20–200 nM) to the perfusion buffer, and perfuse the heart for 15 min while recirculating the buffer (*see* **Note 6**). The TAT–protein is rapidly taken up by all cell types in the heart.
5. Subject the heart to global no-flow ischemia for 30 min by turning off the perfusion system.
6. After 30 min of ischemia, turn on the perfusion system to start reperfusion.
7. Nontransduced TAT–protein is washed out during reperfusion with Krebs-Ringer buffer.

3.3. Detection of TAT–Protein Transduction

Protein transduction and localization can be determined in two ways. The first method is by Western blot analysis using an antibody specific for the TAT fusion protein or the HA tag. The other is by directly labeling the TAT–protein with Texas Red and visualization of uptake by fluorescent microscopy.

3.3.1. Labeling of TAT–Protein With Texas Red

1. Add Texas Red-X succinimidyl ester to the protein at a molar ratio of dye to protein of 1:10.
2. Incubate for 1 h at room temperature.
3. Remove unconjugated dye by gel filtration on Sephadex G-25 columns (equivalent to PD-10 columns).
4. Elute with 3.5 mL of PBS.

3.3.2. Detection of Texas Red-Labeled TAT–Protein by Immuno-fluorescence

1. Fix the heart by perfusing 4% formaldehyde.
2. Remove a 2-mm-thick coronal median slice.
3. Embed the slice in paraffin, and cut sections at a thickness of 3 μm.
4. Deparaffinize in xylene, and rehydrate with graded ethanol.
5. Stain the sections with 30 μg/mL Hoechst 33342 to visualize nuclei.
6. Rinse in PBS.
7. Visualize by fluorescence microscopy.

3.3.3. Detection of TAT–Protein in Heart Tissue by Western Analysis

1. Homogenize the TAT–protein perfused heart by Polytron in lysis buffer.
2. Clear the lysate by centrifugation at 20,000g for 20 min at 4°C.
3. Separate proteins by SDS-PAGE, and transfer to nitrocellulose membrane.
4. Probe for TAT–protein using an antibody (**Fig. 2**).

4. Notes

1. For toxic TAT fusion proteins, use BL21(DE3)pLysS or BL21(DE3)pLysE bacterial strains to express the protein of interest. These strains carry a plasmid with the gene for the T7 lysogen to keep the expression of T7 RNA polymerase low. Chloramphenicol is needed to select for cells that express the lysogen. Use the pLysE strain only for very toxic proteins. This strain expresses higher levels of T7 lysosome than pLysS and will produce a lower level of protein expression after IPTG induction. Also, the T7 RNA polymerase gene is under the expression of the lacUV5 promoter, which is induced by IPTG. However, this is a very leaky promoter, and high levels of basal expression will be present without IPTG present. Glucose (2%) can be added during growth of the bacteria before the induction with IPTG to suppress the lac promoter. This will allow the bacteria to be grown without selection of bacteria that express low levels of the expressed protein.
2. Optimization of protein expression may be required if the protein of interest is not produced in sufficient quantities. Alternatively, a 500-mL culture can be set up overnight without IPTG. The next day, the culture is diluted 1:2, and expression is induced for 2–3 h. We find that this works better for TAT–β-gal, but not TAT–ARC.
3. TAT–fusion proteins have been shown to be taken up by virtually all cell types and tissues including the heart, brain, and bone marrow when they are injected intraperitoneally into mice (4). These proteins cross several biological barriers in vivo including the blood–brain barrier, and thus caution must be used when handling these proteins. However, although the TAT–protein transduction domain was originally isolated from HIV, no infectious agents are known to be contained

A   TAT-β-gal   TAT-ARC

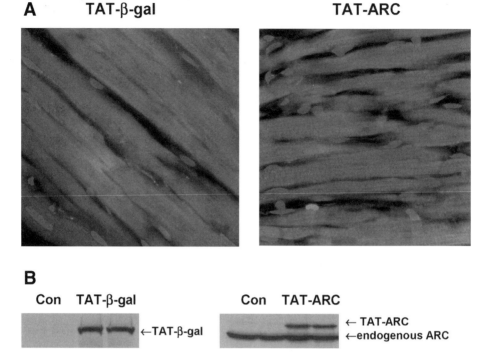

B

Con   TAT-β-gal   Con   TAT-ARC

←TAT-β-gal   ← TAT-ARC
                                        ←endogenous ARC

Fig. 2. Uptake of TAT–β-gal or TAT–ARC in Langendorff-perfused rat hearts. (A) Visualization of Texas-Red–conjugated TAT–β-gal or TAT–ARC using fluorescence microscopy. Nuclei are counterstained with Hoechst 33342. (B) Western blot analysis for TAT fusion proteins in Langendorff perfused rat hearts. Hearts were perfused with or without 20 n*M* TAT–ARC or TAT–β-gal for 15 min, followed by 15 min perfusion to wash out nontransduced TAT protein. Whole-cell lysates were isolated, and TAT proteins were detected by immunoblotting using an antibody specific for the HA tag for TAT–β-gal or an antibody specific for ARC to detect TAT–ARC and endogenous ARC.

in this PTD *(1)*. Because of the high level of transduction efficiency, special consideration must be given when choosing the particular protein of interest to create a TAT fusion protein. It is possible that cytotoxic or proapoptotic proteins could become even more toxic when the TAT PTD is fused to the protein. It has been suggested that NIH Biosafety Level II guidelines for the safe handling of recombinant proteins be followed when working with TAT fusion proteins *(1)*. Complete details of these guidelines can be found on the internet at http:// bmbl.od.nih.gov/sect3bsl2.htm. Dowdy and colleagues *(1)* suggest that TAT fusion proteins should be treated similarly to that of low-level radionucleotides such as ^{35}S. Plastic absorbent pads should be used on benchtops, and latex gloves, goggles, and lab coats should be worn at all times. Spills of concentrated proteins should be digested with 5% Terg-A-Zyme (VWR) at room temperature for at least 10 min. Glassware that is used should be treated with 10% bleach and flushed down the sink with copious amounts of water. Sonication should be performed in a biological safety cabinet if possible to avoid aerosols. Follow local guidelines pertaining to proper disposal procedures for solid waste (*1*).

4. Imidazole at 20 mM in the buffer Z is used as a starting point to reduce the amount of contaminating proteins. If a high background of contaminating bacterial proteins is observed, the imidazole concentration can be increased up to 30 mM.

5. TAT–ARC is stable at 4°C for up to a week or for months at –70°C in PBS. However, the length of time a TAT protein can be stored will be protein-specific and must be determined for that particular protein.

6. The concentration at which the TAT–fusion protein must be administered in vitro must be determined experimentally. In our experience, responses can be seen at 20–200 nM.

Acknowledgments

The authors thank Rick Sayen (The Scripps Research Institute) for technical assistance and discussions. The pTAT-HA vector was a kind gift from Dr. Steven Dowdy (University of California, San Diego). This work was supported in part by grants from the National Institutes of Health (to R.A.G.), Canada Institutes for Health Research, Michael Smith Foundation for Health Research (MSFHR) (to D.J.G.), the St. Paul's Hospital Foundation (to D.J.G.), and the British Columbia Transplant Society (to D.J.G.). D.J.G. is a Canada Research Chair in Cardiovascular Biochemistry and an MSFHR Scholar. A.B.G. is a recipient of an American Heart Association postdoctoral fellowship.

References

1. Becker-Hapak, M., McAllister, S. S., and Dowdy, S. F. (2001) TAT-mediated protein transduction into mammalian cells. *Methods* **24,** 247–256.
2. Wadia, J. S. and Dowdy, S. F. (2002) Protein transduction technology. *Curr. Opin. Biotechnol.* **13,** 52–56.
3. Wadia, J. S. and Dowdy, S. F. (2003) Modulation of cellular function by TAT mediated transduction of full length proteins. *Curr. Protein Pept. Sci.* **4,** 97–104.
4. Schwarze, S. R., Ho, A., Vocero-Akbani, A., and Dowdy, S. F. (1999) In vivo protein transduction: delivery of a biologically active protein into the mouse. *Science* **285,** 1569–1572.
5. Cao, G., Pei, W., Ge, H., et al. (2002) In vivo delivery of a Bcl-xL fusion protein containing the TAT protein transduction domain protects against ischemic brain injury and neuronal apoptosis. *J. Neurosci.* **22,** 5423–5431.
6. Dietz, G. P., Kilic, E., and Bahr, M. (2002) Inhibition of neuronal apoptosis in vitro and in vivo using TAT-mediated protein transduction. *Mol. Cell. Neurosci.* **21,** 29–37.

7. Kilic, U., Kilic, E., Dietz, G. P., and Bahr, M. (2003) Intravenous TAT-GDNF is protective after focal cerebral ischemia in mice. *Stroke* **34,** 1304–1310.

8. Xia, H., Mao, Q., and Davidson, B. L. (2001) The HIV Tat protein transduction domain improves the biodistribution of beta-glucuronidase expressed from recombinant viral vectors. *Nat. Biotechnol.* **19,** 640–644.

9. Gustafsson, A. B., Sayen, M. R., Williams, S. D., Crow, M. T., and Gottlieb, R. A. (2002) TAT protein transduction into isolated perfused hearts: TAT-apoptosis repressor with caspase recruitment domain is cardioprotective. *Circulation* **106,** 735–739.

10. Schwarze, S. R. and Dowdy, S. F. (2000) In vivo protein transduction: intracellular delivery of biologically active proteins, compounds and DNA. *Trends Pharmacol. Sci.* **21,** 45–48.

11. Chen, L., Wright, L. R., Chen, C. H., Oliver, S. F., Wender, P. A., and Mochly-Rosen, D. (2001) Molecular transporters for peptides: delivery of a cardioprotective epsilonPKC agonist peptide into cells and intact ischemic heart using a transport system, R(7). *Chem. Biol.* **8,** 1123–1129.

7

Expression of Human eNOS in Cardiac and Endothelial Cells

Xiuqing Wang, Robert Cade, and Zhongjie Sun

Summary

In this chapter we provide a detailed technique-focused protocol for expression of human endothelial nitric oxide synthase (eNOS) gene delivered by replication-deficient adenovirus. It includes construction of recombinant plasmid with human eNOS gene full-length cDNA (heNOS), packaging of adenovirus with heNOS (Adv-heNOS) in 293 cells, confirmation of Adv-heNOS, amplification of high-titer stock Adv-heNOS, determination of the Adv-heNOS titer, expression of Adv-heNOS in the human abdominal aorta endothelial (HAAE1) cell line and rat heart myoblast cell line (H9C2), and measurement of human eNOS activity and NO production.

Key Words: Recombinant adenovirus; titer; vector; human eNOS; nitric oxide; gene; cloning; gene expression; restriction enzyme; heart cell; endothelial cell; HEK 293 cell; Western blot; PCR; primer; cytopathic effect; plaque formation unit.

1. Introduction

Nitric oxide (NO) is produced in endothelial cells by an enzyme known as endothelial nitric oxide synthase (eNOS), which converts L-arginine to L-citrulline and NO *(1–3)*. Continuous production of endothelium-derived NO in peripheral vessels has been shown to modulate vascular resistance and blood pressure *(4)*. Transient expression of human eNOS protein has been shown to produce a significant reduction in systemic blood pressure *(5)*. The introduction of a foreign gene into somatic cells in culture and in intact organisms is an important investigational technique and holds promise as a therapeutic tool. Recombinant adenoviruses possess several important advantages for direct

From: *Methods in Molecular Medicine, vol. 112: Molecular Cardiology: Methods and Protocols*
Edited by: Z. Sun © Humana Press Inc., Totowa, NJ

introduction of foreign genes into mammalian cells, including high efficiency of gene transfer, broad species and tissue trophism, rapid propagation of recombinant virus to high titers, and simple techniques for the generation of recombinant viral genomes *(6)*. Adenovirus vectors have been used to achieve efficient transfer and expression of recombinant genes in different vasculatures, both ex vivo and in vivo, raising the possibility that this approach may be used to treat cardiovascular disease *(7,8)*. Recombinant adenovirus with human and bovine eNOS genes has proved to be a useful vector for studying the activity and function of eNOS protein *(9–11)*.

We have successfully constructed a replication-deficient adenovirus harboring human eNOS (heNOS) cDNA under the control of the cytomegalovirus (CMV) promoter. In this chapter, we provide a detailed technique-focused protocol for (1) construction of recombinant plasmid with heNOS, (2) packaging of adenovirus (Adv)-heNOS, (3) confirmation of Adv-heNOS, (4) amplification of high-titer stock Adv-heNOS, (5) determination of viral titer, (6) expression of Adv-heNOS in cardiac and endothelial cells, and (7) measurement of heNOS activity and NO production.

2. Materials

1. pET17b vector (Novagen) and pShuttle-Adeno-X system (BD Biosciences Clontech).
2. Endonuclease and T4 DNA ligase (BioLabs).
3. Agarose-gel: dissolve 0.5 g of agarose (powder) in 50 mL of 1XTAE to prepare 1% agarose-gel.
4. TAE agarose-gel running buffer (1X): 40 m*M* Tris-acetate, 1 m*M* EDTA, pH 8.0. Prepare from a 50X stock solution before use. A 50X stock solution can be made by adding 242 g of Tris base to 700 mL of deionized H_2O and then adding 57.1 mL of glacial acetic acid and 100 mL of 500 m*M* EDTA, pH 8.0. Adjust the volume to 1000 mL with deionized H_2O. Store at room temperature.
5. Penicillin (100X): 10,000 U of Penicillin in 1 mL of 0.9% NaCl. Sterilize by filtration through a 0.22-μ filter, then aliquot, and store at –20°C.
6. Streptomycin (100X): dissolve 10 mg of streptomycin in 1 mL of 0.9% NaCl. Sterilize by filtration through a 0.22-μ filter, then aliquot and store at –20°C.
7. Ethidium bromide (EB; 10 mg/mL stock solution): add 1 g of ethidium bromide to 100 mL of deionized H_2O. Stir with a magnetic stirrer for several hours to ensure that the dye is dissolved. Store at room temperature (*see* **Note 1**).
8. NucleoSpin extraction kit (BD Biosciences Clontech).
9. DH5α *E. coli* competent cells (Invitrogen). Store at –80°C.
10. 2.5X Polymerase chain reaction (PCR) mixture (Eppendorf).
11. Plasmid DNA extraction Mini kit (BD Biosciences Clontech).
12. NucleoBond plasmid Midi kit (BD Biosciences Clontech).
13. HEK 293 cells, H9C2 cells, and HAAE1 cells (all from ATCC).

14. Media for cell culture: Dulbecco's modified Eagle's medium (DMEM; Fisher) and F-12k (ATCC).
15. Fetal bovine serum (FBS; ATCC). Store at –70°C.
16. Endothelial cell growth supplement (ECGS) and heparin (100X): dissolve 75 mg ECGS (Sigma) in 10 mL DPBS (Sigma) without calcium and magnesium, with 10 mg heparin (Sigma), then filter as described above, aliquot, and store at –70°C.
17. Gelatin solution (0.1%): add 1 g pig gelatin (Sigma) in 1000 mL of 0.9% NaCl, filter as described above, aliquot, and store at 4°C.
18. Clonfectin™ (BD Biosciences Clontech).
19. Primers: adeno-X forward and reverse primers (BD Biosciences Clontech) and human eNOS-specific primers.
20. Rapid viral titer kit (BD Biosciences Clontech).
21. Lysis buffer: 50 mM Tris-Cl (pH 7.5), 1 mM EDTA, 1% of a protease inhibitor cocktail (Stock solution from Sigma).
22. Sodium dodecyl sulfide (SDS) loading buffer (2X): 100 mM Tris-HCl, pH 6.8, 200 mM dithiothreitol (DTT), 2% SDS, 0.2% bromophenol blue, 20% glycerol (*see* **Note 2**).
23. SDS-polyacrylamide gel electrophoresis (PAGE) running buffer (1X): 25 mM Tris base, 250 mM glycine, 0.1% electrophoresis-grade SDS. Prepare from a 5X stock solution. (A 5X stock solution can be made by dissolving 15.1 g of Tris base and 94 g of glycine in 900 mL of deionized H$_2$O. Then, 50 mL of a 10% [w/ v] stock solution of electrophoresis-grade SDS is added [*see* **Note 3**]. Adjust the volume to 1000 mL with deionized H$_2$O, and store at 4°C.)
24. Transfer buffer (1X): 39 mM glycine, 48 mM Tris base, 0.037% electrophoresis-grade SDS, 20% methanol. To prepare 1 L of transfer buffer, pH 8.3, mix 2.9 g of glycine, 5.8 g of Tris base, 0.37 g of SDS, and 200 mL of methanol. Store at 4°C.
25. TBS-T (or wash) buffer (1X): 100 mM Tris-HCl, pH 7.5, 150 mM NaCl, 0.1% Tween-20 (v/v). Prepare 1000 mL of fresh TBS-T (1X) by adding 100 mL Tris-HCl (10X), 100 mL NaCl (10X), 799 mL of deionized H$_2$O and 1 mL of Tween-20. Stir on a magnetic stirrer for 10 min. (A 10X stock solution of 1 M Tris-HCl, pH 7.5, can be made by dissolving 121.14 g of Tris base in 800 mL of deionized H$_2$O, adjusting the pH to the desired value by using concentrated HCl, then adjust the volume to 1000 mL with deionized H$_2$O. A 10X stock solution of 1.5 M NaCl can be made by dissolving 87 g of NaCl in 1000 mL of deionized H$_2$O, and store at room temperature.)
26. Blocking solution: 5% (w/v) nonfat dried milk in TBS-T buffer (prepare before use).
27. Ampicillin: 50 mg/mL stock solution was made by dissolving 50 mg of ampicillin in 1 mL of 0.9% NaCl. Sterilize by filtration through a 0.22-μm filter, then aliquot, and store at –20°C.
28. Kanamycin: 25 mg/mL stock solution was made by dissolving 25 mg of kanamycin in 1 mL of 0.9% NaCl. Sterilize, aliquot, and store at –20°C.
29. Polyvinylidene difluoride (PVDP) membrane (Osmonics).

30. Mouse anti-human eNOS IgG (BD Transduction Laboratories).
31. Goat anti-mouse IgG horseradish peroxidase (HRP; BD Transduction Laboratories).
32. ECL™ Western Blotting Analysis System (Amersham Biosciences).
33. X-ray film (Kodak).
34. Autoradiography cassette (Fisher).

3. Methods

The methods described below outline (1) construction of recombinant plasmid with heNOS, (2) packaging of Adv-heNOS in HEK 293 cells, (3) confirmation of Adv-heNOS, (4) amplification of high-titer stock Adv-heNOS, (5) determination of Adv-heNOS titer, (6) expression of Adv-heNOS in cardiac and endothelial cells, and (7) measurement of heNOS activity and NO production (**Fig. 1**).

3.1. Construction of Recombinant Plasmid With heNOS

The construction of recombinant plasmid with human eNOS gene full-length cDNA is described in **Subheadings 3.1.1.–3.1.4.** This includes (1) a description of subcloning and cloning vectors, (2) a description of human eNOS gene full length cDNA, (3) the subcloning of pET17b-heNOS for obtaining restriction enzyme sites *Xba*I and *Not*I, and (4) cloning of pShuttle-heNOS for packaging adenovirus with human eNOS full-length cDNA.

3.1.1. pET17b Subcloning Vector and pShuttle Cloning Vector

pET17b is a prokaryotic expression vector (Novagen). It is used to obtain restriction enzyme sites *Xba*I and *Not*I, and to make it easy to insert the target gene into the pShuttle vector for packaging Adv-heNOS. The pShuttle expression system (BD Biosciences Clontech) allows the target gene into a mammalian expression cassette, which consists of the human CMV immediate-early promoter/enhancer($P_{CMV\ IE}$), a multiple cloning site (MCS), and the bovine growth hormone polyadenylation signal (BGH polyA). The entire cassette is flanked by unique I-*Ceu*I and Pl-*Sce*I restriction enzyme sites so that it can be excised and ligated to Adeno-X viral DNA. The vector backbone also possesses the pUC origin (pUC ori) and a kanamycin resistance gene (Kan^r) for propagation and selection in *E. coli*.

3.1.2. Human eNOS Full-Length cDNA

A plasmid (pcDNA3-eNOS) containing heNOS full-length cDNA (heNOS) was kindly donated by Dr. L. Chao (University of South Carolina) *(5)*. It contains the initiation methionine codon followed by 3612 nucleotides coding for a 1204-amino acid human eNOS protein. The coding region for human eNOS was removed from pcDNA3-eNOS by digestion with the restriction enzyme *Eco*RI .

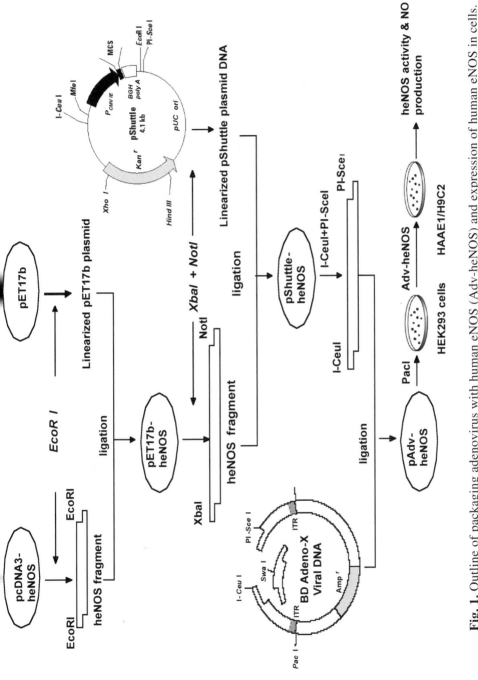

Fig. 1. Outline of packaging adenovirus with human eNOS (Adv-heNOS) and expression of human eNOS in cells.

3.1.3. Subcloning

There is no *Eco*RI enzyme site in the multiple cloning site of the pShuttle vector that will be used for construction of recombinant plasmid pShuttle-heNOS and for further packaging of adenovirus with human eNOS (Adv-heNOS). To obtain the *Xba*I site (upstream) and the *Not*I site (downstream) of heNOS from the pET17b vector, the subcloning step is necessary to avoid blunt-end ligation.

1. Digest both pcDNA3-eNOS *(5)* and pET17b plasmid DNA with *Eco*RI (*see* **Note 4**).
2. Run *Eco*RI-digested pcDNA3-heNOS in agarose-gel (1%) with EB in 1X TAE buffer.
3. Cut the gel, and collect the heNOS fragment DNA from it.
4. Purify the heNOS fragment DNA and *Eco*RI-digested pET17b with a NucleoSpin extraction kit as described by the manufacturer.
5. Ligate heNOS fragments and linearized pET17b with T4 DNA ligase (BioLabs).
6. Transform the ligation product into *E. coli* DH5α competent cells. Smear the transformed *E. coli* DH5α onto LB/agar with ampicillin plates. Incubate at 37°C overnight.
7. Identify the recombinant plasmid by the method of recombinant plasmid fast identification *(13)* or PCR (*see* **Note 5**).
8. Select the correct orientation constructs with restriction enzyme *Bam*HI (BioLabs) digestion (*see* **Note 6**).
9. Extract and purify the recombinant plasmid DNA by using a plasmid DNA extraction kit (BD Biosciences Clontech) for cloning.

3.1.4. Cloning

1. Linearize pShuttle plasmid DNA by double enzyme digestions with *Xba*I and *Not*I (BioLabs).
2. Double-digest the pET17b-heNOS plasmid DNA with *Xba*I and *Not*I.
3. Collect the target DNA fragment and perform ligation, transformation, and plasmid DNA extraction as described in **Subheading 3.1.3.** The only difference is that kanamycin replaces ampicillin.
4. Identify pShuttle-heNOS plasmid with PCR (**Fig. 2A**) and/or restriction enzyme *Bam*HI digestion (**Fig. 2B**).
5. Double-digest the pShuttle-heNOS plasmid DNA with I-*Ceu*I and PI-*Sce*I.
6. Ligate a I-*Ceu*I and PI-*Sce*I expression cassette to the adenovirus backbone (linearized by I-*Ceu*I and PI-*Sce*I; BD Biosciences Clontech).
7. Transform and select the target constructs on LB/ampicillin (100 mg/mL) plates. *E. coli* DH5α containing recombinant adenovirus DNA can be rapidly identified by PCR using the heNOS-specific primers and Adeno-X PCR primers set 2 (BD Biosciences Clontech) (**Fig. 3A,B**).

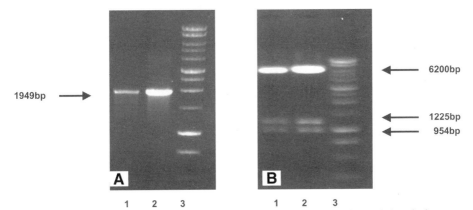

Fig. 2. Identification of pShuttle-heNOS plasmid by PCR (**A**) and restriction enzyme *Bam*HI digestion (**B**). (**A**) Agarose-gel (1%) displays a 1949-bp band of PCR products by using pShuttle-heNOS plasmid DNA (50 ng) as templates and heNOS-specific primers. Lanes 1and 2, 1949-bp heNOS-specific bands; lane 3, DNA ladder. (**B**) Agarose-gel (1%) showed *Bam*HI digestion products of pShuttle-heNOS. There are three *Bam*HI sites (nt 506, nt 1731, and nt 2685 from ATG to TGA) in human eNOS full-length cDNA. The *Bam*HI digestion products contain 954-, 1225-, and 6200-bp bands. Lanes 1 and 2, pShuttle-heNOS DNA digested with *Bam*HI; lane 3, DNA ladder.

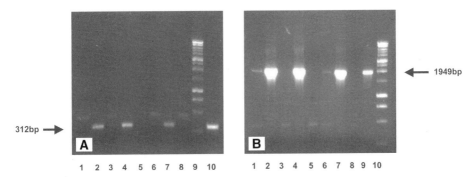

Fig. 3. Identification of pAdv-heNOS plasmids by PCR (1% agarose-gel). (**A**) Use pAdv-heNOS plasmid DNA (lanes 1–8) as templates, Adeno-X forward primer 2 and reverse primer 2 and run PCR; the yield is a 312-bp DNA fragment that spans the pShuttle expression cassette and Adeno-X backbone sequences. There are specific bands (312 bp) in lanes 2, 4, and 7 (plasmid DNA) and no specific band (312 bp) in lanes 1, 3, 5, 6, and 8 (plasmid DNA). Lane 9, DNA ladder; lane 10, 312bp DNA fragments as positive control. (**B**) Use the same plasmid DNA as templates and heNOS-specific primers, and run PCR; the yield is a 1949-bp DNA fragment. Lanes 1, 3, 5, 6, and 8, no 1949-bp band; lanes 2, 4, and 7, 1949-bp bands; lane 9, 1949-bp DNA fragments as positive control; lane 10, DNA ladder.

3.2. Packaging of Adv-heNOS

High quality and quantity of Adv-heNOS plasmid DNA, the lower passage HEK 293 cells were needed for packaging the recombinant Adv-heNOS. The preparation of recombinant pAdv-heNOS plasmid DNA and the packaging of Adv-heNOS in HEK 293 cells that have been transformed with the left end of human adenovirus type 5 DNA *(12)* are described below.

3.2.1. Preparation of Recombinant pAdv-heNOS Plasmid DNA

1. Extract pAdv-heNOS plasmid DNA with a NucleoBond Plasmid Midi Kit (BD Biosciences Clontech) or by the phenol/chloroform/isoamyl alcohol method *(13)* (*see* **Note 7**).
2. Digest the final construct, pAdv-heNOS, by *Pac*I to release the complete linear adenoviral DNA.
3. Purify the *Pac*I-digested product by the phenol/chloroform/isoamyl alcohol method *(13)* (*see* **Note 7**).

3.2.2. Packaging of pAdv-heNOS in HEK 293 Cells

1. Plate HEK 293 cells in a $1-2 \times 10^6$ cells per 60-mm culture plate 12–24 h before transfection.
2. Transfect each 60-mm culture plate with 10 μL (5 μg) of *Pac*I-digested pAdv-heNOS DNA and 10 μL (8 μg) clonfectin using the standard transfection method *(13)* (*see* **Note 8**).
3. Check for cytopathic effect (CPE) (**Fig. 4**) 24 h post transfection (*see* **Note 9**).
4. If no CPE appears after 1 wk of transfection, scrape and transfer the cells to sterile centrifuge tube, centrifuge the suspension at 1000*g* for 5 min at room temperature, and resuspend the pellet in 500 μL of sterile PBS.
5. Lyse cells with three consecutive freeze (dry ice/ethanol bath)-thaw (water bath, <37°C) cycles. Briefly centrifuge the lysate, and store the supernatant at –20°C or use immediately for infecting HEK 293 cells. Repeat the cycles until CPE appears.

3.3. Confirmation of Adv-heNOS

1. Use forward and reverse Adeno-X primers set 2 (BD Biosciences Clontech), which spans the Adeno-X backbone and pShuttle expression cassette and is a quick and efficient way to evaluate Adv-heNOS (**Fig. 5**). The positive Adv-heNOS plaques were used for original stock.
2. PCR cycles are as follows: 94°C for 2 min, 94°C for 15 s, 68°C for 2 min, 30 cycles, 68°C for 3 min.

3.4. Amplification of High-Titer Stock Adv-heNOS

High-titer stock solution was prepared from positive plaques and used to generate high-titer preparation. Viral preparation was produced by infecting a

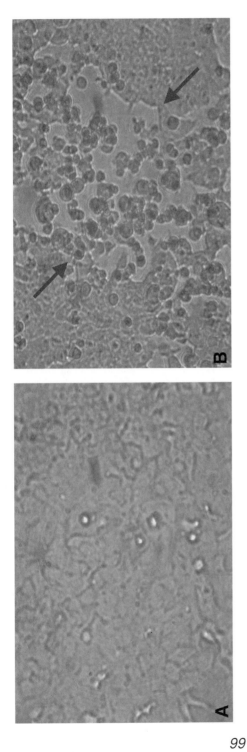

Fig. 4. Typical cytopathic efficiency (CPE) in human embryonic kidney (HEK) 293 cells transfected with Adv-heNOS (original magnification 200X). (**A**) Normal cells. (**B**) Cells transfected with Adv-heNOS. (Arrows show CPE.)

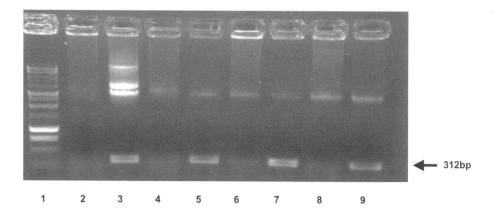

Fig. 5. Confirmation of Adv-heNOS by PCR. After packaging Adv-heNOS in HEK 293 cells, harvest the culture medium (add as template for PCR) and cells, lyse the cell pellet in 1 mL (per T25 flask) of 100 m*M* Tris-HCl (pH 7.4) by three consecutive freeze–thaw cycles, centrifuge the lysate at 12,000*g* for 10 min at 4°C, add 2 μL of supernatant and 4 μL of culture medium as a template for PCR using Adeno-X forward and reverse set 2 primers. Lane 1, DNA ladder; lanes 2, 4, 6, and 8, culture medium as templates yield 312-bp PCR products; lane 3, 5, 7, and 9, supernatant from lysate as templates yield 312-bp PCR products.

confluent monolayer of HEK 293 cells in 75-cm^2 (T75) flasks with viral stock at a multiplicity of infection (MOI) of 10.

1. At 24 h before infection, plate HEK 293 cells in a T75 flask. The cell monolayer will be 50–70% confluent when infected.
2. Incubate cells at 37°C overnight in a humidified atmosphere maintained at 5% CO_2. On the following day, replace the medium with 5 mL of fresh growth medium containing Adv-heNOS.
3. Incubate for 90 min at 37°C in a humidified atmosphere maintained at 5% CO_2.
4. Remove the flask, and added 10 mL of fresh growth medium.
5. Harvest the infected cells (check the CPE) after incubating for 2–4 d at 37°C in a humidified atmosphere maintained at 5% CO_2.
6. Isolate virus using the freeze–thaw method as described in **Subheading 3.2.2.**
7. Aliquot and store the supernatant at –70°C with 15% glycerol (*see* **Note 10**).

3.5. Determining Adv-heNOS Titer

Viral titer can be determined by two methods, the Rapid Adenoviral Titer and the End-Point Dilution Assay. The latter requires 9–10 d and the rapid titer kit requires 3 d.

3.5.1. Rapid Adenoviral Titer

Perform the procedures according to the manufacturer's instructions, which are briefly as follows.

1. Seed HEK 293 cells in 12-well plates (5×10^5 cells/well).
2. Using the cell culture medium (serum-free) as a diluent, dilute Adv-heNOS to 1:10,000 (10^{-4}), 1:100,000(10^{-5}), and 1:1,000,000 (10^{-6}).
3. Add 100 μL of viral dilution to each well. Incubate cells in a humidified 5% CO_2 incubator at 37°C for 48 h.
4. Aspirate medium, and allow cells to dry in hood for 5 min.
5. Fix cells by very gently adding 1 mL ice-cold 100% methanol to each well, and incubate the plate at –20°C for 10 min.
6. Aspirate the methanol, gently rinse the well three times with 1% bovine serum ablumin–phosphate-buffered saline (BSA-PBS).
7. Add mouse anti-Hexon antibody (1:1000 diluted with 1% BSA–PBS) and incubate for 1 h at 37°C (shake three to six times during incubation).
8. Aspirate mouse anti-Hexon antibody, and gently rinse wells three times with 1% BSA–PBS.
9. Add rat antimouse antibody (HRP conjugate, diluted 1:500 with1% BSA–PBS), and incubate for 1 h at 37°C (shake three to six times during incubation).
10. Aspirate rat antimouse antibody, and gently rinse wells three times with 1% BSA–PBS.
11. Add 500 μL diaminobenzidne (DAB) working solution to each well, incubate at room temperature for 10 min.
12. Aspirate DAB, and add 1 mL PBS to each well.
13. Count a minimum of three fields of brown/black positive cells using a microscope with a 20X objective, and calculate the mean number of positive cells in each well.
14. Calculate the formula:

$$\text{Titer (PFU/mL)} = \frac{(\text{infected cells/field}) \times (\text{fields/well})}{\text{volume virus (mL)} \times (\text{dilution factor})}$$

3.5.2. End-Point Dilution Assay

1. Approximately 24 h before the test assay, plate HEK 293 cells in a 96-well plate. Carefully seed all wells at the same density (1×10^4 cells/well) in 100 μL of the growth medium.
2. On the following day, prepare serial dilutions of the Adv-heNOS (10^{-3}–10^{-10}). Add 100 μL of diluted virus to each well in columns 1–10. Add 100 μL of virus-free growth medium to well in columns 11 and 12 as control. Incubate the plate in a humidified 5% CO_2 incubator for 9 d at 37°C.
3. Calculate the fraction of CPE-positive wells in each row, and calculate the viral titer.

4. Calculate the formula:

$$\text{Titer (PFU/mL)} = 10(X + 0.8)$$

where X = the sum of the fractions of CPE-positive wells.

3.6. Expression of Adv-heNOS in Rat Heart Cells and Human Aorta Cells

The entire cassette was flanked by unique I-*Ceu*I and PI-*Sce*I restriction sites containing human CMV immediate-early promoter/enhancer ($P_{CMV\ IE}$), heNOS full-length cDNA, and the bovine growth hormone polyadenylation signal (BGH poly A), which can be expressed in mammalian cells. Two cell lines (human abdominal aorta endothelial cell [HAAE1] and rat heart myoblast cell [H9C2]) were used for expression of Adv-heNOS.

3.6.1. Expression of Adv-heNOS in HAAE1 Cells

1. Culture the HAAE1 cells in 87% F-12k medium, 10% FBS, 1% penicillin and atreptomycin (final concentration: 100 U/mL of penicillin and 100 µg/mL of streptomycin), 1% endothelial cell growth factor (ECGF, final concentration: 75 µg/mL), and 1% heparin (final concentration: 10 µg/mL) at 37°C in a humidified atmosphere maintained at 5% CO_2.
2. Seed the low-passage HAAE1 cells (*see* **Note 11**) in six-well plates (1×10^5 cells/well) 12–24 h before transduction.
3. Add 2×10^7 PFU of Adv-heNOS to each well (200 MOI, i.e., 200 viruses/cell). Incubate at 37°C in a humidified atmosphere maintained at 5% CO2 for 2 d.
4. Aspirate the medium, and harvest the infected cells by adding 300 µL of lysis buffer to each well. Collect the lysate, add 300 µL SDS loading buffer (2×), mix, boil for 5 min, and centrifuge at 12,000g for 5 min at room temperature.
5. Transfer the supernatant to a clean tube, and measure the protein concentration.
6. Detect heNOS protein expression (**Fig. 6**) by Western blotting *(14)*.
   a. Run the samples in 7.5% SDS-PAGE-gel (Bio-Rad) in 1X SDS-PAGE running buffer at 80 V for 30 min, and then increase the voltage to 100 V, and continue running for 1 h at room temperature.
   b. Soak the gel, Whatman filter, and PVDP membrane in transfer buffer for 30 min at room temperature with gentle shaking.
   c. Transfer the protein from the gel to PVDP membrane using the Semi-Dry System (Bio-Rad) at 20 V for 15 min at room temperature.
   d. Block nonspecific proteins by shaking in blocking solution at room temperature for 2 h or at 4°C overnight.
   e. Incubate the PVDP membrane with mouse antihuman eNOS antibody (1:1000 diluted with blocking solution), and shake for 1 h at room temperature.
   f. Wash the membrane four times (5 min two times, 10 min two times) with 100 mL of TBS-T on a shaker.

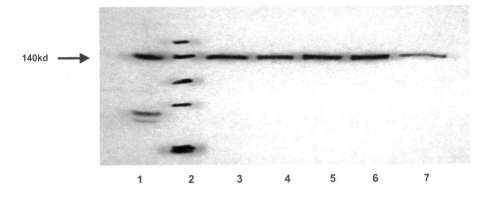

Fig. 6. Western blot analysis of heNOS protein expression in HAAE1 cells transduced with Adv-heNOS (10 µg/lane). Lane 1, positive control of human eNOS protein (10 µg); lane 2, protein marker; lanes 3–6, HAAE1 cells transduced with Adv-heNOS (200 MOI); lane 7, HAAE1 cells transduced with Adv-LacZ (200 MOI). Lane 7 indicates that there is endogenous heNOS expression in HAAE1 cells.

 g. Incubate the PVDP membrane with goat antimouse (HRP-conjugated) antibody (1:2000 diluted with blocking buffer), and shake for 1 h at room temperature.

 h. Repeat **step f**.

 i. Add ECL, incubate at room temperature for 1 min, and expose to X-ray film.

3.6.2. Expression of Adv-heNOS in H9C2 cells

1. Culture H9C2 cells in 89% DMEM with 10% FBS and 1% penicillin and streptomycin at 37°C in a humidified atmosphere maintained at 5% CO_2.
2. Seed H9C2 cells on a six-well plate (1×10^5 cells/well) 12–24 h before transduction.
3. Detect heNOS protein expression in H9C2 cells (**Fig. 7**) by Western blotting (*see* **Subheading 3.6.1, steps 3–6**).

3.7. Measurement of NO Production and heNOS Activity

NO is rapidly changed (by oxidation) to nitrite and nitrate in biological solution, NO is usually determined by measuring total nitrite and nitrate (NOx, index of NO production). NO generated from eNOS has a relatively short half-life and is rapidly converted to NOx. Therefore, measurement of NOx is a good indicator of eNOS activity. In addition, eNOS activity should be measured in cells transduced with the virus to confirm further that heNOS gene transfer results in a functional eNOS gene product.

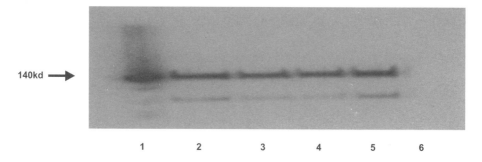

Fig. 7. Western blot analysis of heNOS protein expression in rat H9C2 cells transduced with Adv-heNOS (10 μg/lane). Lane 1, positive control of human eNOS protein (10 μg); lanes 2–5, H9C2 cells transduced with Adv-heNOS (200 MOI); lane 6, H9C2 cells infected with Adv-LacZ (200 MOI). Lane 6 indicates that there is no enogenous heNOS protein expresson in H9C2 cells.

3.7.1. Measurement of NOx **(15)**

1. Seed the cells in a six-well plate 24 h before transduction.
2. Transduce the cells with Adv-heNOS or Adv-LacZ at an MOI of 200.
3. After a 48-h incubation, remove the medium, and wash the cells with PBS.
4. Measure NOx by using a NO analyzing system (Antek Instruments), which includes three components: Nitrite/Nitrate Reducer (model 745), Nitric Oxide Analyzer (model 7020), and a computerized data handling system *(15)*. The Nitrite/Nitrate Reducer rapidly reduces nitrite (room temperature) and nitrate (95°C) to NO with vanadium III. The NO Analyzer has a high sensitivity detector that measures NO based on a gas-phase chemiluminescent reaction between NO and ozone.

3.7.2. heNOS Activity Assay **(9)**

1. Transduce the cells with Adv-heNOS or Adv-LacZ as described in **Subheading 3.7.1.**
2. Harvest the cells after 48 h of transduction; then centrifuge at 20,800g for 10 min, and use the pellet for the assay.
3. Determine total NO synthase (NOS) activity by the conversion of [^{3}H]arginine to [^{3}H]citrulline by using an NOS activity assay kit (Calbiochem) according to the manufacturer's instructions. eNOS activity can be determined by measuring the conversion of [^{3}H]arginine to [^{3}H]citrulline in the presence of the Ca^{2+}-chelating agent EGTA (1 mM) *(16)*.

4. Notes

1. **Caution:** Ethidium bromide is a powerful mutagen and is moderately toxic *(13)*. Wear gloves when preparing EB solution. EB is also a light-sensitive reagent.

Wrap the container with aluminum foil or transfer the solution to a dark bottle. Final concentration is 0.5 µg/mL.

2. 2X SDS gel-loading buffer lacking dithiothreiol (DTT) can be stored at room temperature. DTT (or 10% 2-mercaptoethanol, final concentration) should then be added just before the buffer is used, from a 1 *M* stock solution (dissolve 3.09 g of DTT in 20 mL of 0.01 *M* sodium acetate, pH 5.2. Sterilize by filtration. Dispense into aliquots, and store at –20°C).

3. Wear a mask when weighing SDS, and wipe down the weighing area and balance after use because the fine crystals of SDS disperse easily.

4. Conditions of low ionic strength, high enzyme concentration (>100 U/µg DNA), glycerol concentration >5%, pH > 8.0, or the presence of organic solvents (DMSO and alcohols) may result in star activity. The enzyme reaction buffer offered by company already improved some conditions. The following two points are very important for inhibition of star activity: (1) use as few units as possible to get a complete digestion (this avoids overdigestion and reduces the final glycerol concentration in the reaction and (2) make sure the reaction is free of any organic solvents such as alcohols, which might be present in the DNA preparation.

5. To identify the recombinant plasmid, PCR is a quick and convenient method. Pick up single *E. coli* colonies, and inoculate to 0.5 mL LB/ampicillin. Keep shaking at 37°C for 2 h. Centrifuge 10–50 µL of the shaking product, resuspend the pellet in the proper volume PCR-grade water (use it as the template), and then run PCR using the target-specific primers.

6. Alternatively, PCR can be used to select the correct orientation, inserting constructs if there is no proper enzyme site for use. The specific primers need to be designed according to the plasmid sequence and the target gene sequence.

7. pAdv-heNOS is a large plasmid (>36 kb) that is susceptible to damage and rearrangement in E. coli. For the best results, always use fresh, log-phase cultures for purification of recombinant plasmid DNA. Do not store the culture at room temperature, 4°C, or on ice for long periods (i.e., >24 h) before starting the purification or before incubating a second culture.

8. Cells should be 50 to 70% confluent, display a flat morphology, and adhere well to the plate just prior to transfection. It is also very important to set up a negative control.

9. The time it takes for CPE to appear depends on the transfection efficiency. For the cells with higher transfection efficiency, CPE may appear within 1 wk, wherease CPE may become evident in 2–3 wk for cells with lower transfection efficiency.

10. Replication-competent adenovirus is produced when Adeno-X DNA recombines with E1-containing genomic DNA in HEK 293 cells. Sometimes incompetent adenovirus may be produced during the amplification. Confirm Adv-heNOS after each amplification, and save aliquots of early amplifications already confirmed. Use the stocks to produce additional quantities of Adv-heNOS.

11. The flasks for culture of HAAE1 cells need to be pretreated with 1% gelatin (dissolve 1 g of gelatin in 100 mL of 0.9% NaCl) for at least 10 min at room

temperature. Remove the gelatin solution before the flasks are used. HAAE1 cells are not culture-limitless in vitro. The subculture passages should be recorded. After several passages, the cells cannot be used for transduction (refer to the manufacturer's instructions for limits on passages).

Acknowledgment

This work was supported by the AHA-National, grant 0130387N. We thank Dr. L. Chao for providing us with pcDNA3-eNOS plasmid.

References

1. Palmer, R. M., Ashton, D. S., and Moncada, S. (1988) Vascular endothelial cells synthesize nitric oxide from L-arginine. *Nature* **333,** 664–666.
2. Leone, A. M., Palmer, R. M., Knowles, R. G., Francis, P. L., Ashton, D. S., and Moncada, S. (1991) Constitutive and inducible nitric oxide synthases incorporate molecular oxygen into both nitric oxide and citrulline. *J. Biol. Chem.* **266,** 23,790–23,795.
3. Griffith, O. W. and Stuehr, D. J. (1995) Nitric oxide synthases: properties and catalytic mechanism. *Annu. Rev. Physiol.* **57,** 707–736.
4. Rees, D. D., Palmer, R. M., and Moncada, S. (1989) Role of endothelium-derived nitric oxide in the regulation of blood pressure. *Proc. Natl. Acad. Sci. USA* **86,** 3375–3378.
5. Lin, K. F., Chao, L., and Chao, J.(1997) Prolonged reduction of high blood pressure with human nitric oxide synthase gene delivery. *Hypertension* **30,** 307–313.
6. Robert, D. G. and Robert, S. M. (1995) Adenovirus vectors, in *DNA Cloning 4* (Glover, D. M. and Hames, B. D., eds.), IRL Oxford University, UK.
7. Nabel, E. G. and Nabel, G. J. (1994) Complex models for study of gene function in cardiovascular biology. *Annu. Rev. Physiol.* **56,** 741–761.
8. Schneider, M. D. and French, B. A. (1993) The advent of adenovirus: gene therapy for cardiovascular disease. *Circulation* **88,** 1937–1942.
9. Smith, R. S. Jr., Lin, K. F., Agata, J., Chao, L., and Chao, J. (2002) Human endothelial nitric oxide synthase gene delivery promotes angiogenesis in a rat model of hindlimb ischemia. *Arterioscler. Thrombo. Vasc. Biol.* **22,** 1279–1285.
10. Alexander, M. Y., Brosnan, M. J., Hamilton, C. A., et al. (1999) Gene transfer of endothelial nitric oxide synthase improves nitric oxide-dependent endothelial function in a hypertensive rat model. *Cardiovas. Res.* **43,** 798–807.
11. Shah, V., Chen, A. F., Cao, S., et al. (2000) Gene transfer of recombinant endothelial nitric oxide synthase to liver in vivo and in vitro. *Am. J. Physiol.* **279,** G1023–G1030.
12. Jones, N. and Shenk, T. (1979) Isolation of adenovirus type 5 host range deletion mutants defective for transformation of rat embryo cells. *Cell* **17,** 683–689.
13. Sambrook, J., Fritsch, E. F., and Maniatis, T. (ed.) (1989) *Molecular Cloning, A Laboratory Manual,* Second ed. Cold Spring Harbor, Cold Spring Harbor Laboratory Press, New York.

14. Madamanchi, N. R. and Runge, M. S. (2000) Western blotting, in *Angiotensin Protocols* (Wang, D. H., ed.), Humana, Totowa, NJ, pp. 245–256.

15. Sun, Z., Cade, R., Zhang, Z., Alouidor, J., and Van, H. (2003) Angiotensinogen gene knockout delays and attenuates cold-induced hypertension. *Hypertension* **41,** 322–327.

16. Cernadas, M. R., de Miguel, L. S., Garcia-Duran, M. G., et al. (1998) Expression of constitutive and inducible nitric oxide synthase in the vascular wall of young and aging rats. *Circ. Res.* **83,** 279–286.

8

Strategies of Conditional Gene Expression in Myocardium

An Overview

Heather L. Heine, Hon Sing Leong, Fabio M. V. Rossi, Bruce M. McManus, and Thomas J. Podor

Summary

The use of specialized reporter genes to monitor real-time, tissue-specific transgene expression in animal models offers an opportunity to circumvent current limitations associated with the establishment of transgenic mouse models. The Cre-*lox*P and the tetracycline (Tet)-inducible systems are useful methods of conditional gene expression that allow spatial (cell-type-specific) and temporal (inducer-dependent) control. Most often, the α-myosin heavy chain (α-MHC) promoter is used in these inducible systems to restrict expression of reporter genes and transgenes to the myocardium. An overview of each inducible system is described, along with suggested reporter genes for real-time, noninvasive imaging in the myocardium. Effective gene delivery of the inducible gene expression system is carried out by lentiviral vectors, which offer high transduction efficiency, long-term transgene expression, and low immunogenicity. This chapter outlines the packaging of myocardium-specific inducible expression systems into lentiviral vectors, in which a transgene and a reporter gene are transduced into cardiomyocytes. In doing so, transgene and reporter expression can be monitored/tracked with bioluminescence imaging (BLI) and positron emission tomography (PET).

Key Words: Myocardium; inducible gene expression; positron emission tomography; thymidine kinase; luciferase; bioluminescence imaging; Cre-*lox*P; reverse tetracycline transactivator system; lentiviral vector.

From: *Methods in Molecular Medicine, vol. 112: Molecular Cardiology: Methods and Protocols*
Edited by: Z. Sun © Humana Press Inc., Totowa, NJ

1. Introduction

To understand the activity of gene products within an organism, genes can be inserted or deleted, and the subsequent phenotypic changes observed in an animal can help us understand the effects of those genes. The development of transgenic mice with over/underexpressed transgenes has revolutionized the way we conduct experiments. For the most part, these changes are permanent and may adversely affect the animal during development.

To understand the physiological impact of such genetic alterations, animal tissues are commonly examined histologically postmortem. Reporter molecules such as β-galactosidase (β-gal) *(1)* or fluorescent proteins *(2)* are used to substitute deleted genes or are fused to overexpressed transgenes, permitting monitoring of transgene effects in a visually quantifiable manner. However, postmortem analysis is inconclusive when one is attempting to understand the biological impact of a transgene over time. Such attempts to do so are laborious and time-intensive and may generate ambiguous results. Advances in real-time imaging and the introduction of novel reporter molecules have begun to emerge as effective means of visualizing transgene expression. Currently, transgenes can be monitored in a real-time, noninvasive manner in vivo and can be imaged repeatedly over the course of treatment; in some cases, large scale 3D reconstruction of transgene protein expression can be obtained *(3)*.

The activity of genes can also be more clearly understood if precise control over the place and time of expression is regulated. The use of conditional gene expression systems such as the Cre-*lox*P *(4,5)* and Tet-inducible *(4,6–9)* systems offers inducible control in either a permanent or reversible manner, respectively. Furthermore, placing a transgene under the control of a cell-type-specific promoter, such as the cardiomyocyte specific α-myosin heavy chain (α-MHC) promoter *(10–14)*, ensures transgene expression only in the desired cell type.

Lentiviral vectors offer a promising means of delivering inducible transgenes to the myocardium *(15–18)*. New methods for merging inducible gene expression cassettes into lentiviral vector systems will allow efficient delivery of an inducible transgene expression system to cardiomyocytes. This methodology will circumvent the limitations associated with the development of transgenic mice *(19–21)*. The packaging of conditional expression systems into lentiviral vectors will be discussed so that myocardial transgene and reporter gene expression can be studied in vivo.

2. Reporter Genes That Accompany Conditional Transgene Expression

2.1. Reporter Genes and Transgene Configurations for Image Analysis

Visualization and quantification of transgene expression require a reporter molecule that is expressed in tandem with the transgene. Using reporter genes to follow transgene expression can be achieved by direct or indirect imaging strategies *(22,23)*. In the direct imaging strategy, the reporter molecule is physically fused to the protein of interest. In this configuration, the cDNA of the reporter gene is ligated in frame with the 5' or 3' end of the transgene to generate a fusion protein. Construction of such chimeric genes must account for any potential structural limitations that may promote steric hindrance and a possible interaction between the two components *(24,25)*. The construction of a fusion protein may also necessitate subsequent characterization with respect to functionality, specificity, and stability relative to its equivalent native protein. It should be noted that some reporters, such as the fluorescent proteins, are not as biologically inert as previously thought when coupled to a transgene, and they may have some cytotoxic and protein interference effects *(26)*.

Indirect strategies of reporter gene expression consist of both the transgene and the reporter under the transcriptional control of the same promoter. One indirect configuration features a multicomponent system consisting of the transgene under the control of an inducible promoter and an additional internal ribosomal entry site (IRES) transcriptional element followed by the reporter gene *(27)*. Hence, a typical mRNA transcript would consist of two expression cassettes; the α-MHC promoter-transgene followed by the IRES reporter gene. Note that these two expression cassettes need not be in frame in respect to each other. Another indirect reporter configuration utilizes a bidirectional promoter that can simultaneously initiate transcription of both the transgene and the reporter gene *(4,28)*. This configuration is advantageous, as both the transgene and the reporter can be introduced in a single step. However, difficulties may lie in the selection of a cell-specific bidirectional promoter that will be compatible with the inducible gene expression system used. Overall, both these indirect imaging systems provide a visually quantifiable method of transgene protein expression, while minimizing reporter–transgene protein interference.

Although the "transgene" is the actual gene of interest, the corresponding reporter protein serves as the molecular marker. The *lacZ* gene has historically been used to detect and confirm gene insertion into a vector via blue/white bacterial colony screening *(29)*. In vivo implementation of this reporter gene as well as other reporter genes such as luciferase *(30–33)* and fluorescent proteins *(34,35)* has also shown considerable success, albeit by visual confirmation of postmortem tissues. Real-time in vivo imaging of reporter gene expression is not possible with commonly used reporter genes such as *lacZ* or green fluorescent proteins because of their inability to elicit a detectable and measurable signal that can pass through tissue. Despite these limitations, a new class of reporter genes has been developed to harness the potential of positron emission tomography (PET) and bioluminescence imaging (BLI) technologies *(36–43)*. These technologies permit a noninvasive form of in vivo imaging not previously possible by conventional postmortem techniques, thus allowing investigators to assess and track molecular events with high spatial resolution at any given time point.

2.2. Reporter Genes for Static Postmortem Analysis

2.2.1. The lacZ Reporter Gene

The *lacZ* gene is a commonly used reporter gene for in vitro and in vivo applications and despite its limitations for real-time imaging, it is worth mentioning because of its straightforward implementation *(29)*. The typical length of the *lacZ* gene is approx 3.0 kb, and transcription results in the production of β-gal, which is easily detected colorimetrically either by gross or microscopic examination. A colorimetric change is only observed upon incubation with 5-bromo-4-chloro-3-indolyl-β-D-galactopyranoside (X-gal), which is hydrolyzed by β–gal to form a blue precipitate. In configurations in which a cell-specific promoter will direct the expression of *lacZ* reporter gene and transgene, intracellular accumulation of hydrolyzed X-gal will reflect transgene expression. Despite the strong colorimetric signal generated by hydrolyzed X-gal, this reporter gene does not permit noninvasive, real-time imaging of gene expression with any conventional imaging modality.

2.2.2. Fluorescent Protein Reporter Gene

Fluorescent proteins such as green fluorescent protein (GFP) emit an optical fluorescent signature that allows real-time visualization of cellular and molecular events by fluorescent microscopy. This chromophore protein was originally cloned from the jellyfish *Aequorea victoria (44–47)*. Since then, GFP has been the fluorescent reporter protein of choice, and its advantages as a reporter molecule are numerous *(48,49)*: (1) The protein size is small and compact (<1 kb), (2) it has moderate stability (T_m = 70°C), (3) it has stability through paraformaldehyde fixation, (4) there is no endogenous mammalian protein equivalent, and (5) no substrate is required, only a specific maximum excitation wavelength to induce emission of fluorescence.

Augmentation of the fluorescent properties and robustness of GFP via random and site-directed mutagenesis has ushered in a new progeny of fluorescent proteins, each emitting a different wavelength of light upon maximum excitation with a greater intensity than the original GFP *(50–57)*. To date, there are newly engineered variants of GFP that demonstrate enhanced emission wavelengths of yellow (eYFP), cyan (eCFP), and green (eGFP) colors *(58)*. These efforts have culminated in the availability of multicolored probes with altered excitation and emission wavelengths, enhanced intensity, and improved pH resistance *(59)*. However, the development of dsRed *(60–62)*, a red fluorescent protein isolated from coral (*Discosoma* genus) has been more challenging because of its tetrameric nature and low fluorescent potential. The original dsRed protein shared approximately a 30% protein homology with the GFP family, exhibited nonspecific aggregation into tetramers, and required an initial incubation time of over 30 h at 37°C to generate a steady-state signal. These limitations have now been resolved in genetically engineered forms of dsRed that exhibit minimal nonspecific oligomerization, faster rates of fluorescence maturation, and a decrease in nonspecific emission wavelengths *(60)*. This rainbow of commercially available fluorescent proteins is a powerful tool for cell tracking applications and real-time visualization of molecular events. The DNA sequence of these reporter proteins is typically about 700 bp long, with a corresponding approx 27,000-Dalton protein size *(63)*.

The construction of a GFP fusion vector allows real-time in vitro molecular imaging applications with the use of imaging modalities designed to detect fluorescence *(64,65)*. However, there is limited in vivo utility because conventional fluorescence microscopy does not detect signals beyond a tissue depth of 100 μm, depending on the tissue and the wavelength of light penetrating the sample. Even the most sophisticated fluorescence microscopes, such as multiphoton confocal microscopes, cannot detect fluorescence beyond a tissue depth of several hundred microns *(66–69)*. At best, surgical opening of a skinfold window must be combined with intravital (directed into living tissue) multiphoton laser scanning microscopy for in vivo studies *(70–73)*. Therefore, the use of GFP reporter genes for "dynamic" in vivo work has inherent sampling limitations that do not simulate the capabilities of reporter genes allowing in vivo molecular imaging, such as thymidine kinase for PET imaging or luciferase for BLI.

2.3. Reporter Genes for Dynamic, Noninvasive In Vivo Imaging Analysis

2.3.1. Thymidine Kinase Reporter Gene and PET Imaging

The use of PET as a tool for in vivo reporter molecule imaging is versatile, molecule-specific, and effective *(74–79)*. The basic system consists of a herpes simplex virus type 1 thymidine kinase (HSV1-tk) gene cassette and a transgene cassette that are each controlled by the same upstream promoter element, such as the α-MHC promoter for myocardium-specific expression *(80)*. Intracellular accumulation of HSV1-tk will reflect transgene expression when it phosphorylates an exogenous radiolabeled substrate. This exogenous input of radiolabeled substrate is perfused throughout the animal and actively transported into cells. [^{124}I]- or [^{131}I]-FIAU (2'-fluoro-2'-deoxy-1-β-D-arabinofuranosyl-5-iodouracil) or [^{18}F]-FHBG (9-[4-{^{18}F}fluoro-3-hydroxy methylbutyl]-guanine) given in trace amounts will be phosphorylated by transduced cells that contain the reporter thymidine kinase *(80)*. This phosphoryla-tion reaction "traps" the radiolabeled probe, rendering it immobilized within the cell, thus producing a radioactive signal in a transgene-equivalent quantita-tive manner. Two main thymidine kinase reporter genes are commonly used in conjunction with PET: the wild-type HSV1-tk gene and the mutant HSV1-*sr39tk*, the latter providing greater sensitivity to radiolabeled probe *(74,81,82)*. Although mammalian thymidine kinases exist endogenously, they do not share the same range of substrate specificity as HSV1-tk and HSV1-sr39tk, as they are able to phosphorylate FIAU and FHBG specifically, which leads to probe entrapment and accumulation in transduced/transfected cells *(79)*.

The main advantage of PET imaging is its ability to give quantitative infor-mation on physiological and biochemical processes by recording internal im-ages at predetermined planes within the body sequentially over time in the same animal *(83–85)*. This technology is suitable for animal experimentation because FIAU and FHBG have limited side effects and are already routinely used in the clinic. Although powerful, this radionuclide imaging technology is expensive and requires multidisciplinary expertise *(86)* (e.g., cyclotron and radiochemical resources are needed). Realistic and feasible alternatives to noninvasive in vivo reporter imaging are presently available, such as BLI.

2.3.2. Luciferase Reporter Gene and Bioluminescence Imaging

The phenomenon of bioluminescence was first observed in the ocean as a stressed-induced emission of glowing luminous light from oceanic microor-ganisms. Many organisms also exhibit bioluminescence, including eukaryotic ones such as the North American firefly (*Photinus pyralis*), which is the origin of most luciferase genes (*luc*) *(87–89)*. This luciferase enzyme generates the highest quantum yield known in all luciferases and is commercially available. Bioluminescence is a chemiluminescent reaction between luciferase and its substrate luciferin, which generates light with an emission maximum of 562 nm *(90,91)*. Luciferin, ATP, and O_2 are converted to oxyluciferin, AMP, and PPi by luciferase and an Mg^{2+} cofactor. The luciferase enzyme consists of an approx 1.6-kb sequence encoding a 62,000-Dalton protein *(92–94)*.

Bioluminescence generated by the luciferase reporter reaction can be de-tected with the use of a charge-coupled device camera (CCD), a system that is sensitive to the entire visible spectrum and the near infrared wavelength range. Present CCD camera imaging modalities optimized for in vivo imaging have combined intensified and cooled CCDs that (1) amplify the light signal and (2) minimize background noise (*see* **ref. 95** for a full review on this technology).

The use of CCD cameras for BI may seem crude compared with PET and magnetic resonance imaging (MRI) modalities, but the limitations inherent in BLI technology are mostly owing to light scattering by cell and organelle membranes *(96–98)*, as well as absorption of light by melanins, hemoglobin, and other pigmented macromolecules *(99)*. Transmitted light paths are more diffuse, and spatial resolution is decreased with BLI compared with PET in deep tissue; however, significant amounts of light are still emitted that can be detected externally in small animals *(97)*. Adequate oxygen levels are another requirement for light production by luciferases, and hypoxic conditions may limit the in vivo utility of the *luc* reporter gene. Hence, the sudden loss of light production in vivo may be owing to hypoxic necrotic and apoptotic cells *(100)*. There is typically low background during BLI, as there is no endogenous light production in mammalian cells and tissues *(92)*. In contrast, PET is more problematic because of substrate delivery issues and background noise *(101)*. Biodistribution of luciferin is also uniform throughout the animal, and this substrate can cross the blood–brain barrier *(40,102,103)*. Typically, full biodistribution of luciferin via intraperitoneal and intravenous injection can be achieved in less than 20 min *(40)*. BLI is also advantageous because it is more economical and is also a nonradioactive platform. However, BLI is not capable of 3D imaging and does not offer the same degree of spatial resolution as PET.

2.4. Dual Modality Reporter Imaging Technology

The development of these imaging modalities has eventually led to their combination to address molecular and cellular events specifically and effectively in vivo. The amalgamation of these two modalities will advance in vivo imaging to even greater spatial resolution and temporal specificity. Wu et al. *(42)* have already demonstrated the effectiveness of a dual imaging modality system in cardiac cell transplantation, and exciting prospects are ahead for similar molecular imaging strategies extended to the whole myocardium. Most importantly, this tool will probably soon be used in conjunction with inducible gene expression systems such as the Cre-*lox*P and tetracycline-inducible systems to visualize and confirm conditional transgene expression, allowing real-time, noninvasive in vivo imaging in the myocardium.

3. Inducible Gene Expression Systems
3.1. Introduction

To circumvent the challenges inherent in the developmental biology of transgenic mice models, several novel gene knockout or knockin strategies have been developed within the last decade that allow tissue-specific (spatial) control and the ablation or insertion of a gene product at a specific time. Most of these inducible gene expression strategies are based on a binary system consisting of an *activator* and a *responder* component working in concert. Both of these components can be either injected into the pronuclei of a freshly fertilized oocyte to generate transgenic mice or genetically incorporated into viral vectors for gene delivery. (Lentiviral vector technology will be described in **Subheading 4.**)

The ideal inducible system should have (1) no leaky transgene activity when the system is off; (2) high levels of transcriptional activity when the system is activated; (3) no impact on normal biological processes of the animal; (4) specific induction of targeted cells (no mosaic expression); (5) sustained induction over long periods; (6) induction agents that are readily available, inexpensive, and easy to administer; and (7) reversibility. Two of the most well-characterized and well-developed inducible systems that best meet these criteria, the Cre-*lox*P System and the tetracycline-inducible system, will be described for myocardium-specific applications *(104)*.

3.2. The Cre-loxP System

3.2.1. Overview

The Cre-*lox*P system is based on the recombinant activity of the Cre recombinase enzyme (38,000 Daltons), which is highly specific for *lox*P sites that flank a sequence of interest. Cre originates from bacteriophage P1 *(105,106)*, and upon transcription of the Cre gene, Cre homodimers bind at two 34-bp *lox*P sites, each consisting of two 13-bp inverted repeats and an inverted 8-bp spacer (**Fig. 1**). Cre homodimers will excise out the sequence between two *lox*P sites, thus "bridging" the two ends together. The direction of the 8-bp spacer will determine the direction of recombination *(107)*.

The Cre-*lox*P binary system consists of complementary activator and responder cassettes that are each engineered into two separate lines of transgenic mice. These mice are then crossed to generate progeny containing both activator and responder cassettes. The activator cassette contains Cre, and its expression can be controlled by a tissue-specific promoter such as the myocardium-specific α-MHC promoter. Subsequent expression of Cre in transgenic myocardium can then act on any *lox*P sites in the responder cassette. The Cre-*lox*P system has been used in both gain-of-function and loss-of-function approaches; *lox*P can flank a gene selected for knockout at a particular time, or it can remove a stop sequence between a promoter and a transgene on the responder cassette. For example, in a loss-of-function approach in which a gene of interest is to be knocked out, the sequence is flanked by *lox*P sites (or "floxed") such that the normal function of the gene product is not affected until excision. This is typically accomplished by incorporation of *lox*P sites into the introns surrounding an exon. On the other hand, if the objective is to activate transgene expression, otherwise known as a gain-of-function approach, a floxed transcriptional termination sequence is positioned such that it separates a pro-

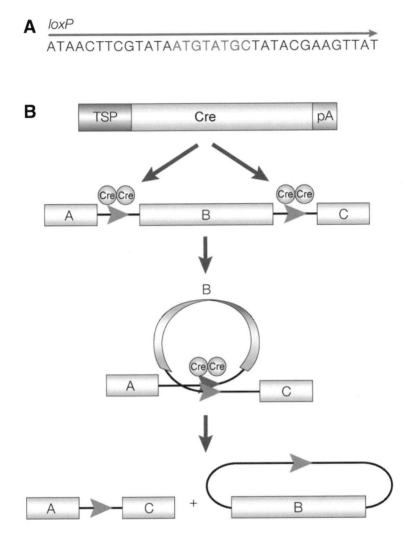

Fig. 1. Cre-*lox*P recombination. (**A**) Site-specific recombination occurs at two *lox*P sites. Each consists of two 13-bp inverted repeats flanking and 8-bp spacer (ATGTATGC), which determines the direction of recombination. (**B**) After transcription is initiated by a tissue-specific promoter, Cre dimers catalyze conservative recombination between two repeated *lox*P sites (arrowheads) resulting in the excision of region B from between regions A and C. If region B is an essential component of a gene, then gene activation occurs. If region B is a stop sequence downstream from a promoter in region A, then recombination would result in gene activation. pA, polyadenylation site; TSP, tissue-specific promoter. (Adapted with permission courtesy of M. Lewandoski from **ref. *104*.**)

moter from the gene of interest *(108)*. In this approach, transgene expression can only be initiated after the stop sequence has been excised by the action of the Cre recombinase.

Inducible Cre-*lox*P systems were initially tested with responder mice containing a floxed stop sequence upstream of the *lacZ* gene *(109,110)*. Eventually, double reporter strains were developed with expression of one reporter before recombination and another reporter after recombination, such as the *lacZ*/GFP double reporter developed by Novak et al. *(111)*. The following website provides a list of many more cell- and tissue-specific Cre activator transgenic mouse lines that have been generated (http://www.mshri.on.ca/nagy/Cre-pub.html).

3.2.2. Cre-ER- and Cre-PR-Inducible Systems

Although conventional Cre-*lox*P-inducible gene expression systems allow spatial control because of the α-MHC promoter, they do not allow precise temporal control of Cre expression. However, Cre-progesterone receptor (Cre-PR) and Cre-estrogen receptor (Cre-ER) systems allow both spatial and temporal control of transgene expression. This system is based on the mechanism of modified estrogen- and progesterone-nuclear hormone receptors, which are inactive in the cytoplasm. Upon activation by either the native estrogen or progesterone hormone, the receptor enters the nucleus and initiates expression of targeted genes. Cre has been fused to modified forms of the Cre-PR *(112–114)* and Cre-ER *(115)* receptors, which are no longer responsive to their endogenous ligands, but instead are responsive to synthetic mifeprestone and tamoxifen, respectively. When the inducer is applied, the receptor will translocate to the nucleus, carrying with it the Cre fusion protein, which can then initiate recombination of floxed target sites. The α-MHC promoter can be used for spatial restriction of the expression of Cre-PR *(112,116–121)* or Cre-ER *(108,112,122–139)* fusion proteins to the myocardium, and temporal control is exercised when a synthetic hormone such as mifeprestone or tamoxifen is added. However, some studies have reported incomplete excision in response to the ligand, or leaky excision occurring independently of the ligand *(112,140)*. Other studies have observed Cre recombinase activity at unforeseen mammalian *lox*P-like sites, causing large chromosomal rearrangements *(141,142)*. Several modified versions of the recombinase *(138,143)*, such as the development of Cre*PR, have reduced unwanted background activity to almost undetectable levels with significantly enhanced recombination activity *(144)*. Additionally, endogenous steroid hormones were found to generate broad background recombination in a variety of organs, which increased over time. To increase the specificity of Cre recombinase, Sohal et al. *(13)* developed a novel Cre-ER type inducible Cre-*lox*P system driven by the α-MHC promoter. A mutated estrogen receptor (Mer) domain flanking the Cre gene permitted endogenous estrogen insensitivity, while only allowing tamoxifen-inducible activity. This MerCreMer fusion was also reported to reduce unwanted Cre activity *(143,145)* and to enhance recombinase activity further.

3.2.3. Cre-loxP in the Heart

Because of the challenges discussed above, relatively few studies have been successful with specific Cre-mediated recombination in the heart since its development (**Table 1**). Early studies utilized the muscle creatine kinase (MCK) promoter, which generated expression in both the heart and skeletal muscle *(146–148)*. Other studies have reported successful Cre-mediated recombination in heart tissue induced by the α-MHC promoter *(117,124,149,150)*, but concerns of premature lethality cast doubt on the over-all effectiveness of this approach because of possible premature expression during embryogenesis and lack of temporal inducibility should recombination occur at these stages.

Most inducible expression approaches consist of a transgene knockin approach, which can be controlled spatially and temporally. The Cre-*lox*P system has been successfully applied in this manner whereby a floxed STOP codon site is situated between a target transgene and a promoter, but an important consideration prior to use of this system is its irreversible nature. Once the floxed fragment has been excised, the responder component will be "on" permanently. This would be undesirable for studies in which graded or reversible expression of transgenes is necessary. The tetracycline-inducible systems offer this added control and thus have considerable advantages over the Cre-*lox*P system.

3.3. The Tetracycline Transactivator Systems

3.3.1. Overview

The tetracycline transactivator (tTA) expression system originates from the genetic elements involved in the regulation of tetracycline resistance gene expression in *Escherichia coli (151)*. The resistance protein tetA functions as a membrane-spanning pump that removes tetracycline from the cell when present and is detrimental to the microorganism when tetracycline is absent. Expression of tetA is constitutively repressed by the tetracycline repressor (tetR), which binds to tetracycline operator (*tet*O) sites upstream of the tetA protein sequence. Should tetracycline enter the cell, it will bind to the repressor tetR and subsequently prevent tetR from binding to the *tet*O sequence, thus promoting expression of the resistance pump.

Table 1
Cre-*loxP*-Induced Gene Expression in the Heart

Cre system	Delivery	Activation molecule	Activation promoter	Activation recombinase	Responder transgene	Phenotype observed in heart	Year	Ref.
Knockin	AdV	None	HSV-TK	Cre	β-gal	Infection of various tissues including heart	1996	*231*
Knockin	Transgenic mice and AdV	None	α-MHC	Cre	β-gal and Luc	Reporter gene expression in the ventricle	1997	*149*
Knockout	Transgenic mice	None	MCK	Cre	IR	Reduction in IR receptor in heart and skeletal muscle	1998	*146*
Knockout	Transgenic mice	None	MLC 2v	Cre	RxRα	Lack of RxRα in ventricular cardiomyocytes	1998	*150*
Knockout	Transgenic mice	None	MCK	Cre	Tfam^*loxP*	Reduced mtDNA and respiratory chain deficiency	1998	*148*
Knockout	Transgenic mice	None	MCK	Cre	Tfam^*loxP*	Respiratory chain deficiency, dilated cardiomyopathy, AV heart conduction blocks	1999	*147*
Knockin	Transgenic mice	None	SmαA and CaαA	Cre	β-gal	Reporter gene expression in heart, aorta and other tissues	2000	*232*
Knockout	Transgenic mice	None	α-MHC	Cre	Tfam^*loxP*	Mitochondrial cardiomyopathy	2000	*124*
Knockin	AdV/ Transgenic mice	None	CAG	Cre	p35	Inhibition of caspase-3 activation and resistance to hypoxia-induced cell death	2000	*233*

Inducible knockin	Transgenic mice	antiprogestin RU486	α-MHC	CrePR1	β-gal	Reporter gene expression in myocardium	2001	*14*
Inducible knockin	Transgenic mice	Tamoxifen	CMV	MerCreMer	β-gal	Reporter gene expression in myocardium	2001	*13*
Knockout	Transgenic mice	None	CMV	Cre	ALK3	Defects in the endocardial cushion, interventricular septum, and trabeculae	2002	*234*
Knockout	Transgenic mice	None	Nkx2-5	IRESCre	β-gal and Z/AP	Reporter gene expression in cardiac progenitor cells and other sites	2002	*235*
Knockin	AdV	None	CMV	Cre	β-gal	Short-term reporter gene delivery	2003	*236*

Abbreviations: AdV, adenovirus; β-gal, β-galactosidase gene; MCK, muscle creatine kinase promoter; expressed at embryonic day 13; Luc, luciferase; MLC 2v, myocin light chain 2v; RxRα, retinoic acid receptor α; IR, insulin receptor; HSV-TK, herpes simplex virus thymidine kinase enhancer/promoter; Tfam^loxP, mitochondrial transcription factor A flanked by *loxP* sites; mtDNA, mitochondrial DNA; AV, atrioventricular; Smoα, human smooth muscle α-actin; Caα, cardiac α-actin; CAG, promoter consisting of cytomegalovirus IE enhancer and chicken β-actin promoter, CrePR1, Cre-progesterone receptor binding domain fusion protein; α-MHC, α-myosin heavy chain, expressed at embryonic day 8; MerCreMer, Cre protein fusion with two mutant estrogen-receptor domains; ALK3, a type IA bone morphogenic protein receptor; CMV, Cytomegalovirus promoter; Nkx2-5, a cardiac homeobox gene; IRESCre, Cre linked at 5′ end to an internal ribosome entry site; Z/AP, double reporter producing β-gal (Z) before Cre excision and human alkaline phosphatase (AP) after Cre excision; AAV, adeno-associated virus.

3.3.2. Tet-Off System (Tetracycline Transactivator)

The efficient use of this prokaryotic system in eukaryotic cells has been permitted by two modifications, resulting in the Tet-Off system. The repressor protein tetR has been transformed from a repressor to a eukaryotic cell activator via fusion with activation domains of the herpes simplex virus VP16 protein, thus producing a new molecule called the tetracycline transactivator (tTA). In addition, a cytomegalovirus (CMV) minimal promoter has been fused with 5–7 *tet*O sequences (the binding sites for tetR) to drive transgene expression upon activation. Thus tTA will naturally bind to *tet*O and activate expression of downstream genes, and when tetracycline (or a derivative like doxycycline, which can more readily pass the blood–brain barrier) is present, it forms a complex with tTA that is then released from *tet*O, turning off expression of downstream transgenes. Thus, upon creation of a transgenic line containing the activator tTA, and crossing to a responder line, a mouse can have transgene expression activated upon removal of Dox (**Fig. 2A**). Disadvantages include the potential toxicity of administering Dox prenatally and throughout development, as well as any effects Dox may have on diseased phenotypes once they have been incurred. An advantage of the system is that tetracycline and its derivatives have already been well established for human therapy, so these compounds are deemed safe for animal experimentation.

3.3.3. Tet-On System (Reverse Tetracycline Transactivator)

The reverse tetracycline transactivator (rtTA) is a mutegenized transactivator that operates in a reverse fashion to tTA, as it binds to *tet*O and activates downstream genes of interest only in the presence of Dox (**Fig. 2B**) *(152)*. Advantages of the system include the more rapid control of transgene induction, as the Tet-Off system can take days to turn off pending the clearance of Dox from the animal *(153)*. Disadvantages include the slight affinity of rtTA for *tet*O even in the absence of Dox, resulting in leaky transgene expression *(154,155)*. In addition, rtTA has a lower affinity for Dox than tTA, and 10 times more Dox is required for maximum activation, a concentration that may be challenging to obtain in some tissues in an in vivo setting *(156)*. Consecutive optimization of the rtTA system has resulted in a transactivator well tolerated by a variety of cell types that is more easily activated by Dox, termed rtTA2S-M2 *(157,158)*. Other advances in responder cassettes have included bidirectional promoters, which allow expression of any two desired transgenes in opposite directions from a modified *tet*O promoter when activated by either tTA or rtTA proteins *(159,160)*.

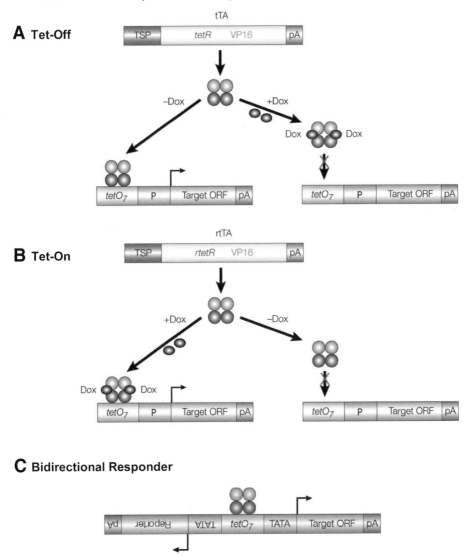

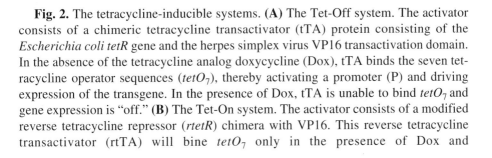

Fig. 2. The tetracycline-inducible systems. **(A)** The Tet-Off system. The activator consists of a chimeric tetracycline transactivator (tTA) protein consisting of the *Escherichia coli tetR* gene and the herpes simplex virus VP16 transactivation domain. In the absence of the tetracycline analog doxycycline (Dox), tTA binds the seven tetracycline operator sequences (*tetO7*), thereby activating a promoter (P) and driving expression of the transgene. In the presence of Dox, tTA is unable to bind *tetO7* and gene expression is "off." **(B)** The Tet-On system. The activator consists of a modified reverse tetracycline repressor (*rtetR*) chimera with VP16. This reverse tetracycline transactivator (rtTA) will bine *tetO7* only in the presence of Dox and

3.3.4. Tetracycline Transcriptional Repressors and Silencers

Other improvements for addressing leaky transgene expression have been the development of tetracycline controlled transcriptional repressors (tTRs) or transcriptional silencers (tTS) that are active only when Dox is absent. To construct these repressors, the domain of tetR involved in dimerization was altered so it would be unable to form dimers with its oppositely modulated cognate rtTA, allowing the two molecules to be used concurrently, one to repress basal activity (tTR or tTS) and the other to move in when the presence of Dox indicates activation is needed (rtTA) *(8,161,162)*. Zhu et al. *(163,164)* were the first to demonstrate tTS suppression of rtTA leakiness in triple transgenic mice, indicating that it completely suppressed basal expression of interleukin (IL)-13 in the lung.

3.3.5. Tetracycline Transactivator System in the Heart

Use of tetracycline-inducible systems in the heart has been exclusively with the Tet-Off system. Most studies reported have used the activator line developed by Fishman et al. *(165–167)* containing the myocardium-specific rat α-MHC promoter (**Table 2**).

The production of the cellular toxin nitric oxide (NO) by immune cells is thought to play a role in controlling invading microorganisms, viruses, and abnormal cells. NO is produced by nitric oxide synthases (NOS). Although NOS has been reported to have a positive ionotropic effect in normal heart tissue, increased inducible nitric oxide synthase (iNOS) has been reported in a variety of pathologies throughout the body *(168–175)*. As humans with cardiac disease have been reported to have increased iNOS, Mungrue et al. *(176)* generated a transgenic mouse conditionally expressing human iNOS in myocardium. The α-MHC promoter was used to drive tTA in the activator cassette with the use of a bidirectional promoter in the responder cassette. In the presence of Dox, no gene expression could occur, and when Dox was absent, expression of both iNOS and β-gal ensued. Overexpression of iNOS seemed to generate significant fatalities compared with the birth success of mothers receiving Dox. Increased iNOS expression upon Dox removal reportedly produced a tenfold increase in total NOS activity and resulting increases in NO in cardiac myocytes over control hearts. Dox was removed at 10-wk of age, and

---

Fig. 2. *(continued)* remains unbound in the absence of Dox. (**C**) The bidirectional responder. Using two minimal promoters, *tetO*$_7$ can be activated by either the tTA or rtTA systems to drive expression on both the reporter gene and the target gene of interest. pA, polyadenylation site; TSP, tissue-specific promoter; ORF, open reading frame. (Adapted with permission courtesy of M. Lewandoski from **ref.** *104*.)

Table 2
Tetracycline-Induced Gene Expression in the Heart

Regulation system	Delivery	Activation promoter	Responder promoter	Responder transgene	Expression phenotype	Year	Ref.
tTA	Plasmid	rat α-MHC	tetO-CMV$_{min}$	Luc	Reporter expression in the heart	1994	*165*
tTA	Transgenic mice	rat α-MHC	tetO-CMV$_{min}$	Id1	Transgene expression in the heart	1994	*166*
tTA	Transgenic mice	rat α-MHC	tetO-CMV$_{min}$	Luc, β-gal	Reporter expression in the heart	1996	*167*
tTA	Transgenic mice	rat α-MHC	tetO-CMV$_{min}$	PKCβ	Hypertrophy	1997	*237*
tTA	Transgenic mice	rat α-MHC	tetO-CMV$_{min}$	Ro-1, lacZ	Decreased heart rate, lethal arrhythmia	1999, 2000, 2002	*238, 239*
tTA	Transgenic mice	rat α-MHC	tetO-CMV$_{min}$	VEGF	Inhibition of endocardial cushion development, long-term improvement in organ perfusion	2001	*177–179*
tTA	Transgenic mice	rat α-MHC	TRE-CMV$_{min}$	HSL	Absence of cardiac lipid accumulation	2001	*240*
tTA	Transgenic mice	rat α-MHC	Bidirectional pBi-1	iNOS and β-gal simultaneously	Cardiomyopathy, bradyarrhythmia, sudden cardiac death	2002	*241*
tTA	Transgenic mice	rat α-MHC	Bidirectional minimal	Antisense mMR and β-gal simultaneously	Severe heart failure and cardiac fibrosis	2002	*242*
tTA	Transgenic mice	rat α-MHC	TRE-CMV$_{min}$	ACVI	Increased cAMP generation and LV contractile function	2002	*243*
tTA	Transgenic mice	mouse α-MHC	MHC$_{min}$^{TetO}	β-gal reporter, ECL1, GSK-3β	Attenuation of hypertrophy	2003	*10*

(continued)

Table 2 (continued)

Regulation system	Delivery	Activation promoter	Responder promoter	Responder transgene	Expression phenotype	Year	Ref.
tTA	Transgenic mice	rat α-MHC	tetO-CMV$_{min}$	Antisense hMR	Half reduction in endogenous hMR	2003	*244*

Abbreviations: tTA, tetracycline transactivator; α-MHC, α-myosin heavy chain; α-gal, β-galactosidase gene; Luc, luciferase; Id1, helix-loop-helix protein serving as a negative regulator of differentiation during skeletal myogenesis; Ro-1, RASSL opioid, no.1, a modified human κ opioid receptor; VEGF, vascular endothelial growth factor; HSL, heart-specific lipase; tetO-CMV$_{min}$, tetracycline operator fused to cytomegalovirus minimal promoter; mMR, mouse mineralocorticoid receptor; TRE-CMV$_{min}$, tetracycline-responsive-element (Clontech, Palo Alto, CA) fused to cytomegalovirus minimal promoter; AC$_{VI}$, adenylcyclase type VI; LV, left ventricular; pBi-1, bidirectional promoter; MHCmin^{TetO}, tetracycline-responsive myosin heavy chain minimal promoter; ECL1, essential myosin light chain; GSK-3β, glycogen synthase kinase-3β; hMR, human mineralocorticoid receptor.

after 30-d cardiac enlargement was observed. These data suggest that iNOS affects cardiac remodeling in ways similar to ventricular dilation and hypertrophy. Cardiac fibrosis and a high incidence of sudden cardiac death from bradyarrhythmia were also observed. The data obtained with this conditional model of cardiac targeted transgene expression were markedly different from those obtained by Heger et al. *(11)*, who in the same year reported that α-MHC-driven overexpression of iNOS had no effect on cardiac structure and function. The direct constitutive knockin animal model employed might have resulted in only the survival of lines without pathological iNOS levels. This is a direct example of the additional information that can be gleaned from conditional transgenic systems.

To address the difficulty in producing nonleaky inducible lines, Sanbe et al. *(10)* have developed a novel tetracycline inducible system whereby both the activator and responder cassettes are driven by mouse α-MHC promoters rather than the rat α-MHC promoter and the CMV minimal promoter typically used. The rat α-MHC promoter fragment used to drive expression of the activator construct is cardiac specific and does not exhibit position-independent or copy number-dependent expression, although it may be differentially expressed in atrial and ventricular cardiomyocytes. In addition, the CMV minimal promoter in the responder line bestows greater risk of activation from outside inputs or from having altered methylation patterns. It is possible that these two issues are responsible for the difficulty in transferring tetracycline inducible technology to the heart. For example, Sanbe et al. *(10)* had to generate between 5 and 20 mouse lines before a successful binary breeding of activator and responder components was achieved. Sanbe et al. attempt to address these issues with the use of a mouse α-MHC promoter in the activator line, combined with an attenuated mouse α-MHC promoter in the responder line. This attenuated α-MHC minimal promoter (MHCmin^{TetO}) was engineered by removing several GATA DNA binding sites and thyroid-responsive elements to reduce its level of cardiac expression. The same group also reported that detectable levels of their modified VP16-tTA fusion protein correlated with a hypertrophic phenotype in all animals; however, those animals producing low levels of tTA owing to aberrant splicing of the transgene were reportedly viable. Surprisingly, they discovered that the VP16-tTA transcript has alternative splice sites and that only small amounts of properly spliced tTA were actually required for adequate activation or repression. This seems to suggest that successively improving the inducibility of the system should not be attempted by increasing the transactivator protein levels. The new activator line, now driven by a murine α-MHC promoter, is reportedly stable in multiple generations and is expressed throughout the adult heart. The responder construct with an attenuated mouse α-MHC promoter seems to conserve its copy number-dependent and position-independent features. This new system was found to work for high- and low-abundance proteins; furthermore, a dramatic reduction was seen in the quantity of animal lines required to produce an efficiently inducible systems, from 5–20 to only 3. This facilitated the more economical and efficient examination of their genes of interest: essential myosin light chain 1 (ELC1) and glycogen synthase kinase-3β (GSK-3β).

To better understand the effects of vascular endothelial growth factor (VEGF)-induced neogenesis, Dor et al. *(177–179)* used transgenic mice expressing the tTA protein driven by heart-specific α-MHC, liver-specific liver-activating protein (LAP) promoter *(180)*, and brain-specific calmodulin kinase II (CamKII) promoter *(181)*. Profiles of strong induction of VEGF were shown in each organ *(178)*. VEGF levels were reported to be fully reversible within a day after tetracycline removal. Extensive disorganized revascularization was observed, accompanied by excessive edema during the VEGF overexpression period. Once VEGF was "switched off," rapid remodeling of the vascular network occurred along with restoration of normal fluid levels. A remarkable finding was that if VEGF overexpression was prematurely withdrawn, most new vessels disappeared; however, if expression was maintained for several weeks, vessels persisted after VEGF withdrawal for many months *(178)*. This discovery was only made possible by the use of the reversible tetracycline switch, and gives indication of the potential usefulness of spatial and temporal controls in biological research.

3.4. Merging the Inducible Gene Expression Systems With Reporter Genes and Lentiviral Vectors

The Cre-*lox*P and tetracycline inducible systems both comprise an activator component (Cre or tTA/rtTA) and a responder component (transgene of interest) that are effective when both are present in the same cell. The development of transgenic mouse lines that carry both the activator and responder components of the Cre-*lox*P or tetracycline-inducible systems is possible by generating a mouse line containing one component and then crossing it with its complementary component. As discussed above, the need to generate multiple animal lines and achieve successful inducible crosses makes this process both time-consuming and laborious. A more practical alternative may be the development of a viral vector-mediated means of gene delivery. Such an alternative would require a vector that can effectively deliver a genetic payload without incurring cytotoxicity, an immunogenic response, or recurrent viral infection. The lentivirus vector can be used to deliver a genetic payload of activator or responder cassettes of inducible transgene/reporter constructs *(182)*. In this approach, lines of mice can be purchased or generated by lentiviral gene delivery that contain the activator cassette. These transgenic mice would then be transduced with lentiviral constructs that contain their transgenic inducible system responder cassette counterpart. For example, the Tet-Off and Tet-On responder cassettes to be transduced could consist of a bidirectional promoter that controls expression of both a transgene and a reporter. This platform allows the researcher to investigate more than one transgene under inducible conditions and circumvents the need to construct multiple lines of crossed transgenic mice. Upon transduction of the complementing responder cassette into cells that already contain the activator cassette, transgene and reporter gene expression can be initiated and controlled depending on the nature of the inducible system employed (**Fig. 2A,B**). The incorporation of the responder cassette into a lentiviral vector for efficient transduction into host cells is described in the next section.

4. In Vivo Gene Delivery of Inducible Gene Expression System

4.1. Introduction

Presently, there are three major avenues of transgene delivery in vivo: (1) direct injection of genetic construct into pronuclei of freshly sterilized murine oocytes to produce transgenic mice; (2) recombinant adenovirus (AdV) or adeno-associated virus (AAV)-based transgene vectors; and (3) lentiviral transgene vectors (*Lentiviridae* genus, retrovirus family). Direct injection of transgenes into oocytes has proved to be the predominant and most trusted technique for gene delivery and development of transgenic animals. However, this technique is very expensive, and not all transgenes are suited for oocyte injection. In addition, the transgene of interest may be embryonic lethal or cause phenotypic alterations via developmental outcomes secondary to the genetic changes implemented (for more pitfalls concerning this technology, *see* **ref. *183***). We propose the use of lentiviral vectors to deliver the transgene payload because of the ability to integrate the transgene and promoter physically into the host cell genome, resulting in more efficient and long-term inducible transgene expression.

4.2. Lentivirus Vector Gene Delivery Systems

The original lentivirus was derived from the HIV virion and consists of a single-stranded RNA genome approx 7–11 kb long *(184,185)*. The lentivirus vector has been developed to become an efficient form of gene delivery that results in long-term transgene expression because of several key features: the ability to integrate into the host genome *(186,187)*, low immunogenicity *(188–190)*, and the ability to integrate into both dividing and nondividing cells with high efficiency *(184,190)*. Previously, adenoviruses (Ad) and AAVs were used for gene delivery, but their popularity has diminished because of immunogenicity issues *(191)* and their inability to integrate viral DNA into the host genome to maintain long-term expression (except for AAV) *(192,193)*.

The success of the lentiviral vector lies in its ability to transduce both dividing and quiescent cells in vivo via its lentiviral preintegration complex (PIC). This viral mechanism facilitates DNA entry into the nucleus via the nucleopore *(194)* and subsequent integration into the host genome. Moreover, most lentivirus vectors currently in use have physically separated the genetic elements required for integration from the rest of the viral genes involved in packaging and replication to prevent replication competent lentivirus (RCL) formation *(195,196)*. Hence, the modern lentiviral vector preparation construct actually consists of two types of vectors: the *transfer vector*, which carries the transgene and regulatory sequences flanked by long terminal repeat (LTR) sequences (**Fig. 3B**), and the *packaging vector*, which contains genes required for virus replication under the control of a heterologous promoter (**Fig. 3A**). Overall, the lentivirus vector only contains the transfer vector and the means to integrate it into the host cell genome—it does not carry the packaging vectors or any other capability of replication and mobilization.

A general scheme of lentivirus vector production is depicted in **Fig. 4**. A packaging cell line that will produce a lentiviral vector titer is cotransfected with the packaging vectors and the transfer vector. These packaging vectors are not replicated, nor are they incorporated into the lentiviral vector because they do not carry the encapsidation signal, Σ. Expressed viral structural proteins and replicated copies of the transfer vector genome will combine to form a lentiviral vector, in which only the transfer vector is encapsidated within the viral structural coat. Most importantly, there are no viral structural genes from the packaging vector encapsidated within the lentiviral vector. The sole purpose of these lentiviral vectors is to incorporate the transfer vector into the host's cell genome.

4.3. Packaging and Transfer Vectors

The genetic maps for vectors involved in lentivirus vector production are illustrated in **Fig. 3A,B**. In addition to viral structural proteins encoded by *gag* and *pol*, the lentiviral genome contains a regulatory element called *rev* that has been placed on a smaller, surrogate vector under the control of a heterologous promoter, in order to decrease the likelihood of RCL. Rev serves to export unspliced mRNA across the nucleus by first binding to the *Rev* response element (RRE) in a multimeric fashion. Consequently, this structure exposes a region within the Rev protein called the nuclear export signal (NES) *(197,198)*. This region of DNA can then bind to nucleopores and receptors, funneling newly synthesized mRNA out to the cytoplasm *(199,200)*. This binding of the NES to the nuclear membrane competes against the host's own splicing mechanisms, while maximizing viral mRNA translation and overriding host mRNA translation. This Rev-mediated series of events allows unspliced mRNA to be

A Packaging Vectors

i)

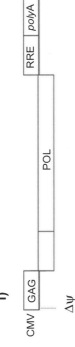

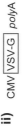

ii) CMV | VSV-G | polyA

iii) RSV | REV | polyA

GAG	Encodes structural polyproteins required for viral packaging and replication (210-213).
POL	Encodes the enzymes *PR* (protease), *RT* (reverse transcriptase), and *IN* (integrase) required for nucleic acid metabolism and viral genome integration into host cell genome (214, 215, 217)
VSV-G	Encodes the surface envelope glycoprotein that determines the tropism or host range that the virus particle can infect (pseudotype) (216)
ψ	Packaging signal, which mediates "encapsidation" of replicated RNA genome into the capsid, the glycoprotein shell or encasement of the virus. This packaging signal, has been muted (Δψ) in order to prevent the encapsidation of replicated RNA genome into virus particles (222).
polyA	Polyadenylation signal on mRNA transcripts increase transgene expression efficiency.
REV	Serves to export unspliced mRNA across the nucleus by binding to *Rev*-response element on the transfer vector (198).
RRE	Rev-response element that allows Rev binding and physical export of mRNA out of the nucleus (219).
CMV/ RSV	Heterologous promoters used to initiate viral protein synthesis or viral genome replication.

Fig. 3. (B) Constructs for lentivirus vector production. **(A)** The packing vectors do not have an encapsidation signal (Π) and therefore cannot be incoporated into the lentiviral vector. i) Viral genes required for structure, reverse transcriptase, and integrase, as described in the text. ii) Viral genes required to encode the pseudotype (host range) of the lentiviral vector. iii) Viral genes required to encode *Rev*, which is essential for nuclear import/export of virally transcribed nucleic acids.

B Transfer Vector

Tet-Off/On Responder cassette

R & U5	Are the two elements that comprise of the 5' LTR (Long Terminal Repeat sequence).
Δgag	A muted form of the sequence that encodes the viral structural proteins (221).
RRE	The Rev-response element helps facilitate the export of the transfer vector out of the nucleus during lentiviral vector formation to prevent aberrant splicing of the RNA viral genome prior to packaging.
SIN-LTR	The 3' end of the transfer vector also contains a self-inactivating signal that prevents mobilization from the host's genome and replication of the transfer vector (204). Reduces possibility of RCL.
WPRE	Incorporation of a post-transcriptional regulatory element of the Woodchuck hepatitis virus (WPRE) increases transgene expression offsetting the effects of the SIN-LTR. It affects the polyadenylation signal and enhances RNA transport out of the nucleus (220).
ψ	Packaging signal or encapsidation signal that allows replicated transfer vector to be incorporated into the capsid, the glycoprotein shell of the virus (222-223).

Fig. 3. (**B**) The transfer vectors are the only nucleic acids packaged into the lentivirus vector as determined by the Π signal downstream of the 5' LTR. Illustrated is a possible Tet-Off or Tet-On responder cassette with a bidirectional promoter in the lentiviral vector.

132

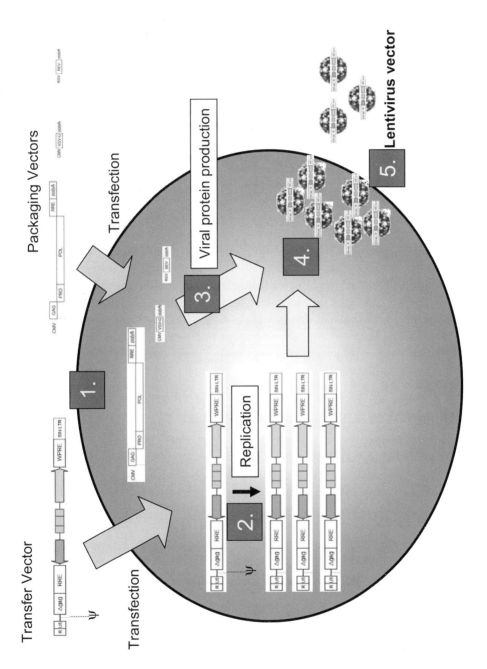

Transfer Vector

Packaging Vectors

Transfection

Transfection

1.

2. Replication

3. Viral protein production

4.

5. Lentivirus vector

133

transported into the cytoplasm, a critical feature required for the translation of *gag, pol*, and foreign transgenes *(201)*.

Virus vector tropism and incorporation into cells is dependent on the membrane envelope encasing the virus and the envelope protein interactions with host cell receptors. The gene that encodes the tropism of the lentiviral vector is also dedicated to another vector under heterologous promoter control. Lentiviral vectors are typically pseudotyped with the VSV-G gene (G-glycoprotein of vesicular stomatitis virus), which is substituted in place of the wild-type *env* gene *(202)*. *env* encodes lentiviral wild-type proteins that form the transmembrane (gp41) and the outer membrane envelope surface (gp120) *(202)*. VSV-G is used because it confers a greater host range and viral particles are more stable and can be concentrated into higher titers (~1 × 10^{10} t.u./mL) *(202)*, thus broadening the infection spectrum of the lentivirus *(202)*. As additional safety measures, SIN *(203)* and WPRE elements that also retain efficient transgene expression have been included in the transfer vector to prevent RCL formation *(204)*. Although the advantages of the lentiviral system are many, lentiviruses do have the potential drawback of causing insertional mutagenesis in important host genes *(205–207)*. We refer the reader to a review by Kafri *(208)* that describes recently developed biosafety measures. This review highlights many of the issues involved in mutagenesis, and assays to assess RCL formation in viral titers.

4.4. Lentiviral Vectors Used in Strategies for Conditional Expression

Development of retroviral vectors for reversible Tet regulation have been generated (**Table 3**) with success and great promise. These vectors allow transduction of a large number of cell types, require relatively minimal effort to prepare, are stable, and can yield populations of regulatable cells within weeks as opposed to months. Kringstein et al. used both the rtTA (Tet-On) and tTA (Tet-Off) systems, carried within a SIN-RetroTet vector *(209)* that was based on the Moloney murine leukemia virus. Tet transactivators were used to provide the first unmistakable evidence that graded transcriptional responses can occur as opposed to more commonly observed all-or-none responses *(27)*.

Fig. 4. *(previous page)* Production of lentivirus vectors. 1, Cotransfection of a cell line with all three packaging vectors and transfer vector; 2, replication of transfer vector; 3, viral protein production from the three packaging lentiviral vectors; 4, the transfer vector and the viral proteins combine to assemble a lentivirus vector; 5, the lentiviral vector will be released out of the cell. These lentiviral vectors have transducing capabilities and are unable to replicate their viral genome.

Table 3
Tetracycline-Inducible Retroviral Vectors

Retrovirus backbone	Regulation system	Location of regulation components	Transgene cassette	Responder transgene(s)	Transduced cell type	Model	Expression phenotype	Year	Ref.
MMLV	tTA Tet-Off	Combination, autoregulatory loop	Bicistronic	lacZ	C57/BL6 primary mouse myoblasts	In vitro	Inducible reporter gene expression	1996	*209*
MMLV	tTA Tet-Off and rtTA Tet-On	Binary	Bicistronic	hGH and GFP	C57 primary mouse myoblasts	In vitro	Graded transcriptional response from inducible reporter gene	1998	*27*
Lentivirus	tTA Tet-Off	Combination, autoregulatory loop	Single-gene	GFP	Human 293 cells, rat brain in vivo	In vitro and in vivo	Inducible reporter gene expression	2000	*18*
Lentivirus	rtTA Tet-On	Binary and combination	Single gene, bicistronic, and multigene	eGFP, HAS, neomycin phosphor-transferase	Human skin fibroblasts	In vitro	Coexpression of regulated transgenes	2000	*224*
Lentivirus	rtTA Tet-On	Combination, autoregulatory loop	Viral genome	Viral genes	SupT1 T-cell, C33A cells	In vitro	Inducible replication of HIV virus	2001	*225*
MMLV	tTA Tet-Off	Combination,	Bicistronic	BCR-ABL	IL-3-dependent murine Ba/F3 cell line	In vitro and in vivo	Inducible BCR-ABL gene expression	2001	*226*
RSV	rtTA Tet-On	Binary autoregulatory loop	Single-gene	eGFP	Chick embryo	In vivo	Inducible reporter gene expression	2002	*227*

(continued)

Table 3 (continued)

Retrovirus backbone	Regulation system	Location of regulation components	Transgene cassette	Responder transgene(s)	Transduced cell type	Model	Expression phenotype	Year	Ref.
Lentivirus	tTA2s Tet-Off	Binary and combination	Bicistronic	GFP and Luc	Cord blood CD34+ cells	In vitro and ex vivo	Inducible long-term reporter gene expression	2002	*182*
Lentivirus	rtTA Tet-On with tTS	Combination	Bidirectional	GDNF and eGFP	HiB5 cells	In vitro and in vivo	Inducible transgene expression	2002	*16*
Lentivirus	tTA Tet-Off	Binary	Single-gene	CNTF, GFP, YFP, *lacZ*	Rat striatal neurons	In vivo	Neuroprotective effect associated with the production of CNTF	2002	*228*
Lentivirus-adenovirus	rtTA Tet-On	Combination, autoregulatory loop	Single-gene	Viral genome and GFP	Human T-cell leukemia cell line	In vitro	Efficient gene transfer from adenovector and stable integration from lentivector. Efficient and stable expression of inducible reporter gene	2003	*15*
Lentivirus	tTR-KRAB	Combination	Bicistronic	GFP, interfering RNA, dsRed	HeLa cells, MCF-7sc cell	In vitro	Efficient inducible knockdown of cellular genes	2003	*229*

| Lentivirus | rtTA2s-M2 Tet-On | Binary | Single-gene | *lacZ* | Cotransfection of Chinese hamster ovary and human endothelial hybridoma cells | In vitro and in vivo | Inducible reporter gene expression in vivo and in vitro | 2003 | *230* |

Abbreviations: tTA, tetracycline transactivator; rtTA, reverse tetracycline transactivator; tTS, tetracycline transcriptional repressor; rtTA2s-M2, mutated reverse tetracycline transactivator; MMLV, Moloney murine leukemia virus; hGH, human growth hormone; GFP, green fluorescent protein; eGFP, enhanced green fluorescent protein; HAS, heat-stable antigen; PBMCs, peripheral blood mononuclear cells; YFP, yellow fluorescent protein; *lacZ*, β-galactosidase gene; Luc, luciferase; CNTF, ciliary neurotrophic factor; BCR-ABL, molecular marker of human chronic myelogenous leukemia; tTR-KRAB, tetracycline repressor from *Escherichia coli* Tn*10*, fused to the KRAB domain of human Kox1.

The use of lentiviral vectors to transduce cells with both the activator and responder cassettes has been done either sequentially or simultaneously. Although the separation of these two cassettes allows more transgene DNA to be packaged, mosaic effects and dose problems may occur if more than one of each component is inserted within a cell. To stably transduce dividing and nondividing cells with regulatable transgenes, Kafri et al. *(18)* reported the packaging of the entire Tet system into a single lentiviral vector.

5. Discussion

The goal of this chapter was to describe a strategy in which transgene expression can be spatially and temporally induced and confirmed by reporter gene expression without undergoing the establishment of a transgenic mouse line. In other words, we propose a real-time method of transgenic animal investigation of the myocardium using the tools described. It is now possible to couple a transgene of interest to a reporter gene and drive expression under the direction of the α-MHC promoter. In this model, both genes are only expressed when transduced into host cardiomyocytes, and real-time imaging and monitoring of both proteins by either PET or BLI will allow molecular imaging of the transgene protein and perhaps its interplay within the cell at all phases of development and disease. Spatial and temporal control of transgenes offered by the Cre-*lox*P and tetracycline-inducible systems offers easily controlled transgene expression and has been steadily improved to offer greater inducibility, reduced background expression, greater tissue penetration, and cell specificity. The use of lentiviral vector delivery systems to bring together one or more components of these systems is slowly emerging as the new alternative to transgenic mouse development, and use of both the Cre-*lox*P and Tet systems will accelerate discovery. Although it has been slow but sure, the application of these techniques in vivo to further our understanding of the heart and its diseases is beginning to bear fruit.

Acknowledgments

The authors thank Mark Lewandoski for permission to use his figures. This work was funded by operating grants from the Canadian Institutes of Health Research (CIHR), St. Paul's Hospital Foundation, and the Heart and Stroke Foundation of BC and Yukon (HSBCY) to Dr. Tom Podor and Dr. Bruce McManus. The authors also extend their apologies to investigators whose work was not recognized or adequately presented.

References

1. Cui, C., Wani, M. A., Wight, D., Kopchick, J., and Stambrook, P. J. (1994) Reporter genes in transgenic mice. *Transgenic Res.* **3,** 182–194.

2. Reddi, P. P., Kallio, M., and Herr, J. C. (1999) Green fluorescent protein as a reporter for promoter analysis of testis-specific genes in transgenic mice. *Methods Enzymol.* **302,** 272–284.

3. Weissleder, R. and Ntziachristos, V. (2003) Shedding light onto live molecular targets. *Nat. Med.* **9,** 123–128.

4. Chtarto, A., Bender, H. U., Hanemann, C. O., Kemp, T., Lehtonen, E., Levivier, M., et al. (2003) Tetracycline-inducible transgene expression mediated by a single AAV vector. *Gene Ther.* **10,** 84–94.

5. Hoess, R. H. and Abremski, K. (1984) Interaction of the bacteriophage P1 recombinase Cre with the recombining site loxP. *Proc. Natl. Acad. Sci. USA* **81,** 1026–1029.

6. Yao, F., Svensjo, T., Winkler, T., Lu, M., Eriksson, C., and Eriksson, E. (1998) Tetracycline repressor, tetR, rather than the tetR-mammalian cell transcription factor fusion derivatives, regulates inducible gene expression in mammalian cells. *Hum. Gene Ther.* **9,** 1939–1950.

7. Rossi, F. M. and Blau, H. M. (1998) Recent advances in inducible gene expression systems. *Curr. Opin. Biotechnol.* **9,** 451–456.

8. Rossi, F. M., Guicherit, O. M., Spicher, A., Kringstein, A. M., Fatyol, K., Blakely, B. T., and Blau, H. M. (1998) Tetracycline-regulatable factors with distinct dimerization domains allow reversible growth inhibition by p16. *Nat. Genet.* **20,** 389–393.

9. Mizuguchi, H., Xu, Z. L., Sakurai, F., Mayumi, T., and Hayakawa, T. (2003) Tight positive regulation of transgene expression by a single adenovirus vector containing the rtTA and tTS expression cassettes in separate genome regions. *Hum. Gene Ther.* **14,** 1265–1277.

10. Sanbe, A., Gulick, J., Hanks, M. C., Liang, Q., Osinska, H., and Robbins, J. (2003) Reengineering inducible cardiac-specific transgenesis with an attenuated myosin heavy chain promoter. *Circ. Res.* **92,** 609–616.

11. Heger, J., Godecke, A., Flogel, U., Merx, M. W., Molojavyi, A., Kuhn-Velten, W. N., and Schrader, J. (2002) Cardiac-specific overexpression of inducible nitric oxide synthase does not result in severe cardiac dysfunction. *Circ. Res.* **90,** 93–99.

12. Okamoto, Y., Chaves, A., Chen, J., et al. (2001) Transgenic mice with cardiac-specific expression of activating transcription factor 3, a stress-inducible gene, have conduction abnormalities and contractile dysfunction. *Am. J. Pathol.* **159,** 639–650.

13. Sohal, D. S., Nghiem, M., Crackower, M. A., et al. (2001) Temporally regulated and tissue-specific gene manipulations in the adult and embryonic heart using a tamoxifen-inducible Cre protein. *Circ. Res.* **89,** 20–25.

14. Minamino, T., Gaussin, V., DeMayo, F. J., and Schneider, M. D. (2001) Inducible gene targeting in postnatal myocardium by cardiac-specific expression of a hormone-activated Cre fusion protein. *Circ. Res.* **88,** 587–592.

15. Kubo, S. and Mitani, K. (2003) A new hybrid system capable of efficient lentiviral vector production and stable gene transfer mediated by a single helper-dependent adenoviral vector. *J. Virol.* **77,** 2964–2971.

16. Johansen, J., Rosenblad, C., Andsberg, K., Moller, A., Lundberg, C., Bjorlund, A., and Johansen, T. E. (2002) Evaluation of Tet-on system to avoid transgene down-regulation in ex vivo gene transfer to the CNS. *Gene Ther.* **9,** 1291–1301.

17. Pacchia, A. L., Adelson, M. E., Kaul, M., Ron, Y., and Dougherty, J. P. (2001) An inducible packaging cell system for safe, efficient lentiviral vector production in the absence of HIV-1 accessory proteins. *Virology* **282,** 77–86.

18. Kafri, T., van Praag, H., Gage, F. H., and Verma, I. M. (2000) Lentiviral vectors: regulated gene expression. *Mol. Ther.* **1,** 516–521.

19. Punzon, I., Criado, L. M., Serrano, A., Serrano, F., and Bernad, A. (2003) Highly efficient lentiviral-mediated human cytokine transgenesis on the NOD/scid background. *Blood* **103,** 580–582.

20. Tiscornia, G., Singer, O., Ikawa, M., and Verma, I. M. (2003) A general method for gene knockdown in mice by using lentiviral vectors expressing small interfering RNA. *Proc. Natl. Acad. Sci. USA* **100,** 1844–1848.

21. Hamra, F. K., Gatlin, J., Chapman, K. M., Grellhesl, D. M., Garcia, J. V., Hammer, R. E., and Garbers, D. L. (2002) Production of transgenic rats by lentiviral transduction of male germ-line stem cells. *Proc. Natl. Acad. Sci. USA* **99,** 14,931–14,936.

22. Blasberg, R. G. and Gelovani, J. (2002) Molecular-genetic imaging: a nuclear medicine-based perspective. *Mol. Imaging* **1,** 280–300.

23. Blasberg, R. G. and Gelovani-Tjuvajev, J. (2002) In vivo molecular-genetic imaging. *J. Cell Biochem. Suppl.* **39,** 172–183.

24. Hoffmann, M. M. and Stoffel, W. (1996) Construction and functional characterization of recombinant fusion proteins of human lipoprotein lipase and apolipoprotein CII. *Eur. J. Biochem.* **237,** 545–552.

25. Peng, S., Zhou, J., and Frazer, I. H. (1999) Construction and production of fluorescent papillomavirus-like particles. *J. Tongji. Med. Univ.* **19,** 170–174, 180.

26. Torbett, B. E. (2002) Reporter genes: too much of a good thing? *J. Gene Med.* **4,** 478,479.

27. Kringstein, A. M., Rossi, F. M., Hofmann, A., and Blau, H. M. (1998) Graded transcriptional response to different concentrations of a single transactivator. *Proc. Natl. Acad. Sci. USA* **95,** 13,670–13,675.

28. Schuettengruber, B., Doetzlhofer, A., Kroboth, K., Wintersberger, E., and Seiser, C. (2003) Alternate activation of two divergently transcribed mouse genes from a bidirectional promoter is linked to changes in histone modification. *J. Biol. Chem.* **278,** 1784–1793.

29. Pauly, G. T., Hughes, S. H., and Moschel, R. C. (1991) A sectored colony assay for monitoring mutagenesis by specific carcinogen-DNA adducts in Escherichia coli. *Biochemistry* **30,** 11,700–11,706.

30. He, Q., Wang, D., Yang, X. P., Carretero, O. A., and LaPointe, M. C. (2001) Inducible regulation of human brain natriuretic peptide promoter in transgenic mice. *Am. J. Physiol. Heart Circ. Physiol.* **280,** H368–376.

31. LaPointe, M. C., Yang, X. P., Carretero, O. A., and He, Q. (2002) Left ventricular targeting of reporter gene expression in vivo by human BNP promoter in an adenoviral vector. *Am. J. Physiol. Heart Circ. Physiol.* **283,** H1439–1445.

32. Chen, X., Cui, Z., Zhang, F., Chang, W., Chen, L., and Liu, L. (2002) Angiotensin II and cAMP regulate AT(1)-mRNA expression in rat cardiomyocytes by transcriptional mechanism. *Eur. J. Pharmacol.* **448,** 1–9.

33. He, Q., Mendez, M., and LaPointe, M. C. (2002) Regulation of the human brain natriuretic peptide gene by GATA-4. *Am. J. Physiol. Endocrinol. Metab.* **283,** E50–57.

34. Laing, J. G., Tadros, P. N., Green, K., Saffitz, J. E., and Beyer, E. C. (1998) Proteolysis of connexin43-containing gap junctions in normal and heat-stressed cardiac myocytes. *Cardiovasc. Res.* **38,** 711–718.

35. Petrich, B. G., Molkentin, J. D., and Wang, Y. (2003) Temporal activation of c-Jun N-terminal kinase in adult transgenic heart via cre-loxP-mediated DNA recombination. *FASEB J.* **17,** 749–751.

36. Jenkins, D. E., Oei, Y., Hornig, Y. S., Yu, S. F., Dusich, J., Purchio, T., and Contag, P. R. (2003) Bioluminescent imaging (BLI) to improve and refine traditional murine models of tumor growth and metastasis. *Clin. Exp. Metastasis* **20,** 733–744.

37. Zhang, W., Purchio, A. F., Chen, K., Wu, J., Lu, L., Coffee, R., Contag, P. R., and West, D. B. (2003) A transgenic mouse model with a luciferase reporter for studying in vivo transcriptional regulation of the human CYP3A4 gene. *Drug Metab. Dispos.* **31,** 1054–1064.

38. Zhang, W., Contag, P. R., Madan, A., Stevenson, D. K., and Contag, C. H. (1999) Bioluminescence for biological sensing in living mammals. *Adv. Exp. Med. Biol.* **471,** 775–784.

39. Contag, P. R., Olomu, I. N., Stevenson, D. K., and Contag, C. H. (1998) Bioluminescent indicators in living mammals. *Nat. Med.* **4,** 245–247.

40. Contag, C. H., Spilman, S. D., Contag, P. R., et al. (1997) Visualizing gene expression in living mammals using a bioluminescent reporter. *Photochem. Photobiol.* **66,** 523–531.

41. Wu, J. C., Chen, I. Y., Sundaresan, G., et al. (2003) Molecular imaging of cardiac cell transplantation in living animals using optical bioluminescence and positron emission tomography. *Circulation* **108,** 1302–1305.

42. Wu, J. C., Inubushi, M., Sundaresan, G., Schelbert, H. R., and Gambhir, S. S. (2002) Optical imaging of cardiac reporter gene expression in living rats. *Circulation* **105,** 1631–1634.

43. Ray, P., Wu, A. M., and Gambhir, S. S. (2003) Optical bioluminescence and positron emission tomography imaging of a novel fusion reporter gene in tumor xenografts of living mice. *Cancer Res.* **63,** 1160–1165.

44. Prasher, D. C., Eckenrode, V. K., Ward, W. W., Prendergast, F. G., and Cormier, M. J. (1992) Primary structure of the Aequorea victoria green-fluorescent protein. *Gene* **111,** 229–233.

45. Haseloff, J., Siemering, K. R., Prasher, D. C., and Hodge, S. (1997) Removal of a cryptic intron and subcellular localization of green fluorescent protein are required to mark transgenic Arabidopsis plants brightly. *Proc. Natl. Acad. Sci. USA* **94,** 2122–2127.

46. Prasher, D. C. (1995) Using GFP to see the light. *Trends Genet.* **11**, 320–323.
47. Chalfie, M., Tu, Y., Euskirchen, G., Ward, W. W., and Prasher, D. C. (1994) Green fluorescent protein as a marker for gene expression. *Science* **263**, 802–805.
48. Yu, Y. A., Oberg, K., Wang, G., and Szalay, A. A. (2003) Visualization of molecular and cellular events with green fluorescent proteins in developing embryos: a review. *Luminescence* **18**, 1–18.
49. Tavare, J. M., Fletcher, L. M., and Welsh, G. I. (2001) Using green fluorescent protein to study intracellular signalling. *J. Endocrinol.* **170**, 297–306.
50. Heim, R., Prasher, D. C., and Tsien, R. Y. (1994) Wavelength mutations and posttranslational autoxidation of green fluorescent protein. *Proc. Natl. Acad. Sci. USA* **91**, 12,501–12,504.
51. Delagrave, S., Hawtin, R. E., Silva, C. M., Yang, M. M., and Youvan, D. C. (1995) Red-shifted excitation mutants of the green fluorescent protein. *Biotechnology* **13**, 151–154.
52. Ehrig, T., O'Kane, D. J., and Prendergast, F. G. (1995) Green-fluorescent protein mutants with altered fluorescence excitation spectra. *FEBS Lett.* **367**, 163–166.
53. Heim, R., Cubitt, A. B., and Tsien, R. Y. (1995) Improved green fluorescence. *Nature* **373**, 663,664.
54. Cubitt, A. B., Heim, R., Adams, S. R., Boyd, A. E., Gross, L. A., and Tsien, R. Y. (1995) Understanding, improving and using green fluorescent proteins. *Trends Biochem. Sci.* **20**, 448–455.
55. Crameri, A., Whitehorn, E. A., Tate, E., and Stemmer, W. P. (1996) Improved green fluorescent protein by molecular evolution using DNA shuffling. *Nat. Biotechnol.* **14**, 315–319.
56. Yang, T. T., Cheng, L., and Kain, S. R. (1996) Optimized codon usage and chromophore mutations provide enhanced sensitivity with the green fluorescent protein. *Nucleic Acids Res.* **24**, 4592,4593.
57. Li, X., Zhao, X., Fang, Y., Jiang, X., Duong, T., Fan, C., Huang, C. C., and Kain, S. R. (1998) Generation of destabilized green fluorescent protein as a transcription reporter. *J. Biol. Chem.* **273**, 34,970–34,975.
58. Nagai, T., Ibata, K., Park, E. S., Kubota, M., Mikoshiba, K., and Miyawaki, A. (2002) A variant of yellow fluorescent protein with fast and efficient maturation for cell-biological applications. *Nat. Biotechnol.* **20**, 87–90.
59. Griesbeck, O., Baird, G. S., Campbell, R. E., Zacharias, D. A., and Tsien, R. Y. (2001) Reducing the environmental sensitivity of yellow fluorescent protein. Mechanism and applications. *J. Biol. Chem.* **276**, 29,188–29,194.
60. Terskikh, A. V., Fradkov, A. F., Zaraisky, A. G., Kajava, A. V., and Angres, B. (2002) Analysis of DsRed Mutants. Space around the fluorophore accelerates fluorescence development. *J. Biol. Chem.* **277**, 7633–7636.
61. Bevis, B. J., and Glick, B. S. (2002) Rapidly maturing variants of the Discosoma red fluorescent protein (DsRed). *Nat. Biotechnol.* **20**, 83–87.
62. Campbell, R. E., Tour, O., Palmer, A. E., Steinbach, P. A., Baird, G. S., Zacharias, D. A., and Tsien, R. Y. (2002) A monomeric red fluorescent protein. *Proc. Natl. Acad. Sci. USA* **99**, 7877–7882.

63. Inc, C. L. (2002) Invitrogen, Inc.
64. Arndt-Jovin, D. J., Robert-Nicoud, M., and Jovin, T. M. (1990) Probing DNA structure and function with a multi-wavelength fluorescence confocal laser microscope. *J. Microsc.* **157**, 61–72.
65. Lechleiter, J. D., Lin, D. T., and Sieneart, I. (2002) Multi-photon laser scanning microscopy using an acoustic optical deflector. *Biophys. J.* **83**, 2292–2299.
66. Mitsiades, C. S., Mitsiades, N. S., Bronson, R. T., et al. (2003) Fluorescence imaging of multiple myeloma cells in a clinically relevant SCID/NOD in vivo model: biologic and clinical implications. *Cancer Res.* **63**, 6689–6696.
67. Wack, S., Hajri, A., Heisel, F., et al. (2003) Feasibility, sensitivity, and reliability of laser-induced fluorescence imaging of green fluorescent protein-expressing tumors in vivo. *Mol. Ther.* **7**, 765–773.
68. Hoffman, R. M. (2001) Visualization of GFP-expressing tumors and metastasis in vivo. *Biotechniques* **30**, 1016–1022, 1024–1026.
69. Bennett, J., Duan, D., Engelhardt, J. F., and Maguire, A. M. (1997) Real-time, noninvasive in vivo assessment of adeno-associated virus-mediated retinal transduction. *Invest. Ophthalmol. Vis. Sci.* **38**, 2857–2863.
70. Huang, Q., Shan, S., Braun, R. D., et al. (1999) Noninvasive visualization of tumors in rodent dorsal skin window chambers. *Nat. Biotechnol.* **17**, 1033–1035.
71. Jain, R. K., Munn, L. L., and Fukumura, D. (2002) Dissecting tumour pathophysiology using intravital microscopy. *Nat. Rev. Cancer* **2**, 266–276.
72. Padera, T. P., Stoll, B. R., So, P. T., and Jain, R. K. (2002) Conventional and high-speed intravital multiphoton laser scanning microscopy of microvasculature, lymphatics, and leukocyte-endothelial interactions. *Mol. Imaging.* **1**, 9–15.
73. Brown, E. B., Campbell, R. B., Tsuzuki, Y., Xu, L., Carmeliet, P., Fukumura, D., and Jain, R. K. (2001) In vivo measurement of gene expression, angiogenesis and physiological function in tumors using multiphoton laser scanning microscopy. *Nat. Med.* **7**, 864–868.
74. Tjuvajev, J. G., Finn, R., Watanabe, K., et al. (1996) Noninvasive imaging of herpes virus thymidine kinase gene transfer and expression: a potential method for monitoring clinical gene therapy. *Cancer Res.* **56**, 4087–4095.
75. Gambhir, S. S., Barrio, J. R., Wu, L., et al. (1998) Imaging of adenoviral-directed herpes simplex virus type 1 thymidine kinase reporter gene expression in mice with radiolabeled ganciclovir. *J. Nucleic Med.* **39**, 2003–2011.
76. Gambhir, S. S., Barrio, J. R., Phelps, M. E., et al. (1999) Imaging adenoviral-directed reporter gene expression in living animals with positron emission tomography. *Proc. Natl. Acad. Sci. USA* **96**, 2333–2338.
77. Brust, P., Haubner, R., Friedrich, A., et al. (2001) Comparison of [18F]FHPG and [124/125I]FIAU for imaging herpes simplex virus type 1 thymidine kinase gene expression. *Eur. J. Nucleic Med.* **28**, 721–729.
78. Tjuvajev, J. G., Doubrovin, M., Akhurst, T., et al. (2002) Comparison of radiolabeled nucleoside probes (FIAU, FHBG, and FHPG) for PET imaging of HSV1-tk gene expression. *J. Nucleic Med.* **43**, 1072–1083.
79. Min, J. J., Iyer, M., and Gambhir, S. S. (2003) Comparison of [(18)F]FHBG and

[(14)C]FIAU for imaging of HSV1-tk reporter gene expression: adenoviral infection vs stable transfection. *Eur. J. Nucl. Med. Mol. Imag.* **30**, 1547–1560.

80. Tjuvajev, J. G., Avril, N., Oku, T., et al. (1998) Imaging herpes virus thymidine kinase gene transfer and expression by positron emission tomography. *Cancer Res.* **58**, 4333–4341.

81. Tjuvajev, J. G., Stockhammer, G., Desai, R., Uehara, H., Watanabe, K., Gansbacher, B., and Blasberg, R. G. (1995) Imaging the expression of transfected genes in vivo. *Cancer Res.* **55**, 6126–6132.

82. Gambhir, S. S., Bauer, E., Black, M. E., et al. (2000) A mutant herpes simplex virus type 1 thymidine kinase reporter gene shows improved sensitivity for imaging reporter gene expression with positron emission tomography. *Proc. Natl. Acad. Sci. USA* **97**, 2785–2790.

83. Cherry, S. R. and Gambhir, S. S. (2001) Use of positron emission tomography in animal research. *Ilar. J.* **42**, 219–232.

84. Pearson, T. A. (2002) New tools for coronary risk assessment: what are their advantages and limitations? *Circulation* **105**, 886–892.

85. Weber, D. A. and Ivanovic, M. (1999) Ultra-high-resolution imaging of small animals: implications for preclinical and research studies. *J. Nucleic Cardiol.* **6**, 332–344.

86. Beanlands, R. (1996) Positron emission tomography in cardiovascular disease. *Can. J. Cardiol.* **12**, 875–883.

87. Park, J. B. (2001) Concurrent measurement of promoter activity and transfection efficiency using a new reporter vector containing both Photinus pyralis and Renilla reniformis luciferase genes. *Anal. Biochem.* **291**, 162–166.

88. Bonin, A. L., Gossen, M., and Bujard, H. (1994) Photinus pyralis luciferase: vectors that contain a modified luc coding sequence allowing convenient transfer into other systems. *Gene* **141**, 75–77.

89. Gal, D., Weir, L., Leclerc, G., Pickering, J. G., Hogan, J., and Isner, J. M. (1993) Direct myocardial transfection in two animal models. Evaluation of parameters affecting gene expression and percutaneous gene delivery. *Lab. Invest.* **68**, 18–25.

90. Wang, Y., Yu, Y. A., Shabahang, S., Wang, G., and Szalay, A. A. (2002) Renilla luciferase- Aequorea GFP (Ruc-GFP) fusion protein, a novel dual reporter for real-time imaging of gene expression in cell cultures and in live animals. *Mol. Genet. Genomics* **268**, 160–168.

91. Hakkila, K., Maksimow, M., Karp, M., and Virta, M. (2002) Reporter genes lucFF, luxCDABE, gfp, and dsred have different characteristics in whole-cell bacterial sensors. *Anal. Biochem.* **301**, 235–242.

92. de Wet, J. R., Wood, K. V., DeLuca, M., Helinski, D. R., and Subramani, S. (1987) Firefly luciferase gene: structure and expression in mammalian cells. *Mol. Cell. Biol.* **7**, 725–737.

93. de Wet, J. R., Wood, K. V., Helinski, D. R., and DeLuca, M. (1986) Cloning firefly luciferase. *Methods Enzymol.* **133**, 3–14.

94. de Wet, J. R., Wood, K. V., Helinski, D. R., and DeLuca, M. (1985) Cloning of firefly luciferase cDNA and the expression of active luciferase in Escherichia coli. *Proc. Natl. Acad. Sci. USA* **82**, 7870–7873.

95. Oshiro, M. (1998) Cooled CCD versus intensified cameras for low-light video—applications and relative advantages. *Methods Cell Biol.* **56,** 45–62.

96. Tuchin, V. V., Xu, X., and Wang, R. K. (2002) Dynamic optical coherence tomography in studies of optical clearing, sedimentation, and aggregation of immersed blood. *Appl. Opt.* **41,** 258–271.

97. Rice, B. W., Cable, M. D., and Nelson, M. B. (2001) In vivo imaging of light-emitting probes. *J. Biomed. Opt.* **6,** 432–440.

98. Grentzmann, G., Ingram, J. A., Kelly, P. J., Gesteland, R. F., and Atkins, J. F. (1998) A dual-luciferase reporter system for studying recoding signals. *RNA* **4,** 479–486.

99. Tromberg, B. J., Shah, N., Lanning, R., Cerussi, A., Espinoza, J., Pham, T., Svaasand, L., and Butler, J. (2000) Non-invasive in vivo characterization of breast tumors using photon migration spectroscopy. *Neoplasia* **2,** 26–40.

100. Contag, C. H., Contag, P. R., Mullins, J. I., Spilman, S. D., Stevenson, D. K., and Benaron, D. A. (1995) Photonic detection of bacterial pathogens in living hosts. Mol. Microbiol. **18,** 593–603.

101. Mandl, S., Schimmelpfennig, C., Edinger, M., Negrin, R. S., and Contag, C. H. (2002) Understanding immune cell trafficking patterns via in vivo bioluminescence imaging. *J. Cell Biochem. Suppl.* **39,** 239–248.

102. Reynolds, J. S., Troy, T. L., Mayer, R. H., et al. (1999) Imaging of spontaneous canine mammary tumors using fluorescent contrast agents. *Photochem. Photobiol.* **70,** 87–94.

103. Rehemtulla, A., Stegman, L. D., Cardozo, S. J., Gupta, S., Hall, D. E., Contag, C. H., and Ross, B. D. (2000) Rapid and quantitative assessment of cancer treatment response using in vivo bioluminescence imaging. *Neoplasia* **2,** 491–495.

104. Lewandoski, M. (2001) Conditional control of gene expression in the mouse. *Nat. Rev. Genet.* **2,** 743–755.

105. Sauer, B. and Henderson, N. (1988) Site-specific DNA recombination in mammalian cells by the Cre recombinase of bacteriophage P1. *Proc. Natl. Acad. Sci. USA* **85,** 5166–5170.

106. Sternberg, N. and Hamilton, D. (1981) Bacteriophage P1 site-specific recombination. I. Recombination between loxP sites. *J. Mol. Biol.* **150,** 467–486.

107. Garcia, E. L. and Mills, A. A. (2002) Getting around lethality with inducible Cre-mediated excision. *Semin. Cell. Dev. Biol.* **13,** 151–158.

108. Zheng, B., Zhang, Z., Black, C. M., de Crombrugghe, B., and Denton, C. P. (2002) Ligand-dependent genetic recombination in fibroblasts : a potentially powerful technique for investigating gene function in fibrosis. *Am. J. Pathol.* **160,** 1609–1617.

109. Soriano, P. (1999) Generalized lacZ expression with the ROSA26 Cre reporter strain. *Nat. Genet.* **21,** 70,71.

110. Mao, X., Fujiwara, Y., and Orkin, S. H. (1999) Improved reporter strain for monitoring Cre recombinase-mediated DNA excisions in mice. *Proc. Natl. Acad. Sci. USA* **96,** 5037–5042.

111. Novak, A., Guo, C., Yang, W., Nagy, A., and Lobe, C. G. (2000) Z/EG, a double reporter mouse line that expresses enhanced green fluorescent protein upon Cre-mediated excision. *Genesis* **28,** 147–155.

112. Kellendonk, C., Tronche, F., Casanova, E., Anlag, K., Opherk, C., and Schutz, G. (1999) Inducible site-specific recombination in the brain. *J. Mol. Biol.* **285,** 175–182.

113. Ngan, E. S., Schillinger, K., DeMayo, F., and Tsai, S. Y. (2002) The mifepristone-inducible gene regulatory system in mouse models of disease and gene therapy. *Semin. Cell. Dev. Biol.* **13,** 143–149.

114. Kellendonk, C., Tronche, F., Monaghan, A. P., Angrand, P. O., Stewart, F., and Schutz, G. (1996) Regulation of Cre recombinase activity by the synthetic steroid RU 486. *Nucleic Acids Res.* **24,** 1404–1411.

115. Feil, R., Brocard, J., Mascrez, B., LeMeur, M., Metzger, D., and Chambon, P. (1996) Ligand-activated site-specific recombination in mice. *Proc. Natl. Acad. Sci. USA* **93,** 10,887–10,890.

116. Tsujita, M., Mori, H., Watanabe, M., Suzuki, M., Miyazaki, J., and Mishina, M. (1999) Cerebellar granule cell-specific and inducible expression of Cre recombinase in the mouse. *J. Neurosci.* **19,** 10,318–10,323.

117. Minamino, T., Gaussin, V., DeMayo, F. J., and Schneider, M. D. (2001) Inducible gene targeting in postnatal myocardium by cardiac-specific expression of a hormone-activated Cre fusion. *Protein Circ Res.* **88,** 587–592.

118. Kitayama, K., Abe, M., Kakizaki, T., et al. (2001) Purkinje cell-specific and inducible gene recombination system generated from C57BL/6 mouse ES cells. *Biochem. Biophys. Res. Commun.* **281,** 1134–1140.

119. Zhou, Z., Wang, D., Wang, X. J., and Roop, D. R. (2002) In utero activation of K5.CrePR1 induces gene deletion. *Genesis* **32,** 191,192.

120. Wan, Y. and Nordeen, S. K. (2002) Identification of genes differentially regulated by glucocorticoids and progestins using a Cre/loxP-mediated retroviral promoter-trapping strategy. *J. Mol. Endocrinol.* **28,** 177–192.

121. Ghoumari, A. M., Dusart, I., El-Etr, M., Tronche, F., Sotelo, C., Schumacher, M., and Baulieu, E. E. (2003) Mifepristone (RU486) protects Purkinje cells from cell death in organotypic slice cultures of postnatal rat and mouse cerebellum. *Proc. Natl. Acad. Sci. USA* **100,** 7953–7958.

122. Herceg, Z., Hulla, W., Gell, D., Cuenin, C., Lleonart, M., Jackson, S., and Wang, Z. Q. (2001) Disruption of Trrap causes early embryonic lethality and defects in cell cycle progression. *Nat. Genet.* **29,** 206–211.

123. Imai, T., Jiang, M., Chambon, P., and Metzger, D. (2001) Impaired adipogenesis and lipolysis in the mouse upon selective ablation of the retinoid X receptor alpha mediated by a tamoxifen-inducible chimeric Cre recombinase (Cre-ERT2) in adipocytes. *Proc. Natl. Acad. Sci. USA* **98,** 224–228.

124. Li, H., Wang, J., Wilhelmsson, H., Hansson, A., Thoren, P., Duffy, J., Rustin, P., and Larsson, N. G. (2000) Genetic modification of survival in tissue-specific knockout mice with mitochondrial cardiomyopathy. *Proc. Natl. Acad. Sci. USA* **97,** 3467–3472.

125. Imai, T. (2003) Functional genetic dissection of nuclear receptor signalling in obesity, diabetes and liver regeneration using spatiotemporally controlled somatic mutagenesis in the mouse. *Keio. J. Med.* **52,** 198–203.

126. Badea, T. C., Wang, Y., and Nathans, J. (2003) A noninvasive genetic/pharmacologic strategy for visualizing cell morphology and clonal relationships in the mouse. *J. Neurosci.* **23,** 2314–2322.

127. Weber, P., Schuler, M., Gerard, C., Mark, M., Metzger, D., and Chambon, P. (2003) Temporally controlled site-specific mutagenesis in the germ cell lineage of the mouse testis. *Biol. Reprod.* **68,** 553–559.

128. Casanova, E., Fehsenfeld, S., Lemberger, T., Shimshek, D. R., Sprengel, R., and Mantamadiotis, T. (2002) ER-based double iCre fusion protein allows partial recombination in forebrain. *Genesis* **34,** 208–214.

129. Guo, C., Yang, W., and Lobe, C. G. (2002) A Cre recombinase transgene with mosaic, widespread tamoxifen-inducible action. *Genesis* **32,** 8–18.

130. Gu, G., Dubauskaite, J., and Melton, D. A. (2002) Direct evidence for the pancreatic lineage: NGN3+ cells are islet progenitors and are distinct from duct progenitors. *Development* **129,** 2447–2457.

131. Hayashi, S. and McMahon, A. P. (2002) Efficient recombination in diverse tissues by a tamoxifen-inducible form of Cre: a tool for temporally regulated gene activation/inactivation in the mouse. *Dev. Biol.* **244,** 305–318.

132. Loonstra, A., Vooijs, M., Beverloo, H. B., et al. (2001) Growth inhibition and DNA damage induced by Cre recombinase in mammalian cells. *Proc. Natl. Acad. Sci. USA* **98,** 9209–9214.

133. Chiba, H., Chambon, P., and Metzger, D. (2000) F9 embryonal carcinoma cells engineered for tamoxifen-dependent Cre-mediated site-directed mutagenesis and doxycycline-inducible gene expression. *Exp. Cell. Res.* **260,** 334–339.

134. Indra, A. K., Li, M., Brocard, J., Warot, X., et al. (2000) Targeted somatic mutagenesis in mouse epidermis. *Horm. Res.* **54,** 296–300.

135. Vallier, L., Mancip, J., Markossian, S., et al. (2001) An efficient system for conditional gene expression in embryonic stem cells and in their in vitro and in vivo differentiated derivatives. *Proc. Natl. Acad. Sci. USA* **98,** 2467–2472.

136. Fuhrmann-Benzakein, E., Garcia-Gabay, I., Pepper, M. S., Vassalli, J. D., and Herrera, P. L. (2000) Inducible and irreversible control of gene expression using a single transgene. *Nucleic Acids Res.* **28,** E99.

137. Li, M., Indra, A. K., Warot, X., Brocard, J., Messaddeq, N., Kato, S., Metzger, D., and Chambon, P. (2000) Skin abnormalities generated by temporally controlled RXRalpha mutations in mouse epidermis. *Nature* **407,** 633–636.

138. Indra, A. K., Warot, X., Brocard, J., Bornert, J. M., Xiao, J. H., Chambon, P., and Metzger, D. (1999) Temporally-controlled site-specific mutagenesis in the basal layer of the epidermis: comparison of the recombinase activity of the tamoxifen-inducible Cre-ER(T) and Cre-ER(T2) recombinases. *Nucleic Acids Res.* **27,** 4324–4327.

139. Metzger, D., Clifford, J., Chiba, H., and Chambon, P. (1995) Conditional site-specific recombination in mammalian cells using a ligand-dependent chimeric Cre recombinase. *Proc. Natl. Acad. Sci. USA* **92,** 6991–6995.

140. Schwenk, F., Kuhn, R., Angrand, P. O., Rajewsky, K., and Stewart, A. F. (1998) Temporally and spatially regulated somatic mutagenesis in mice. *Nucleic Acids Res.* **26,** 1427–1432.

141. Schmidt, E. E., Taylor, D. S., Prigge, J. R., Barnett, S., and Capecchi, M. R. (2000) Illegitimate Cre-dependent chromosome rearrangements in transgenic mouse spermatids. *Proc. Natl. Acad. Sci. USA* **97,** 13,702–13,707.

142. Thyagarajan, B., Guimaraes, M. J., Groth, A. C., and Calos, M. P. (2000) Mammalian genomes contain active recombinase recognition sites. *Gene* **244,** 47–54.

143. Zhang, Y., Riesterer, C., Ayrall, A. M., Sablitzky, F., Littlewood, T. D., and Reth, M. (1996) Inducible site-directed recombination in mouse embryonic stem cells. *Nucleic Acids Res.* **24,** 543–548.

144. Wunderlich, F. T., Wildner, H., Rajewsky, K., and Edenhofer, F. (2001) New variants of inducible Cre recombinase: a novel mutant of Cre-PR fusion protein exhibits enhanced sensitivity and an expanded range of inducibility. *Nucleic Acids Res.* **29,** E47.

145. Verrou, C., Zhang, Y., Zurn, C., Schamel, W. W., and Reth, M. (1999) Comparison of the tamoxifen regulated chimeric Cre recombinases MerCreMer and CreMer. *Biol. Chem.* **380,** 1435–1438.

146. Bruning, J. C., Michael, M. D., Winnay, J. N., et al. (1998) A muscle-specific insulin receptor knockout exhibits features of the metabolic syndrome of NIDDM without altering glucose tolerance. *Mol. Cell* **2,** 559–569.

147. Wang, J., Wilhelmsson, H., Graff, C., et al. (1999) Dilated cardiomyopathy and atrioventricular conduction blocks induced by heart-specific inactivation of mitochondrial DNA gene expression. *Nat. Genet.* **21,** 133–137.

148. Larsson, N. G., Wang, J., Wilhelmsson, H., et al. (1998) Mitochondrial transcription factor A is necessary for mtDNA maintenance and embryogenesis in mice. *Nat. Genet.* **18,** 231–236.

149. Agah, R., Frenkel, P. A., French, B. A., Michael, L. H., Overbeek, P. A., and Schneider, M. D. (1997) Gene recombination in postmitotic cells. Targeted expression of Cre recombinase provokes cardiac-restricted, site-specific rearrangement in adult ventricular muscle in vivo. *J. Clin. Invest.* **100,** 169–179.

150. Chen, J., Kubalak, S. W., and Chien, K. R. (1998) Ventricular muscle-restricted targeting of the RXRalpha gene reveals a non-cell-autonomous requirement in cardiac chamber morphogenesis. *Development* **125,** 1943–1949.

151. Yamamoto, A., Hen, R., and Dauer, W. T. (2001) The ons and offs of inducible transgenic technology: a review. *Neurobiol. Dis.* **8,** 923–932.

152. Gossen, M., Freundlieb, S., Bender, G., Muller, G., Hillen, W., and Bujard, H. (1995) Transcriptional activation by tetracyclines in mammalian cells. *Science* **268,** 1766–1769.

153. Ryding, A. D., Sharp, M. G., and Mullins, J. J. (2001) Conditional transgenic technologies. *J. Endocrinol.* **171,** 1–14.

154. Keyvani, K., Baur, I., and Paulus, W. (1999) Tetracycline-controlled expression but not toxicity of an attenuated diphtheria toxin mutant. *Life Sci.* **64,** 1719–1724.

155. Imhof, M. O., Chatellard, P., and Mermod, N. (2000) A regulatory network for the efficient control of transgene expression. *J. Gene Med.* **2,** 107–116.

156. Corbel, S. Y. and Rossi, F. M. (2002) Latest developments and in vivo use of the Tet system: ex vivo and in vivo delivery of tetracycline-regulated genes. *Curr. Opin. Biotechnol.* **13,** 448–452.

157. Lamartina, S., Roscilli, G., Rinaudo, C. D., et al. (2002) Stringent control of gene expression in vivo by using novel doxycycline-dependent trans-activators. *Hum. Gene Ther.* **13**, 199–210.

158. Urlinger, S., Baron, U., Thellmann, M., Hasan, M. T., Bujard, H., and Hillen, W. (2000) Exploring the sequence space for tetracycline-dependent transcriptional activators: novel mutations yield expanded range and sensitivity. *Proc. Natl. Acad. Sci. USA* **97**, 7963–7968.

159. Yamamoto, A., Lucas, J. J., and Hen, R. (2000) Reversal of neuropathology and motor dysfunction in a conditional model of Huntington's disease. *Cell* **101**, 57–66.

160. Krestel, H. E., Mayford, M., Seeburg, P. H., and Sprengel, R. (2001) A GFP-equipped bidirectional expression module well suited for monitoring tetracycline-regulated gene expression in mouse. *Nucleic Acids Res.* **29**, E39.

161. Deuschle, U., Meyer, W. K., and Thiesen, H. J. (1995) Tetracycline-reversible silencing of eukaryotic promoters. *Mol. Cell. Biol.* **15**, 1907–1914.

162. Freundlieb, S., Schirra-Muller, C., and Bujard, H. (1999) A tetracycline controlled activation/repression system with increased potential for gene transfer into mammalian cells. *J. Gene Med.* **1**, 4–12.

163. Zhu, Z., Ma, B., Homer, R. J., Zheng, T., and Elias, J. A. (2001) Use of the tetracycline-controlled transcriptional silencer (tTS) to eliminate transgene leak in inducible overexpression transgenic mice. *J. Biol. Chem.* **276**, 25,222–25,229.

164. Zheng, T., Zhu, Z., Wang, Z., et al. (2000) Inducible targeting of IL-13 to the adult lung causes matrix metalloproteinase- and cathepsin-dependent emphysema. *J. Clin. Invest.* **106**, 1081–1093.

165. Fishman, G. I., Kaplan, M. L., and Buttrick, P. M. (1994) Tetracycline-regulated cardiac gene expression in vivo. *J. Clin. Invest.* **93**, 1864–1868.

166. Passman, R. S. and Fishman, G. I. (1994) Regulated expression of foreign genes in vivo after germline transfer. *J. Clin. Invest.* **94**, 2421–2425.

167. Yu, Z., Redfern, C. S., and Fishman, G. I. (1996) Conditional transgene expression in the heart. *Circ. Res.* **79**, 691–697.

168. Shimabukuro, M., Ohneda, M., Lee, Y., and Unger, R. H. (1997) Role of nitric oxide in obesity-induced beta cell disease. *J. Clin. Invest.* **100**, 290–295.

169. Guslandi, M. (1998) Nitric oxide and inflammatory bowel diseases. *Eur. J. Clin. Invest.* **28**, 904–907.

170. Wong, M. L., Rettori, V., al-Shekhlee, A., et al. (1996) Inducible nitric oxide synthase gene expression in the brain during systemic inflammation. *Nat. Med.* **2**, 581–584.

171. Balligand, J. L., Ungureanu-Longrois, D., Simmons, W. W., et al. (1994) Cytokine-inducible nitric oxide synthase (iNOS) expression in cardiac myocytes. Characterization and regulation of iNOS expression and detection of iNOS activity in single cardiac myocytes in vitro. *J. Biol. Chem.* **269**, 27,580–27,588.

172. de Belder, A. J., Radomski, M. W., Why, H. J., et al. (1993) Nitric oxide synthase activities in human myocardium. *Lancet* **341**, 84,85.

173. Haywood, G. A., Tsao, P. S., von der Leyen, et al. (1996) Expression of inducible nitric oxide synthase in human heart failure. *Circulation* **93**, 1087–1094.

174. Lewis, N. P., Tsao, P. S., Rickenbacher, P. R., et al. (1996) Induction of nitric oxide synthase in the human cardiac allograft is associated with contractile dysfunction of the left ventricle. *Circulation* **93,** 720–729.

175. Nathan, C. (1997) Inducible nitric oxide synthase: what difference does it make? *J. Clin. Invest.* **100,** 2417–2423.

176. Mungrue, I. N., Gros, R., You, X., et al. (2002) Cardiomyocyte overexpression of iNOS in mice results in peroxynitrite generation, heart block, and sudden death. *J. Clin. Invest.* **109,** 735–743.

177. Dor, Y., Djonov, V., and Keshet, E. (2003) Induction of vascular networks in adult organs: implications to proangiogenic therapy. *Ann. NY Acad. Sci.* **995,** 208–216.

178. Dor, Y., Djonov, V., Abramovitch, R., Itin, A., Fishman, G. I., Carmeliet, P., Goelman, G., and Keshet, E. (2002) Conditional switching of VEGF provides new insights into adult neovascularization and pro-angiogenic therapy. *EMBO J.* **21,** 1939–1947.

179. Dor, Y., Camenisch, T. D., Itin, A., Fishman, G. I., McDonald, J. A., Carmeliet, P., and Keshet, E. (2001) A novel role for VEGF in endocardial cushion formation and its potential contribution to congenital heart defects. *Development* **128,** 1531–1538.

180. Kistner, A., Gossen, M., Zimmermann, F., Jerecic, J., Ullmer, C., Lubbert, H., and Bujard, H. (1996) Doxycycline-mediated quantitative and tissue-specific control of gene expression in transgenic mice. *Proc. Natl. Acad. Sci. USA* **93,** 10,933–10,938.

181. Mayford, M., Bach, M. E., Huang, Y. Y., Wang, L., Hawkins, R. D., and Kandel, E. R. (1996) Control of memory formation through regulated expression of a CaMKII transgene. *Science* **274,** 1678–1683.

182. Vigna, E., Cavalieri, S., Ailles, L., Geuna, M., Loew, R., Bujard, H., and Naldini, L. (2002) Robust and efficient regulation of transgene expression in vivo by improved tetracycline-dependent lentiviral vectors. *Mol. Ther.* **5,** 252–261.

183. Corbel, S. Y. and Rossi, F. M. (2002) Latest developments and in vivo use of the Tet system: ex vivo and in vivo delivery of tetracycline-regulated genes. *Curr. Opin. Biotechnol.* **13,** 448–452.

184. Gould, D. J. and Favorov, P. (2003) Vectors for the treatment of autoimmune disease. *Gene Ther.* **10,** 912–927.

185. Lori, F., di Marzo Veronese, F., de Vico, A. L., Lusso, P., Reitz, M. S., Jr., and Gallo, R. C. (1992) Viral DNA carried by human immunodeficiency virus type 1 virions. *J. Virol.* **66,** 5067–5074.

186. Blomer, U., Naldini, L., Kafri, T., Trono, D., Verma, I. M., and Gage, F. H. (1997) Highly efficient and sustained gene transfer in adult neurons with a lentivirus vector. *J. Virol.* **71,** 6641–6649.

187. Weinberg, J. B., Matthews, T. J., Cullen, B. R., and Malim, M. H. (1991) Productive human immunodeficiency virus type 1 (HIV-1) infection of nonproliferating human monocytes. *J. Exp. Med.* **174,** 1477–1482.

188. Baekelandt, V., Eggermont, K., Michiels, M., Nuttin, B., and Debyser, Z. (2003) Optimized lentiviral vector production and purification procedure prevents immune response after transduction of mouse brain. *Gene Ther.* **10,** 1933–1940.

189. Giannoukakis, N., Mi, Z., Gambotto, A., Eramo, A., Ricordi, C., Trucco, M., and Robbins, P. (1999) Infection of intact human islets by a lentiviral vector. *Gene Ther.* **6,** 1545–1551.

190. Thomas, C. E., Ehrhardt, A., and Kay, M. A. (2003) Progress and problems with the use of viral vectors for gene therapy. *Nat. Rev. Genet.* **4,** 346–358.

191. Marshall, E. (1999) Gene therapy death prompts review of adenovirus vector. *Science* **286,** 2244,2245.

192. Ferrari, F. K., Samulski, T., Shenk, T., and Samulski, R. J. (1996) Second-strand synthesis is a rate-limiting step for efficient transduction by recombinant adeno-associated virus vectors. *J. Virol.* **70,** 3227–3234.

193. Fisher, K. J., Choi, H., Burda, J., Chen, S. J., and Wilson, J. M. (1996) Recombinant adenovirus deleted of all viral genes for gene therapy of cystic fibrosis. *Virology* **217,** 11–22.

194. Whittaker, G. R., Kann, M., and Helenius, A. (2000) Viral entry into the nucleus. *Annu. Rev. Cell. Dev. Biol.* **16,** 627–651.

195. Otto, E., Jones-Trower, A., Vanin, E. F., Stambaugh, K., Mueller, S. N., Anderson, W. F., and McGarrity, G. J. (1994) Characterization of a replication-competent retrovirus resulting from recombination of packaging and vector sequences. *Hum. Gene Ther.* **5,** 567–575.

196. Chong, H., Starkey, W., and Vile, R. G. (1998) A replication-competent retrovirus arising from a split-function packaging cell line was generated by recombination events between the vector, one of the packaging constructs, and endogenous retroviral sequences. *J. Virol.* **72,** 2663–2670.

197. Fischer, U., Huber, J., Boelens, W. C., Mattaj, I. W., and Luhrmann, R. (1995) The HIV-1 Rev activation domain is a nuclear export signal that accesses an export pathway used by specific cellular RNAs. *Cell* **82,** 475–483.

198. Meyer, B. E. and Malim, M. H. (1994) The HIV-1 Rev trans-activator shuttles between the nucleus and the cytoplasm. *Genes Dev.* **8,** 1538–1547.

199. Bogerd, H. P., Fridell, R. A., Madore, S., and Cullen, B. R. (1995) Identification of a novel cellular cofactor for the Rev/Rex class of retroviral regulatory proteins. *Cell* **82,** 485–494.

200. Fritz, C. C., Zapp, M. L., and Green, M. R. (1995) A human nucleoporin-like protein that specifically interacts with HIV. *Rev. Nature* **376,** 530–533.

201. Pollard, V. W. and Malim, M. H. (1998) The HIV-1 Rev protein. *Annu. Rev. Microbiol.* **52,** 491–532.

202. Burns, J. C., Friedmann, T., Driever, W., Burrascano, M., and Yee, J. K. (1993) Vesicular stomatitis virus G glycoprotein pseudotyped retroviral vectors: concentration to very high titer and efficient gene transfer into mammalian and nonmammalian cells. *Proc. Natl. Acad. Sci. USA* **90,** 8033–8037.

203. Iwakuma, T., Cui, Y., and Chang, L. J. (1999) Self-inactivating lentiviral vectors with U3 and U5 modifications. *Virology* **261,** 120–132.

204. Zufferey, R., Dull, T., Mandel, R. J., Bukovsky, A., Quiroz, D., Naldini, L., and Trono, D. (1998) Self-inactivating lentivirus vector for safe and efficient in vivo gene delivery. *J. Virol.* **72,** 9873–9880.

205. Connolly, J. B. (2002) Lentiviruses in gene therapy clinical research. *Gene Ther.* **9,** 1730–1734.
206. Faust, E. A., Acel, A., Udashkin, B., and Wainberg, M. A. (1995) Human immunodeficiency virus type 1 integrase stabilizes a linearized HIV-1 LTR plasmid in vivo. *Biochem. Mol. Biol. Int.* **36,** 745–758.
207. Woods, N. B., Muessig, A., Schmidt, M., et al. (2003) Lentiviral vector transduction of NOD/SCID repopulating cells results in multiple vector integrations per transduced cell: risk of insertional mutagenesis. *Blood* **101,** 1284–1289.
208. Kafri, T. (2004) Gene delivery by lentivirus vectors an overview. *Methods Mol. Biol.* **246,** 367–390.
209. Hofmann, A., Nolan, G. P., and Blau, H. M. (1996) Rapid retroviral delivery of tetracycline-inducible genes in a single autoregulatory cassette. *Proc. Natl. Acad. Sci. USA* **93,** 5185–5190.
210. Hill, C. P., Worthylake, D., Bancroft, D. P., Christensen, A. M., and Sundquist, W. I. (1996) Crystal structures of the trimeric human immunodeficiency virus type 1 matrix protein: implications for membrane association and assembly. *Proc. Natl. Acad. Sci. USA* **93,** 3099–3104.
211. Gamble, T. R., Yoo, S., Vajdos, F. F., et al. (1997) Structure of the carboxyl-terminal dimerization domain of the HIV-1 capsid protein. *Science* **278,** 849–853.
212. Schmalzbauer, E., Strack, B., Dannull, J., Guehmann, S., and Moelling, K. (1996) Mutations of basic amino acids of NCp7 of human immunodeficiency virus type 1 affect RNA binding in vitro. *J. Virol.* **70,** 771–777.
213. Huang, M., Orenstein, J. M., Martin, M. A., and Freed, E. O. (1995) p6Gag is required for particle production from full-length human immunodeficiency virus type 1 molecular clones expressing protease. *J. Virol.* **69,** 6810–6818.
214. Kaplan, A. H., Manchester, M., and Swanstrom, R. (1994) The activity of the protease of human immunodeficiency virus type 1 is initiated at the membrane of infected cells before the release of viral proteins and is required for release to occur with maximum efficiency. *J. Virol.* **68,** 6782–6786.
215. Peliska, J. A. and Benkovic, S. J. (1992) Mechanism of DNA strand transfer reactions catalyzed by HIV-1 reverse transcriptase. *Science* **258,** 1112–1118.
216. Li, X., Mukai, T., Young, D., Frankel, S., Law, P., and Wong-Staal, F. (1998) Transduction of CD34+ cells by a vesicular stomach virus protein G (VSV-G) pseudotyped HIV-1 vector. Stable gene expression in progeny cells, including dendritic cells. *J. Hum. Virol.* **1,** 346–352.
217. Katz, R. A. and Skalka, A. M. (1994) The retroviral enzymes. *Annu. Rev. Biochem.* **63,** 133–173.
218. Arya, S. K., Zamani, M., and Kundra, P. (1998) Human immunodeficiency virus type 2 lentivirus vectors for gene transfer: expression and potential for helper virus-free packaging. *Hum. Gene Ther.* **9,** 1371–1380.
219. Zemmel, R. W., Kelley, A. C., Karn, J., and Butler, P. J. (1996) Flexible regions of RNA structure facilitate co-operative Rev assembly on the Rev-response element. *J. Mol. Biol.* **258,** 763–777.
220. Schambach, A., Wodrich, H., Hildinger, M., Bohne, J., Krausslich, H. G., and

Baum, C. (2000) Context dependence of different modules for posttranscriptional enhancement of gene expression from retroviral vectors. *Mol. Ther.* **2**, 435–445.

221. Trono, D., Feinberg, M. B., and Baltimore, D. (1989) HIV-1 Gag mutants can dominantly interfere with the replication of the wild-type virus. *Cell* **59**, 113–120.

222. Clever, J. L. and Parslow, T. G. (1997) Mutant human immunodeficiency virus type 1 genomes with defects in RNA dimerization or encapsidation. *J. Virol.* **71**, 3407–3414.

223. McBride, M. S. and Panganiban, A. T. (1996) The human immunodeficiency virus type 1 encapsidation site is a multipartite RNA element composed of functional hairpin structures. *J. Virol.* **70**, 2963–2973.

224. Reiser, J., Lai, Z., Zhang, X. Y., and Brady, R. O. (2000) Development of multigene and regulated lentivirus vectors. *J. Virol.* **74**, 10,589–10,599.

225. Verhoef, K., Marzio, G., Hillen, W., Bujard, H., and Berkhout, B. (2001) Strict control of human immunodeficiency virus type 1 replication by a genetic switch: Tet for Tat. *J. Virol.* **75**, 979–987.

226. Dugray, A., Geay, J. F., Foudi, A., et al. (2001) Rapid generation of a tetracycline-inducible BCR-ABL defective retrovirus using a single autoregulatory retroviral cassette. *Leukemia* **15**, 1658–1662.

227. Sato, N., Matsuda, K., Sakuma, C., Foster, D. N., Oppenheim, R. W., and Yaginuma, H. (2002) Regulated gene expression in the chicken embryo by using replication-competent retroviral vectors. *J. Virol.* **76**, 1980–1985.

228. Regulier, E., Pereira de Almeida, L., Sommer, B., Aebischer, P., and Deglon, N. (2002) Dose-dependent neuroprotective effect of ciliary neurotrophic factor delivered via tetracycline-regulated lentiviral vectors in the quinolinic acid rat model of Huntington's disease. *Hum. Gene Ther.* **13**, 1981–1990.

229. Wiznerowicz, M. and Trono, D. (2003) Conditional suppression of cellular genes: lentivirus vector-mediated drug-inducible RNA interference. *J. Virol.* **77**, 8957–8961.

230. Koponen, J. K., Kankkonen, H., Kannasto, J., Wirth, T., Hillen, W., Bujard, H., and Yla-Herttuala, S. (2003) Doxycycline-regulated lentiviral vector system with a novel reverse transactivator rtTA2S-M2 shows a tight control of gene expression in vitro and in vivo. *Gene Ther.* **10**, 459–466.

231. Wang, Y., Krushel, L. A., and Edelman, G. M. (1996) Targeted DNA recombination in vivo using an adenovirus carrying the cre recombinase gene. *Proc. Natl. Acad. Sci. USA* **93**, 3932–3936.

232. Miwa, T., Koyama, T., and Shirai, M. (2000) Muscle specific expression of Cre recombinase under two actin promoters in transgenic mice. *Genesis* **26**, 136–138.

233. Araki, T., Shibata, M., Takano, R., et al. (2000) Conditional expression of anti-apoptotic protein p35 by Cre-mediated DNA recombination in cardiomyocytes from loxP-p35-transgenic mice. *Cell Death Differ.* **7**, 485–492.

234. Gaussin, V., Van de Putte, T., Mishina, Y., et al. (2002) Endocardial cushion and myocardial defects after cardiac myocyte-specific conditional deletion of the bone morphogenetic protein receptor ALK3. *Proc. Natl. Acad. Sci. USA* **99**, 2878–2883.

235. Stanley, E. G., Biben, C., Elefanty, A., et al. (2002) Efficient Cre-mediated deletion in cardiac progenitor cells conferred by a 3'UTR-ires-Cre allele of the homeobox gene Nkx2-5. *Int. J. Dev. Biol.* **46,** 431–439.

236. Iwatate, M., Gu, Y., Dieterle, T., et al. (2003) In vivo high-efficiency transcoronary gene delivery and Cre-LoxP gene switching in the adult mouse heart. *Gene Ther.* **10,** 1814–1820.

237. Bowman, J. C., Steinberg, S. F., Jiang, T., Geenen, D. L., Fishman, G. I., and Buttrick, P. M. (1997) Expression of protein kinase C beta in the heart causes hypertrophy in adult mice and sudden death in neonates. *J. Clin. Invest.* **100,** 2189–2195.

238. Redfern, C. H., Degtyarev, M. Y., Kwa, A. T., et al. (2000) Conditional expression of a Gi-coupled receptor causes ventricular conduction delay and a lethal cardiomyopathy. *Proc. Natl. Acad. Sci. USA* **97,** 4826–4831.

239. Redfern, C. H., Coward, P., Degtyarev, M. Y., et al. (1999) Conditional expression and signaling of a specifically designed Gi-coupled receptor in transgenic mice. *Nat. Biotechnol.* **17,** 165–169.

240. Suzuki, J., Shen, W. J., Nelson, B. D., et al. (2001) Absence of cardiac lipid accumulation in transgenic mice with heart-specific HSL overexpression. *Am. J. Physiol. Endocrinol. Metab.* **281,** E857–866.

241. Mungrue, I. N., Husain, M., and Stewart, D. J. (2002) The role of NOS in heart failure: lessons from murine genetic models. *Heart Fail. Rev.* **7,** 407–422.

242. Beggah, A. T., Escoubet, B., Puttini, S., et al. (2002) From the Cover: Reversible cardiac fibrosis and heart failure induced by conditional expression of an antisense mRNA of the mineralocorticoid receptor in cardiomyocytes. *Proc. Natl. Acad. Sci. USA* **99,** 7160–7165.

243. Gao, M. H., Bayat, H., Roth, D. M., et al. (2002) Controlled expression of cardiac-directed adenylylcyclase type VI provides increased contractile function. *Cardiovasc. Res.* **56,** 197–204.

244. Ouvrard-Pascaud, A. and Jaisser, F. (2003) Pathophysiological role of the mineralocorticoid receptor in heart: analysis of conditional transgenic models. *Pflugers Arch.* **445,** 477–481.

9

Gene Silencing Using Adenoviral RNAi Vector in Vascular Smooth Muscle Cells and Cardiomyocytes

Hideko Kasahara and Hiroki Aoki

Summary

RNA interference (RNAi) is a new and rapidly progressing technology for facilitating functional gene silencing. To perform highly efficient RNAi in cardiomyocytes, vascular smooth muscle cells, and vascular endothelial cells, which are known to have very low transfection efficiency, adenovirus-mediated RNAi was employed. The effects of RNAi on GAPDH transcripts were successfully reduced by nearly 90% in the primary cultured cells, indicating that adenovirus-mediated gene silencing is a promising technique for gene silencing in cardiovascular studies. This chapter describes general guidelines for selecting RNAi target sites, construction of a shuttle vector encoding short hairpin RNAi, and generation of recombinant adenovirus.

Key Words: Adenovirus; RNA interference; RNAi; gene silencing; transcription; heart; vascular; cardiomyocytes; vascular smooth muscle; short hairpin RNA; infection; cloning; U6 promoter.

1. Introduction

The recently developed technique of RNA interference (RNAi) is a breakthrough method to silence the gene of interest. RNAi in mammalian cells is introduced by double-stranded RNA molecules of 21 nt in length with 2-nt 3' overhands (short interfering RNA [siRNA]) or by hairpin-forming 45–50-mer RNA molecules (short hairpin RNA [shRNA]) that are complementary to the gene of interest through plasmid transfection or adenovirus infection. In primary cultured cardiomyocytes, vascular smooth muscle cells, and endothelial cells, efficient transfection of siRNA or the plasmid encoding shRNA is not

From: *Methods in Molecular Medicine, vol. 112: Molecular Cardiology: Methods and Protocols*
Edited by: Z. Sun © Humana Press Inc., Totowa, NJ

expected. Therefore we examined the feasibility of adenoviral RNAi application in these cells.

The major barrier preventing the wide use of adenovirus-based gene deliveries in applications is the difficulty in making new adenovirus. Hardy et al. *(1)* developed a method for creating recombinant adenoviruses without plaque assays using HEK 293 cells stably expressing Cre recombinase (CRE8 cells), a shuttle vector pAdlox, and a special adenovirus called Ψ5. In Ψ5 adenovirus, the packaging site is flanked by two loxP sites that will be deleted in the presence of Cre recombinase. Therefore, Cre-mediated recombination deletes the intervening packaging sequence in Ψ5, producing an unpackageable viral genome in CRE8 cells and promoting recombination between the pAdlox shuttle vector and Ψ5 genome. After three passages of this negative selection, only 0.2% of donor Ψ5 virus is detected in CRE8 cells; therefore plaque assays for purifying recombinant adenovirus from Ψ5 are not necessary *(1)*. We have generated various adenoviruses using this method, typically within 3 wk after construction of the shuttle vector *(2–4)*. To apply this method in adenoviral RNAi production, we recently modified the pAdlox shuttle vector [provided by S. Hardy and described in **ref.** *1*] by replacing the cytomegalovirus (CMV) promoter–polylinker fragment of the pAdlox vector with the U6 promoter–polylinker fragment of pSilencer1.0-U6 shRNA expression vector *(5)* (Ambion). The resulting shuttle vector was named pAdloss (*see* **Fig. 1** and **Note 1**).

We will describe the general guidelines for selecting the RNAi target site (**Subheading 3.1.**) and designing an oligonucleotide duplex encoding a hairpin shRNA (**Subheading 3.2.1.** and **Fig. 2**) that will be subcloned into the pAdloss shuttle vector (**Subheading 3.2.2.**). Then generation of adenovirus (**Subheading 3.3.**), purification, and titer check, (**Subheading 3.4.**), followed by examination of RNAi effects (**Subheading 3.5.**) will also be described (*see* **Note 2**).

As an example, rat GAPDH RNAi was produced, and its gene silencing efficiency in rat cardiomyocytes and vascular smooth muscle cells was examined. We found more than 90% reduction of GAPDH RNA expression within 48 h after adenoviral infection in these cells, indicating the efficiency of gene silencing using this new system in cardiovascular research (**Fig. 3**).

2. Materials

2.1. Selection of the Target Sites

1. Annealing buffer: 100 m*M* potassium acetate, 30 m*M* HEPES-KOH, 2 m*M* magnesium acetate, pH 7.4.
2. Dulbecco's modified Eagle's medium (DMEM) without serum or antibiotics.
3. DMEM with 10% fetal bovine serum (FBS) containing appropriate antibiotics.

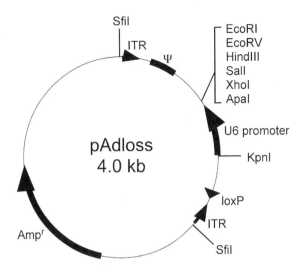

Fig. 1. Schematic of the pAdloss–adenoviral U6 siRNA shuttle vector.

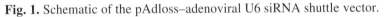

```
       Sense      Loop     Antisense
5'-        N(19) TTCAAGAGA N(19) TTTTTT    -3' (53 bases)
3'-CCGG N(19) AAGTTCTCT N(19) AAAAAATTAA-5' (61 bases)
   ApaI                              EcoRI
```

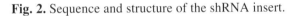

Fig. 2. Sequence and structure of the shRNA insert.

4. DMEM with 30% FBS containing appropriate antibiotics.
5. TE: 10 m*M* Tris-HCl, pH 8.0, 1 m*M* EDTA.
6. A10 rat aortic smooth muscle cell line (ATCC).
7. siRNA for GAPDH (*see* **Note 3**):
   5'-GUGGACAUUGUUGCCAUCAdTdT-3'
   5'-UGAUGGCAACAAUGUCCACdTdT-3'.
8. Oligofectamine (Invitrogen).

2.2. Construction of shRNA Template in the Shuttle Vector pAdloss

1. pAdloss shuttle vector (**Fig. 1**).
2. Oligonucleotides (**Fig. 2**).
3. Restriction enzymes (*Apa*I, *Eco*RI, *Hin*dIII), T4 DNA ligase.
4. Standard materials for agarose gel electrophoresis.
5. *E. coli* competent cells (e.g., DH5α).
6. LB broth, LB plate, LB plus ampicillin plates.
7. Ampicillin.

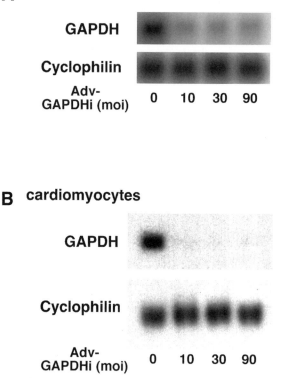

Fig. 3. Silencing effects of adenoviral GAPDH RNAi in primary cultured rat vascular smooth muscle cells **(A)** and cardiomyocytes **(B)**.

8. Sequencing primers:
   U6 sequence primer: 5'-GCACAAAAGGAAACTCACCCTAAC-3'.
   pAdloss reverse sequence primer: 5'-CACTCTTGAGTGCCAGCGAGTAG-3'.
9. A10 rat aortic smooth muscle cell line (ATCC).
10. DMEM with 10% FBS containing appropriate antibiotics.
11. DMEM without serum or antibiotics.
12. FuGene 6 (Roche).

2.3. Generation of Recombinant Adenovirus

1. Adenovirus Ψ5 backbone *(1)*.
2. Recombinant pAdloss shuttle vector.
3. Restriction enzyme, *Sfi*I.
4. Saturated phenol/chloroform.
5. 3 *M* Sodium acetate, pH 5.2.

6. 100% and 70% ethanol stored at -20°C.
7. CRE8 cells (HEK 293 cells stably expressing Cre recombinase) *(1)*.
8. DMEM with 10% newborn calf serum containing appropriate antibiotics.
9. Calcium phosphate transfection reagent: 2 *M* $CaCl_2$, HEPES 2X buffered saline, e.g., ProFection Mammalian Transfection Systems (Promega).
10. PBS: 136 m*M* NaCl, 2.7 m*M* KCl, 10 m*M* Na_2HPO_4, 1.8 m*M* KH_2PO_4, pH 8.1. Sterilize.
11. Adenovirus storage buffer *(6)*: 10 m*M* Tris-HCl, 2 m*M* $MgCl_2$, 4% sucrose, 12.5 mg/L phenol red, pH 8.1. Filter-sterilize.
12. Adenovirus lysis buffer: 10 m*M* Tris-HCl, 1.5 mg/L phenol red, pH 8.1 (*see* **Note 4**). Filter-sterilize.

2.4. Purification and Titration of Recombinant Adenovirus

2.4.1. Purification of Recombinant Adenovirus

1. Adenovirus lysis buffer: 10 m*M* Tris-HCl, 1.5 mg/L phenol red, pH 8.1 (*see* **Note 4**).
2. Light CsCl/Tris: 263 g/L CsCl, 10 m*M* Tris-HCl, pH 8.1, $\rho = 1.20$ g/mL.
3. Heavy CsCl/Tris: 610 g/L CsCl, 10 m*M* Tris-HCl, pH 8.1, $\rho = 1.45$ g/mL.
4. Adenovirus storage buffer (*see* **Subheading 2.3.**).
5. Appropriate ultracentrifuge equipment and rotors.
6. Ultra-Clear centrifuge tube no. 344058 (SW28, BECKMAN) or equivalent.
7. Ultra-Clear centrifuge tube no. 344059 (SW41, BECKMAN) or equivalent.
8. 18-Gage needles and 5- and 2.5-mL syringes.
9. Desalting column, e.g., EconoPack 10DG (Bio-Rad).
10. 0.45-μm Syringe-driven cellulose acetate filter.

2.4.2. Titration of Recombinant Adenovirus

1. HEK 293 cells.
2. DMEM with 10% newborn calf serum containing appropriate antibiotics.
3. 8-Channel pipetor.
4. 96-Well flat-bottomed tissue culture plates.
5. Filtered pipet tips (one pack for each 96-well plate).
6. Inverted microscope.

2.5. Examination of RNAi Effect by Northern Blotting (see Note 5)

1. Primary cultured cells, e.g., cardiomyocytes, vascular smooth muscle cells (*see* **Note 6**).
2. TRIzol reagent (Invitrogen), RNeasy (Qiagen), or equivalent materials for RNA extraction.
3. 1 L 10X MOPS: 83.7 g MOPS-free acid, 13.6 g sodium acetate trihydrate, 20 mL 0.5 *M* EDTA, pH 7.0.
4. 100 mL 1% agarose gel: 1 g agarose, 10 mL 10X MOPS, 84.5 mL H_2O, 5.5 mL formaldehyde (37%).
5. Nylon membrane, e.g., Hybond™-*N* (Amersham).

6. 20X SSC 1 L: 175 g sodium chloride, 88 g sodium citrate, pH 7.0.
7. Random prime DNA labeling kit (Invitrogen) or equivalent materials for DNA labeling.
8. α[^{32}P]dCTP.
9. 100 mL 50X Denhardt solution: 1 g Ficoll 400, 1 g polyvinylpyrrolidone, 1 g bovine serum albumin (fraction V).
10. Hybridization buffer: 50% formamide, 0.5% sodium dodecyl sulfate (SDS), 6X SSC, 5X Denhardt's solution, salmon sperm 40 μg/mL DNA.
11. Wash buffer 1: 2X SSC, 0.1% SDS.
12. Wash buffer 2: 0.1X SSC, 0.1% SDS.
13. GAPDH and cyclophilin probes (*see* **Note 7**).

3. Methods
3.1. Selection of the Target Sites

Selection of the effective target site is the most critical step in RNAi experiments. However, the mechanistic basis underlying the effective vs noneffective target site has not been fully elucidated. Therefore, it is advisable to choose several, preferably four or more, target sites for a single gene. Several companies claim to have developed a proprietary algorithm for the selection of target sites with a better success rate. Usually, selection of the target site with such algorithms is an option in designing and purchasing synthetic siRNA. Alternatively, ready-made siRNA may be purchased. Ready-made siRNA is usually guaranteed to suppress the target mRNA level to a certain extent. Using commercially available services is one of the options, provided that the sequence information is available upon the purchase of siRNA.

3.1.1. General Guidelines for Selecting of the Target Sites

The guideline described here is based on the rule proposed by Elbashir et al. *(7)* (*see* **Note 8**). Several manufacturers provide free access for designing siRNA (Qiagen: http://siRNA.qiagen.com/Index.jsp and Ambion: http://www.ambion.com/techlib/misc/siRNA_finder.html).

1. Search for AA dinucleotide sequences in the coding region of the transcript. AA and following 19-nt sequences are potential target sites.
2. Select sequences with a 30 to 50% GC content.
3. Avoid sequences with four or more consecutive As or Ts, which will terminate the transcription by RNA polymerase III.
4. Perform a BLAST search (http://www.ncbi.nlm.nih.gov/blast) for the potential target sites in the database of the same species as the target cells. When the selected target sequence shows more than 16–17 contiguous base pairs of homology with known transcripts in the target species, the selected target sequence should be disregarded. Select several target sites scattering along the coding region (*see* **Note 9**).

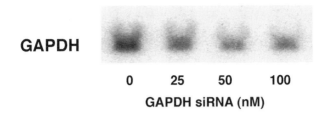

GAPDH

0   25   50   100
GAPDH siRNA (nM)

Fig. 4. Silencing effects of GAPDH siRNA in the A10 rat vascular smooth muscle cell line.

3.1.2. Examination of Synthetic siRNA Effect in Cell Lines

The RNAi effect of the target site can be examined by transfection of synthetic siRNA when cells with high transfection efficiency are available. Note that the cell line should be derived from the same species as the selected target sites, because even a single base mismatch may reduce the RNAi efficiency. In this section, we describe an example of RNAi effects of rat GAPDH in the A10 rat vascular smooth muscle cell line.

1. Design the target site(s). For RNAi of rat GAPDH, following target site was chosen: 5'-AAGTGGACATTGTTGCCATCA-3'.
2. Dissolve two oligonucleotides (5'-GUGGACAUUGUUGCCAUCAdTdT-3'; 5'-UGAUGGCAACAAUGUCCACdTdT-3', *see* **Subheading 2.1.5.**) in the RNase-free annealing buffer. The final concentration is 20 μ*M* for each oligonucleotide.
3. Heat the oligonucleotide solution at 90°C for 1 min, followed by 37°C for 60 min.
4. The annealed siRNA solution can be stored at –20°C.
5. Plate A10 cells at a density of 2.0×10^5 cells/well in 6-well plates 1 d before transfection.
6. Replace culture media with serum-free DMEM before transfection.
7. Set up the following mixture:
   A: 1.25–5 μL oligonucleotide solution (20 μ*M* stock) and 180 μL serum-free DMEM. Adjust the final volume to 185 μL with the annealing buffer.
   B: 4 μL Oligofectamine in 15 μL serum-free DMEM (*see* **Note 10**).
8. Add mixture B to mixture A, mix gently, and incubate at room temperature for 20 min to form siRNA/Oligofectamine complex.
9. Aspirate serum-free DMEM from the culture plates.
10. Add 800 μL serum-free DMEM to each well.
11. Add 200 μL of complex to each well.
12. Incubate the cells for 4 h at 37°C in a CO_2 incubator.
13. Add 500 μL DMEM with 30% FBS.
14. Isolate RNA at 48 hr after the transfection to analyze GAPDH mRNA expression (**Fig. 4**) (*see* **Subheading 3.5.**).

3.2. Construction of pAdloss Shuttle Vector Encoding shRNA

The selected RNAi target sequences (*see* **Subheading 3.1.**) are utilized for generation of adenoviral shuttle vector encoding shRNA.

3.2.1. Design Sense and Antisense DNA Oligonucleotides Encoding a Hairpin siRNA

Insert 19 bp of the 3'-end of the sequence in the sense N(19) site and the corresponding antisense oligonucleotides in the antisense N(19) site to generate two oligonucleotides encoding a hairpin structure (**Figs. 2** and **5**). An example of sense and antisense oligonucleotides of GAPDH RNAi (5'-AA<u>GTGGACATTGTTGCCATCA</u>-3'; 19 bp is underlined) is shown in **Fig. 5**.

3.2.2. Cloning of Double-Stranded Oligonucleotide Into pAdloss Shuttle Vector

After annealing of 53 and 61 bp of oligonucleotides (**Fig. 5**), the double-stranded oligonucleotides are inserted in the *Apa*I and *Eco*RI sites of the multicloning site (MCS) in the pAdloss vector (**Fig. 1**) using standard subcloning methods.

1. Dissolve two oligonucleotides for the siRNA insert in H_2O at a concentration of 1 µg/µL. Mix 2 µL of each oligonucleotide, 0.5 µL of 1 *M* $MgCl_2$ and 47.5 µL of H_2O into a 1.5-mL tube (total 80 ng/µL).
2. Heat the tube at 95°C for 5 min, and then place it into a 65°C heat block. Place the heat block at room temperature until it slowly cools down to the room temperature. The annealed siRNA insert can be used directly in a ligation reaction or stored at –20°C until needed.
3. Digest 10 µg pAdloss vector with *Apa*I and *Eco*RI, and purify the linearized pAdloss at a concentration of 100 ng/µL.
4. Mix 1 µL of the annealed oligonucleotides (80 ng), 1 µL of *Apa*I-*Eco*RI–digested pAdloss vector (100 ng), 1 µL of 10X T4 DNA ligase buffer, 1 µL of T4 DNA ligase and 6 µL of H_2O. Incubate the ligation mixture at 16°C overnight.
5. Optional: Ethanol-precipitate the ligated sample, and dissolve the pellet with 9 µL of H_2O. Add 1 µL of 10X *Hin*dIII enzyme buffer, 0.1 µL of *Hin*dIII restriction enzyme. Incubate 30 min at 37°C to eliminate self ligated or undigested pAdloss plasmid.
6. Transform the ligation mixture into competent *E. coli*. Plate *E. coli* on the LB-ampicillin plates.
7. Perform miniprep to confirm the presence of the shRNA template insert (*see* **Note 11**).
8. Sequence the insert from both directions (*see* **Note 12**).

Sense   Loop   Antisense

5'- **GTGGACATTGTTGCCATCA** TTCAAGAGA **TGATGGCAACAATGTCCAC** TTTTTT -3' (53 bases)

3'-CCGG **CACCTGTAACAACGGTAGT** AAGTTCTCT **ACTACCGTTGTTACAGGTG** AAAAAATTAA-5' (61 bases)

ApaI   **EcoRI**

Fig. 5. Sequence of shRNA insert of GAPDH RNAi.

3.2.3. Examination of pAdloss-shRNA Effect in Cell Lines (Optional)

When cells with high transfection efficiency are available, the RNAi effect of the target site can be examined by transfection of the pAdloss–shRNA shuttle vector. A negative control is designed with a randomized sequence of the same composition as the target sequence that shows no homology with known genes. A one- or two-base mismatch construct is not recommended as a negative control because it may interfere with translation even though it may not degrade target mRNA. In this section, we describe an example of RNAi of rat GAPDH in the A10 rat vascular smooth muscle cell line by transfection of pAdloss–GAPDHi.

1. Plate A10 cells at a density of 2.0×10^5 cells/well in a 6-well plate 1 d before the transfection.
2. Replace the culture media with fresh serum-containing DMEM just before transfection.
3. Aliquot 100 µL DMEM without serum or antibiotics in microcentrifuge tubes.
4. Add 3 µL FuGENE 6 to each tube (*see* **Note 13**).
5. Add 0.05–1.0 µg pAdloss–GAPDHi to each tube, mix gently, and incubate at room temperature for 20 min to form the complex.
6. Add FuGENE 6 and plasmid complex to each well.
7. Incubate the cells for 48 h at 37°C in a CO_2 incubator.
8. Isolate the RNA at 48 h after the transfection to analyze GAPDH mRNA expression (*see* **Subheading 3.5.**).

3.3. Generation of Recombinant Adenovirus

Recombinant adenovirus is generated by cotransfecting Ψ5 backbone and pAdloss shuttle vector into CRE8 cells, which stably express Cre recombinase that will facilitate generation of recombinant adenovirus and will eliminate nonrecombinant Ψ5 virus. As described in the Introduction (**Subheading 1.**), more than 99% of virus detected in CRE8 cells is expected to be recombinant after three passages (generation 3 [G3]) of this negative selection. We normally perform it on a small scale (using cells in 35- or 60-mm culture plates) up to G3 adenovirus generation, followed by G4 adenovirus generation in a 150-mm plate. G4 virus is infected into a total of 20 150-mm plates for large-scale virus production.

3.3.1. Transfection of Linearized Shuttle Vector and Adenoviral Ψ5 Backbone Into CRE8 Cells

1. Digest 10 µg of the cloned pAdloss shuttle vector with *Sfi*I at 50°C overnight. Extract once with phenol/chloroform. Ethanol precipitate the plasmid, and resuspend it in 50 µL of H_2O under sterile conditions (conc. 0.2 µg/µL).

2. 24 h before transfection, plate 0.5×10^6 CRE8 cells per 35-mm plate in DMEM with 10% newborn calf serum.
3. Transfect CRE8 cells with 1 µg of Ψ5 viral backbone and 1 µg (5 µL) of the *Sfi*I-digested pAdloss construct using standard calcium phosphate methods.
4. After 4 h, change the culture medium.
5. Incubate the cells for 7–10 d at 37°C in a CO_2 incubator with addition of fresh medium every 2–3 d.

3.3.2. Recombinant Virus Production

1. Harvest cultures when about 50% of the cells have become infected and detached from the culture plate. Cells are easily detached from the plate by pipeting up and down.
2. Collect cells by centrifugation ($150g$) for 5 min. Remove culture medium, resuspend cells in 0.5 mL of adenovirus storage buffer, and transfer cells into a 1.5-mL tube. Freeze the cells in liquid nitrogen, and thaw at 37°C with occasional mixing to lyse the cells. Repeat freeze/thaw treatment twice more for a total of three freeze/thaw treatments. Centrifuge the cell lysates at $1500g$.
3. Add 75 µL of cell lysates to tissue culture medium with CRE8 cells plated on a 60-mm dish at 60–70% of confluence. Keep the remaining cell lysates as a first generation of adenovirus (G1) at –80°C.
4. Incubate for 2–3 d until 50% of the cells have detached from the culture plate. Repeat the cell harvest and freeze/thaw cycles described in **Subheading 3.3.2.2.**
5. Add 25 µL (5%) of cell lysates in CRE8 cells plated on a 60-mm plate at 60 to 70% of confluence. Keep the remaining cell lysates as a second generation of virus at –80°C (G2).
6. Incubate for 1–2 d until 50% of the cells have detached from the culture plate. Repeat cell harvest and freeze/thaw cycles as described in **Subheading 3.3.2.2.**
7. Add 75 µL of cell lysates to CRE8 cells plated on a 150-mm plate at 60 to 70% of confluence. Keep the remaining cell lysates as a third generation of virus at –80°C (G3).
8. Incubate for 1–2 d until 50% of the cells have detached from the culture plate. Repeat the cell harvest, resuspension of cells in 1 mL of adenovirus storage buffer, and freeze/thaw cycles (G4 virus).

3.3.3. Virus Expansion

1. Plate 1.2×10^7 CRE8 cells per 150-mm plate. Prepare 20 plates for each viral construct 1 d before infection.
2. Add about 40 µL of G4 adenovirus to a 150-mm plate when CRE8 cells are about 90% confluent. Repeat for a total of 20 plates.
3. Harvest cells into several 50-mL tubes when about 50% of the cells have become infected and detached from the culture plate.
4. Collect cells by centrifugation ($150g$) for 5 min. Remove the culture medium and resuspend the cells in 10 mL PBS/tube. Collect cells by centrifugation ($150g$) for

5 min. Discard PBS without disturbing the pellet. Resuspend the pellet in 2 mL PBS, and put all the cells into a single 50-mL tube.

5. Collect cells by centrifugation (150*g*) for 5 min. Discard PBS without disturbing the pellet.
6. If the crude virus can be directly used for the experiments, resuspend cells in 10 mL of adenovirus storage buffer. If further virus purification is desired, resuspend cells in 10 mL of adenovirus lysis buffer.
7. Lyse the cells by three freeze/thaw cycles.
8. Centrifuge the infected cell lysates at 1500*g* for 10 min.
9. Transfer the supernatant to a fresh tube (supernatant 1).
10. Resuspend the pellet in 5 mL of the adenovirus storage buffer or lysis buffer described in **Subheading 3.3.6.** Centrifuge and combine the supernatant with supernatant 1. This is the crude recombinant adenovirus.

3.4. Purification and Titration of Recombinant Adenovirus

The crude recombinant adenovirus is now ready to be titrated directly (**Subheading 3.4.2.**) or purified using standard cesium chloride gradients (**Subheading 3.4.1.**).

3.4.1. Purification of Recombinant Adenovirus

There are three steps in the adenovirus purification, which usually takes 2 d. The first step is to remove most of the cellular contaminants and defective viral particles by discontinuous CsCl gradient. The second step is to separate infectious viral particles from defective ones completely by continuous CsCl gradient. The third step is to remove CsCl by a desalting column.

1. Pour 10 mL light CsCl/Tris into an SW28 ultracentrifuge tube.
2. Pipet 10 mL heavy CsCl/Tris below the light CsCl/Tris layer using a 10-mL pipet without disturbing the interface of heavy and light CsCl solutions.
3. Overlay all the crude virus lysate on top of the CsCl gradient.
4. Top with adenovirus lysis buffer. Check balance.
5. Ultracentrifuge at 52,000*g*, 14°C, 2 h.
6. At the end of the centrifugation, virus should be visible as an opaque white band. Puncture the tube under the virus band with an 18-gage needle attached to a 5-mL syringe, and collect the virus. Avoid band(s) above the main band.
7. Dilute the virus solution with an equal volume of adenovirus lysis buffer.
8. Relay onto 8 mL CsCl gradient (4 mL heavy CsCl/Tris, 4 mL light CsCl/Tris) in SW41 tube (up to 3.5 mL).
9. Top with adenovirus lysis buffer. Check balance.
10. Ultracentrifuge at 50,000*g*, 14°C, overnight.
11. Puncture the tube under the virus band with an 18-gage needle attached to a 2.5-mL syringe, and collect the virus. Avoid band(s) above the main band.
12. Prepare Bio-Rad EconoPack 10DG desalting column.
13. Equilibrate the desalting column with adenovirus storage buffer.

14. Measure virus suspension volume (should be <3 mL).
15. Apply virus suspension to the column, and allow the entire sample to enter the column.
16. Apply an additional adenovirus storage buffer to make the total volume to 3 mL (e.g., when the virus suspension volume is 2.5 mL, apply 0.5 mL of adenovirus storage buffer).
17. Allow the entire buffer to enter the column. Discard the effluent.
18. Add 1.5X sample volume or 4 mL of adenovirus storage buffer (whichever is less).
19. Collect this fraction as the desalted virus fraction.
20. Filter the purified virus through a 0.45-µm cellulose acetate filter.

3.4.2. Titration of Recombinant Adenovirus

Viral particle titer can be measured using either physically (by measuring the OD 260 nm) or biologically. Of the several biological assays, we describe the method called *tissue culture infectious dose 50* ($TCID_{50}$). First, 293 cells in 96-well plates are infected with serially diluted viruses, and then the cytopathic effect in each well is determined after 10–14 d of incubation.

1. Dilute the viral stock by 10^{-4} with DMEM (without serum). Dilution can be easily performed by serial dilution. Dispense 0.9 mL of DMEM into 1.5-mL tubes (four tubes for each construct). Add 0.1 mL of the viral stock into the first tube (10^{-1} dilution). Shake the tube well. Transfer 0.1 mL of 10^{-1} dilution into the second tube (10^{-2} dilution). Transfer 0.1 mL of 10^{-2} dilution into the third tube (10^{-3} dilution). Transfer 0.1 mL of 10^{-3} dilution into the fourth tube (10^{-4} dilution).
2. Dispense 50 µL of DMEM with serum into all the wells of 96-well tissue culture plates by using an eight-channel pipetor. Prepare one plate for each viral stock that needs to be titrated (e.g., prepare four plates for four different viral constructs).
3. Dispense 25 µL of 10^{-4}-diluted virus into the first lane (a total of eight wells; **Fig. 6**, lane 1).
4. Pipet up and down five times to mix, using an eight-channel pipetor.
5. Transfer 25 µL of the mixture from the first lane to the second lane. Pipet up and down five times.
6. Change pipet tips. Transfer 25 µL of the second lane into the third lane.
7. Repeat dilution up to the 11th lane. Change tips between the lanes.
8. Prepare 6–7 mL of the HEK 293 cell suspension in DMEM with serum at $\approx 10^5$ cells/mL, and dispense 50 µL ($\approx 5 \times 10^3$ cells) per well into all 96 wells.
9. Add 50 µL of DMEM with serum every 3–4 d. Leave the plates at 37°C in a CO_2 incubator for 10–14 d until a cytopathic effect is evident.
10. Read the plates using an inverted microscope. A well is counted as positive even if only a small spot or a few cells show cytopathic effect. If it is hard to determine, compare the well with the negative control (**Fig. 6**, lane 12, no viral infection).

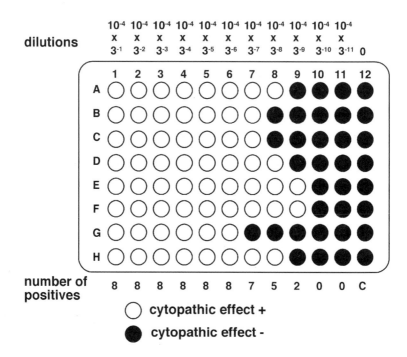

Fig. 6. An example of $TCID_{50}$ measured on a 96-well plate.

11. Determine $TCID_{50}$ using the Kärber statistical method. In this example (**Fig. 6**), 100% of the wells are positive for cytopathic effects (8/8 wells) up to dilution $10^{-4} \times 3^{-6}$ (lane 6), whereas 0% of the wells are positive at dilution $10^{-4} \times 3^{-10}$ (lane 10).

12. $TCID_{50} = 10X$

$X = \log a - [(\text{the sum of positive ratios}) - 0.5] \times \log (\text{dilution ratio between the lanes})$

a = dilution of the first lane ($10^{-4} \times 3^{-1}$); the dilution ratio in this example = 3

The sum of positive ratios = 8/8 + 8/8 + 8/8 + 8/8 + 8/8 + 8/8 + 7/8 + 5/8 + 2/8 = 7.75

$$X = \log (10^{-4} \times 3^{-1}) - (7.75 - 0.50) \times \log 3$$

$$= \log (10^{-4} \times 3^{-1} \times 3^{-6.75}) = -4 - 6.75 \log 3 = -7.22$$

$TCID_{50} = 10^{-7.22}$ (for a 50-μL aliquot of virus) ($10^{-7.22}$ times dilution of the 50 μL of viral stock is considered 1 PFU)

Viral titer = 1 mL/0.05 mL/$10^{-7.22}$ = $20 \times 10^{7.22}$ = 3.32×10^{8} (PFU/mL).

3.5. Examination of RNAi Effect

Evidence of gene silencing can be obtained by measuring a reduction in mRNA levels, protein levels, or both (*see* **Note 14**). In this section, we demonstrate an example of the effects using adenoviral RNAi to silence GAPDH expression in vascular smooth muscle cells and cardiomyocytes (**Fig. 3**). The method most appropriate for each gene in different cell systems needs to be optimized individually. We recommend generating multiple candidate hairpin sequences and testing for their gene silencing efficiency, particularly when screening of siRNA or pAdloss–RNAi transfection are not applicable. Once good silencing effects are observed in at least one candidate construct, another virus containing the scrambled sequence can be generated as a negative control to specify the silencing effects further.

3.5.1. Optimization of the Amount of Recombinant Adenovirus

1. Plate neonatal cardiomyocytes purified by differential centrifugation through a discontinuous Percoll gradient per 100-mm dish in culture medium 1 d before infection with the appropriate density (*see* **Note 6**). For vascular smooth muscle cells, plate the cells a few days prior to the experiments and use them when their growth is at the appropriate density.
2. Change the media prior to the infection, and then directly add GAPDH-RNAi crude or purified virus into the media at 10, 30, and 90 multiplicity of infection (MOI; *see* **Note 15**).
3. After 3 h of incubation, remove the media containing the virus, and replace it with normal tissue culture media.
4. Incubate for additional 45 h (total 48 h after virus infection).
5. Isolate RNA at 48 h after the transfection to analyze GAPDH mRNA expression. Use 5–20 µg of total RNA extracted from each sample and examine their levels of expression by Northern blotting with a GAPDH probe and a cyclophilin probe as control (*see* **Note 7**).

4. Notes

1. The pAdloss shuttle vector was constructed as follows: a *Kpn*I-*Sac*I fragment was isolated from pSilencer1.0-U6 containing the U6 promoter (Ambion) and the MCS. The *Kpn*I-*Sac*I fragment was inserted into the pAdlox backbone at the *Kpn*I-*Xho*I sites.
2. Investigators handling adenovirus should refer to the appropriate institutional office for the regulation, safety precaution, appropriate handling, and disposal of the infectious materials.
3. Many companies offer custom siRNA synthesis service. We purchased HPP grade siRNA from Qiagen.
4. Phenol red is added to monitor the pH. Lower pH (<7.0) may cause virus aggregation and drastic loss of virus infectivity (*6*). Do not include phenol red in CsCl to make the adenovirus band visible.

5. A detailed protocol for Northern analysis can be found in laboratory textbooks such as *Current Protocols in Molecular Biology.*

6. Refer to the literature including ours for preparation of primary cultured rat neonatal cardiomyocytes *(4)* and vascular smooth muscle cells *(8)*.

7. Probe was generated by reverse transcriptase-polymerase chain reaction (RT-PCR) with GAPDH-specific primers (forward, 5'-TTCATTGACCTCAACTACAT-3'; reverse, 5'-GTGGCAGTGATGGCATGGAC-3'; 450 bp) and cyclophilin-specific primers (forward, 5'-GCAGACAAAGTTCCAAAGACAG-3'; reverse, 5'-GAGAGCAGAGATTACAGGGTATTG-3'; 523 bp)

8. As RNAi is a new and rapidly progressing technology, new concepts are continuously introduced. For example, recent reports have provoked several precautions regarding the nonspecific effect of siRNA or shRNA. Although initially it was thought that short double-strand RNA can circumvent the interferon response, introduction of 21-bp siRNA *(9)* or expression of shRNA *(10)* may still induce an interferon response in mammalian cells. RNAi is mediated by an RNA-induced silencing complex (RISC) that incorporates an antisense strand of siRNA as a guide for the selection of target mRNA. Part of the nonspecific or "off-target" effect of siRNA may be induced by the opposite (sense) strand of the siRNA. This problem can be potentially avoided by designing asymmetrical siRNA. Recent studies reported that lower thermal stability of the 5' end of the antisense strand facilitates incorporation of the antisense strand into the RISC complex while suppressing the incorporation of the sense strand *(11,12)*. These points need to be considered in designing and validating RNAi experiments.

9. Because of mRNA structure or RNA binding proteins, the 5' or 3' untranslated regions (UTRs) or those near the start AUG may not be accessible to the RISC complex. Therefore, these sites are usually avoided as potential target sites.

10. Many companies offer various transfection reagents for siRNA. We successfully used Oligofectamine (Invitrogen), but other reagents may work as well. Optimal transfection conditions, including the transfection reagent, should be determined individually.

11. Digest the plasmids with *Xba*I. Two *Xba*I sites spanning multicloning sites. Thus, the insert-less plasmid will show 400 bp of *Xba*I digested fragment vs. insert-plus 457 bp. Alternatively, screening can be performed by PCR using the primer set spanning the multicloning sites (5'-GCACAAAAGGAAACTCACCCTAAC-3'; 5'-CACTCTTGAGTGCCAGCGAGTAG-3'). The insert-positive colonies will show 264-bp PCR products.

12. Because of the hairpin structure of the plasmid, the sequence reaction needs to be optimized, by increasing the initial denature temperature and time, the addition of dimethyl sulfoxide, and increasing plasmid and primer concentration.

13. Other transfection reagents may work as well. Optimal transfection conditions need to be determined individually.

14. siRNA or shRNA suppresses expression of the target protein by several mechanisms. First, they degrade the target mRNA by RNA interference. Second, they may suppress translation of the target mRNA in the same way as miRNA *(13)*.

Third, they may cause epigenetic silencing of the target gene, although this phenomenon has not been reported in mammalian cells (*see* **ref.** *14* for a recent review). Therefore, the effect of siRNA or shRNA may be examined at the mRNA level and/or the protein level.

15. In neonatal cardiomyocytes and vascular smooth muscle cells, all three viral concentration (10, 30, and 90 MOI) of GAPDH-RNAi reduced GAPDH mRNA expression by more than 90% (**Fig. 3**). However, in adult cardiomyocytes, a higher viral concentration (>30 MOI) is necessary to reduce the GAPDH transcripts (data not shown). The infection conditions need to be optimized individually.

References

1. Hardy, S., Kitamura, M., Harris-Stansil, T., Dai, Y., and Phipps, M. L. (1997) Construction of adenovirus vectors through Cre-lox recombination. *J. Virol.* **71,** 1842–1849.
2. Kasahara, H., Usheva, A., Ueyama, T., Aoki, H., Horikoshi, N., and Izumo, S. (2001) Characterization of homo- and heterodimerization of cardiac Csx/Nkx2.5 homeoprotein. *J. Biol. Chem.* **276,** 4570–4580.
3. Aoki, H., Kang, P.M., Hampe, J., et al. (2002) Direct activation of mitochondrial apoptosis machinery by c-Jun N-terminal kinase in adult cardiac myocytes. *J. Biol. Chem.* **277,** 10,244–10,250.
4. Kasahara, H., Ueyama, T., Wakimoto, H., et al. (2003) Nkx2.5 homeoprotein regulates expression of gap junction protein connexin 43 and sarcomere organization in postnatal cardiomyocytes. *J. Mol. Cell Cardiol.* **35,** 243–256.
5. Brummelkamp, T. R., Bernards, R., and Agami, R. (2002) A system for stable expression of short interfering RNAs in mammalian cells. *Science* **296,** 550–553.
6. Nyberg-Hoffman, C. and Aguilar-Cordova, E. (1999) Instability of adenoviral vectors during transport and its implication for clinical studies. *Nat. Med.* **5,** 955–957.
7. Elbashir, S. M., Martinez, J., Patkaniowska, A., Lendeckel, W., and Tuschl, T. (2001) Functional anatomy of siRNAs for mediating efficient RNAi in *Drosophila melanogaster* embryo lysate. *EMBO J.* **20,** 6877–6888.
8. Adachi, M., Katsumura, K. R., Fujii, K., Kobayashi, S., Aoki, H., and Matsuzaki. M. (2003) Proteasome-dependent decrease in Akt by growth factors in vascular smooth muscle cells. *FEBS Lett.* **554,** 77–80.
9. Sledz, C. A., Holko, M., de Veer, M. J., Silverman R. H., and Williams B. R. (2003) Activation of the interferon system by short-interfering RNAs. *Nat. Cell Biol.* **5,** 834–839.
10. Bridge, A. J., Pebernard, S., Ducraux, A., Nicoulaz, A. L., and Iggo, R. (2003) Induction of an interferon response by RNAi vectors in mammalian cells. *Nat. Genet.* **34,** 263,264.
11. Khvorova, A. Reynolds, A., and Jayasena, S. D. (2003) Functional siRNAs and miRNAs exhibit strand bias. *Cell* **115,** 209–216.
12. Schwarz, D. S,. Hutvagner, G., Du, T., Xu, Z., Aronin, N., and Zamore, P. D. (2003) Asymmetry in the assembly of the RNAi enzyme complex. *Cell* **115,** 199–208.

13. Doench, J. G., Petersen, C. P., and Sharp, P. A. (2003) siRNAs can function as miRNAs. *Genes Dev.* **17,** 438–442.
14. Grewal, S. I. and Moazed, D. (2003) Heterochromatin and epigenetic control of gene expression. *Science* **301,** 798–802.

III

STEM CELL THERAPY FOR CARDIOVASCULAR DISEASE

10

Cardiac Commitment of Embryonic Stem Cells for Myocardial Repair

Dana Zeineddine, Evangelia Papadimou, Annabelle Mery, Claudine Ménard, and Michel Pucéat

Summary

Embryonic stem (ES) cells represent a source for cell-based regenerative therapies of heart failure. The pluripotency and the plasticity of ES cells allow them to be committed to a cardiac lineage following treatment with growth factors of the transforming growth factor (TGF)-β superfamily. We describe a protocol designed to turn on expression of cardiac-specific genes in undifferentiated murine ES cells stimulated with BMP2 and/or TGF-β. Cell commitment results in a significant improvement in spontaneous cardiac differentiation of ES cells both in vitro and in vivo.

Key Words: Embryonic stem cell; cell commitment; cardiomyocyte.

1. Introduction

Heart failure has become a world-wide epidemic. Most chronic heart diseases develop after cardiac stroke, cardiomyopathies, and muscle myopathies *(1)*. The clinical picture of these diseases is nonspecific and includes degenerative myocytes and increased interstitial fibrosis *(2,3)*. Pharmacology-based treatment of heart failure is still limited, opening an avenue to new therapeutic strategies including regenerative cell therapies.

From: *Methods in Molecular Medicine, vol. 112: Molecular Cardiology: Methods and Protocols*
Edited by: Z. Sun © Humana Press Inc., Totowa, NJ

1.1. Cell-Based Therapeutic Approaches and Requirement for Commitment of Stem Cells

To replace the degenerative myocytes in ischemic myocardium, different cell types have been grafted into the heart, including myoblasts, cardioblasts, and fetal or neonatal cardiomyocytes *(4–9)*. The low dividing capacity of already differentiated muscle cells *(10)* and the lack of electrical coupling of such grafted cells within the myocardium *(11,12)* have limited their therapeutic benefit. Adult stem cells including hematopoietic stem cells or mesemchymal cells represent another cell source for cardiac repair *(13–15)*. Bone marrow stem cells transplanted into infarcted heart differentiated into smooth muscle cells, cardiomyocytes, and endothelial cells. The functional benefit of these cells was modest *(16)*, and this phenomenon may be a rare event *(17)*.

Mesenchymal stem cells (MSCs) or marrow stromal cells are noncirculating multipotent cells *(18)*, isolated from the cavity of adult bone marrow. They have the potentiality to differentiate along various mesenchymal lineages including bone, muscle, and possibly heart both in vitro *(19,20)* and in vivo *(21)*. They were also engrafted into the myocardium, where they transdifferentiated into cardiac-like cells *(22)*. However, to differentiate into cardiac-like cells, the MSCs have to be treated with 5-azacytidine, a drug that interferes with the synthesis of nucleic acids and with gene expression by causing demethylation of the DNA. Although such treatment was shown to induce a mesodermal cell lineage *(23)* including skeletal muscle, it remains unclear whether it may specifically commit MSCs to the cardiac lineage and what could be the long-term effect of such epigenetic modifications of the genome.

A subpopulation of mesemchymal stem cells, referred as to mesodermal progenitor cells (MPCs) *(24)* has recently been isolated from bone marrow of 2- to 50-yr-old individuals. However, like MSC, 5-azacytidine is required to differentiate them into cardiomyocytes. Infused intravenously into mice, they do not contribute to cardiac muscle *(25)*.

Alternatively, the use of pluripotent embryonic stem or germinal cells (ES or EG cells) may turn out to be promising. Pluripotential cells in the embryo are capable of giving rise to different progeny representative of the three embryonic layers, the endoderm, the mesoderm, and the ectoderm. In 1981, the first pluripotent ES cell line was derived from a mouse blastocyst *(26)*. In 1995 and then in 1998, primate *(27)* and human ES cell lines *(28)* were generated. The ES cells share with the EG and carcinoma cells the properties of self-renewal, absence of senescent crisis and of contact inhibition when cultured in vitro, and the ability to differentiate in any cell type (including germline cells *[29]*) but the placental cells. They proliferate rapidly (6–8 h) and a clonal population can be easily initiated. The plasticity of ES cells makes them a very attractive cell population to be used for clinical purposes in the near future. However, their high proliferative capability calls for strategies to commit stem cells specifically to the cardiac lineage before injection into a diseased myocardium.

1.2. Lineage-Specific Commitment of Embryonic Stem Cells

Cell commitment or specification is a process by which an undifferentiated cell enters a developmental pathway *(30)*. This is triggered following cell stimulation with growth factors or morphogens or "form-producing" substances *(31)*. During embryogenesis, cardiac cell specification occurs before primitive streak formation. ES cells from the inner cell mass of the blastocyst respond to morphogens to give rise to all tissues of the embryo except the placenta. Heart precursors are found very early in the lateral posterior epiblast, at the early primitive streak *(32)*. Nodal, a member of the transforming growth factor (TGF)-β superfamily, plays a crucial role in the cardiogenic cell determination process *(33)*. We thus reasoned that the cardiogenic factors of the TGF-β superfamily should commit the ES cells to a cardiac lineage. In this chapter, we describe a protocol designed in our laboratory to reach this aim.

2. Materials

1. CGR8 ES cells *(34)*.
2. BHK21 cell culture medium (Eurobio, Les Ullis, France).
3. Nonessential amino acids (Eurobio CSTAANOO-OU).
4. Na pyruvate (Eurobio CSTVTOO-OU).
5. Glutamine (Eurobio CSTGLUOO-OU).
6. Penicillin/streptomycin (Eurobio CABPESO1-OU).
7. Propagation medium: 500 mL BHK21 medium, 100X 5 mL nonessential amino acids, 5 mL 100 mM Na Pyruvate, 10,000 U penicillin/10 mg/mL streptomycin (5 mL), 5 mL 200 mM glutamine, 0.5 mL 1×10^{-4} M mercaptoethanol (Sigma, cat. no. M7154) (in phosphate-buffered saline [PBS], stable for 1 mo, stored at 4°C), 35 mL fetal calf serum (Hyclone, Perbio France CH30160.03), 0.05 mL leukemia inhibitory factor (LIF)-D conditioned medium (1:1000), 0.05 mL Plasmocin (In vivogen).
8. Differentiation Medium: 400 mL BHK21 medium, 5 mL 100 X nonessential amino acids, 5 mL 100 mM Na pyruvate, 10,000 U penicillin/10 mg/mL streptomycin (5 ml), 5 mL 200 mM glutamine, 0.5 mL 1×10^{-4} M mercaptoethanol, 100 mL FCS (Hyclone, Perbio France, cat. no. CH30160.03), 0.05 mL stock 170 mg/L Na selenite (Sigma, cat. no. S5261).
9. LIF produced from LIF-D cells *(35)*.
10. 0.05% Trypsin/0.02% EDTA in PBS.
11. 0.1% Gelatin (Sigma, cat. no. P4170) in PBS. Sterilize, coat the sterile dishes for 1 h at room temperature, aspirate the gelatin, and let it dry for 2–3 min in the hood.

12. CHO cells-expressed recombinant human bone morphogenetic protein 2 (BMP2) (RnDSystem Europe).
13. CHO cells-expressed recombinant human TGF-β1 (RnDSystem Europe).

3. Methods
3.1. Cell Culture and Cell Treatment With Morphogens

1. ES cells are thawed out and passed twice prior to treatment with BMP2 or TGF-β (*see* **Note 1**).
2. For trypsinization, cells are washed once with PBS, trypsinized for 5 min at 37°C, collected as an isolated cell suspension, and spun down for 6 min at 1000*g*.
3. After resuspension in the propagation medium, 400,000 cells/10-cm gelatin-coated dish are plated prior to growth factor stimulation (*see* **Note 2**).
4. ES cells are treated for 24 h after replating with 5 ng/mL BMP2 or 2.5 ng/mL TGF-β or 2.5 ng/mL TGF-β + 1 ng/mL BMP2 for 24 h in the presence of LIF (*see* **Note 3**).
5. At 24 h later, cells are trypsinized, collected in cold PBS, spun down, and lysed with RNA lysis buffer. RNA is extracted using a commercially available kit (Zymo Research, Orange, CA).

3.2. Quantitative Real-Time PCR

1. After reverse transcription, 10 ng cDNA is used for real-time quantitative polymerase chain reaction (PCR), performed with a Lightcycler and the SYBR Green fast start kit (Roche, Germany).
2. Primers used in real-time PCR are as follows: Brachyury forward 5'-GACTTCGTGACGGCTGACAA-3' and reverse 5'-CGAGTCTGGGTGGAT GTAG-3'; MEF2C forward 5'-AGATACCCACAACACACCACGCGCC-3' and reverse 5'-ATCCTTCAGAGAGTCGCATGCGCTT-3'; Nkx2.5 forward 5'-CATTTTACCCGGGAGCCTACGGTG-3' and reverse 5'-GCTTTCCGTCGC CGCCGTGCGCGTG-3'; β-tubulin forward 5'-CCGGACAGTGTGGCAACC AGATCGG-3' and reverse 5'-TGGCCAAAAGGACCTGAGCGAACGG-3'.
3. The PCR reaction contains 10 μL of Master SYBR Green I mix (Taq DNA polymerase, buffer, deoxynucleoside trisphosphate mix, and SYBR Green I dye) diluted 1:10 with nuclease-free H_2O, 3 m*M* $MgCl_2$, and 0.5 μ*M* of each primer. Then 2 μL of diluted cDNA is added to the PCR mix in the light cycler capillary.
4. Results are expressed as a function of the level of expression of the gene of interest in control uncommitted stem cells using a previously described mathematical model *(36)*. Data are normalized using β-tubulin as an index of cDNA content after reverse transcription.
5. Amplification includes an initial denaturation step at 95°C for 8 min, 40 cycles of denaturation at 95°C for 3 s, annealation at 65°C for 10 s, and extension at 72°C for 10 s performed at a temperature transition rate of 20°C/s. Fluorescence is measured at the end of each extension step. After amplification, a melting curve is acquired by heating the product to 95°C, cooling to and maintaining at 70°C

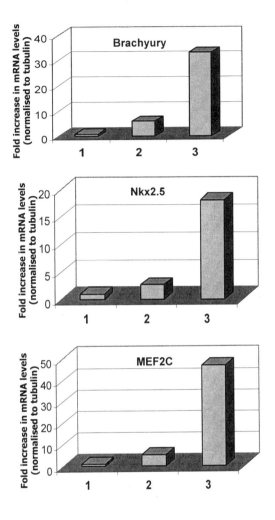

Fig. 1. Fold stimulation in mRNA expression (normalized to tubulin expression) following cell stimulation with: 1, none, control ES cells; 2, TGF-β; 3, TGF-β + BMP ($n = 2$).

for 20 s, and then slowly (0.3°C/s) heating to 95°C. Examples of results obtained on cardiac-committed cells are shown in **Fig. 1**.

Cardiac commitment of ES cells with growth factors of the TGF-β super-family has translated into a significant improvement in cardiac cell differentiation in vitro and to a spontaneous in vivo differentiation of the cells into contractile myocytes, when they are transplanted into a diseased heart *(37)*. Regeneration of tissue with stem cells clearly holds promise as a novel therapeutic approach to cure degenerative diseases. With all the limitations of differentiated cells in mind, a cell-committed progenitor, proliferating in a growth factor-regulated manner, is likely to be the most appropriate therapeutic cell. To exploit this clinical potential, numerous studies must be devoted toward an understanding of the basic biology of the cell. More specifically, the molecular mechanisms underlying the switch between the undifferentiated state and the lineage committed progenitor including the changes in its cell cycle regulation have to be fully elucidated.

4. Notes

1. The number of cell passages after thawing out the cells prior to treatment with morphogens is important. Do not keep ES cells in culture for too many passages (no more than three).
2. The confluency of cells at the beginning of cell treatment with growth factors is critical and influences the cell response to these factors. Thus, 400,000 plated cells 24 h before addition of growth factors should not lead to more than a 30–40% confluency of the dish the next day.
3. The culture propagation medium should be changed 24 h after replating the cells and prior to growth factor stimulation. Then add the growth factors at least 3 h after the change of medium. Adding fresh medium with fresh LIF overstimulates signal transducer amd activator of transcription (STAT)3 phosphorylation *(38)*, which may affect the cell response to growth factors.

Acknowledgments

We are grateful to Atta Behfar (CNRS, Montpellier and Mayo Clinic, Rochester, MN) and Dr. Andre Terzic (Mayo Clinic,) for their contributions to early steps of this work. This work was funded by the Fondation de France and Association Francaise contre les Myopathies. E.P. is a fellow of the Marie Curie program of the European Community. C.M. is a fellow of the Groupe de Recherches et Reflexion sur la Recherche Cardiovasculaire. M.P. is a established investigator at INSERM.

References

1. Megeney, L. A., Kablar, B., Perry, R. L., Ying, C., May, L. and Rudnicki, M. A. (1999) Severe cardiomyopathy in mice lacking dystrophin and MyoD. *Proc. Natl. Acad. Sci. USA* **96,** 220–225.
2. Schonberger, J., et al. (2001) Many roads lead to a broken heart: the genetics of dilated cardiomyopathy. *Am. J. Hum. Genet.* **69,** 249–260.
3. Cox, G. and Kunkel, L. (1997) Dystrophies and heart disease. *Curr. Opin. Cardiol.* **12,** 229–343.
4. Scorsin, M., Marotte, F., Sabri, A., Le Dref, O., Demirag, M., Samuel, J. L., Rappaport, L., and Menasche, P. (1996) Can grafted cardiomyocytes colonize peri-infarct myocardial areas? *Circulation* **94,** II337–1340.

5. Klug, M. G., Soonpaa, M. H., Koh, G. Y. and Field, L. J. (1996) Genetically selected cardiomyocytes from differentiating embronic stem cells form stable intracardiac grafts. *J. Clin. Invest.* **98**, 216–224.
6. Leor, J., Patterson, M., Quinones, M. J., Kedes, L. H., and Kloner, R. A. (1996) Transplantation of fetal myocardial tissue into the infarcted myocardium of rat. A potential method for repair of infarcted myocardium? *Circulation* **94**, II332–336.
7. Kessler, P. D. and Byrne, B. J. (1999) Myoblast cell grafting into heart muscle: cellular biology and potential applications. *Annu. Rev. Physiol.* **61**, 219–242.
8. Roell, W., et al. (2002) Cellular cardiomyoplasty improves survival after myocardial injury. *Circulation* **105**, 2435–2441.
9. Rubart, M., Pasumarthi, K. B., Nakajima, H., Soonpaa, M. H., Nakajima, H. O., and Field, L. J. (2003) Physiological coupling of donor and host cardiomyocytes after cellular transplantation. *Circ. Re.s* **92**, 1217–1224.
10. Beltrami, A. P., et al. (2001) Evidence that human cardiac myocytes divide after myocardial infarction. *N. Engl. J. Med.* **344**, 1750–1757.
11. Scorsin, M., et al. (2000) Comparison of the effects of fetal cardiomyocyte and skeletal myoblast transplantation on postinfarction left ventricular function. *J. Thorac. Cardiovasc. Surg.* **119**, 1169–1175.
12. Zhang, M., Methot, D., Poppa, V., Fujio, Y., Walsh, K., and Murry, C. E. (2001) Cardiomyocyte grafting for cardiac repair: graft cell death and anti-death strategies. *J. Mol. Cell. Cardiol.* **33**, 907–921.
13. McDonald, J. W., Liu, X. Z., Qu, Y., Liu, S., Mickey, S. K., Turetsky, D., Gottlieb, D. I., and Choi, D. W. (1999) Transplanted embryonic stem cells survive, differentiate and promote recovery in injured rat spinal cord. *Nat. Med.* **5**, 1410–1412.
14. Brazelton, T. R., Rossi, F. M., Keshet, G. I., and Blau, H. M. (2000) From marrow to brain: expression of neuronal phenotypes in adult mice. *Science* **290**, 1775–1779.
15. Lagasse, E., et al. (2000) Purified hematopoietic stem cells can differentiate into hepatocytes in vivo. *Nat. Med.* **6**, 1229–1234.
16. Orlic, D., et al. (2001) Bone marrow cells regenerate infarcted myocardium. *Nature* **410**, 701–705.
17. Reinecke, H. and Murry, C. E. (2002) Taking the death toll after cardiomyocyte grafting: a reminder of the importance of quantitative biology. *J. Mol. Cell. Cardiol.* **34**, 251–253.
18. Friedenstein, A. J., Petrakova, K. V., Kurolesova, A. I., and Frolova, G. P. (1968) Heterotopic of bone marrow. Analysis of precursor cells for osteogenic and hematopoietic tissues. *Transplantation* **6**, 230–247.
19. Prockop, D. J. (1997) Marrow stromal cells as stem cells for nonhematopoietic tissues. *Science* **276**, 71–74.
20. Pittenger, M. F., et al. (1999) Multilineage potential of adult human mesenchymal stem cells. *Science* **284**, 143–147.
21. Liechty, K. W., MacKenzie, T. C., Shaaban, A. F., Radu, A., Moseley, A. M., Deans, R., Marshak, D. R. and Flake, A. W. (2000) Human mesenchymal stem cells engraft and demonstrate site-specific differentiation after in utero transplantation in sheep. *Nat. Med.* **6**, 1282–1286.

22. Wang, J. S., Shum-Tim, D., Galipeau, J., Chedrawy, E., Eliopoulos, N. and Chiu, R. C. (2000) Marrow stromal cells for cellular cardiomyoplasty: feasibility and potential clinical advantages. *J. Thorac. Cardiovasc. Surg.* **120,** 999–1005.

23. Konieczny, S. F. and Emerson, C. P., Jr. (1984) 5-Azacytidine induction of stable mesodermal stem cell lineages from 10T1/2 cells: evidence for regulatory genes controlling determination. *Cell* **38,** 791–800.

24. Reyes, M. and Verfailler, C. M. (2001) Characterization of multipotent adult progenitor cells, a subpopulation of mesenchymal stem cells. *Ann. NY Acad. Sci.* **938,** 233–235.

25. Jiang, Y. E. A. (2002) Pluripotency of mesechymal stem cells derived from adult marrow *Nature* **870,** 1–9.

26. Evans, M. J. and Kaufman, M. H. (1981) Establishment in culture of pluripotential cells from mouse embryos *Nature* **292,** 154–156.

27. Thomson, J. A., Kalishman, J., Golos, T. G., Durning, M., Harris, C. P., Becker, R. A., and Hearn, J. P.(1995) Isolation of a primate embryonic stem cell line *Proc. Natl. Acad. Sci. USA* **92,** 7844–7848.

28. Thomson, J. A., Itskovitz-Eldor, J., Shapiro, S. S., Waknitz, M. A., Swiergiel, J. J., Marshall, V. S., and Jones, J. M. (1998) Embryonic stem cell lines derived from human blastocysts *Science* **282,**1145–1147.

29. Hübner, K., et al. (2003) Derivation of oocytes from mouse embryonic stem cells. *Science* **300,** 1251–1256.

30. Slack, J. (1991) *From Egg to Embryo: Reginal specification in Early Development,* 2nd ed., Cambridge University Press, Cambridge, England.

31. Wolpert, L. (1989) Positional information revisited. *Development* **107,** 3–12.

32. Tam, P. P. L. and Schoenwolf, G. (1999) Cardiac fate map: lineage, allocation, morphogenetic movement and cell commitment, in *Heart Development* (Harvey, R. P. and Rosenthal, N., eds.), pp. 3–18.

33. Whitman, M. (2001) Nodal signaling in early vertebrate embryos: themes and variations. *Dev. Cell* **1,** 605–617.

34. Smith, A. G. (1991) Culture and differentiation of embryonic stem cells. *J. Tiss. Cult. Meth.* **13,** 89–94.

35. Meyer, N., Jaconi, M., Ladopoulou, A., Fort, P., and Puceat, M. (2000) A fluorescent reporter gene as a marker for ventricular specification in ES-derived cardiac cells. *FEBS Lett.* **478,** 151–158.

36. Pfaffl, M. W. (2001) A new mathematical model for relative quantification in real-time RT-PCR. *Nucleic Acids Res.* **9,** e45.

37. Behfar, A., Zingman, L., Hodgson, D., Rauzier, J., Kane, G., Terzic, A., and Pucéat, M. (2002) Stem cell differentiation requires a paracrine pathway in the heart. *FASEB J.* **16,** 1558–1566.

38. Boeuf, H., et al. (2001) The ribosomal S6 kinases, cAMP-responsive element-binding, and STAT3 proteins are regulated by different leukemia inhibitory factor signaling pathways in mouse embryonic stem cells. *J. Biol. Chem.* **276,** 46,204–46,211.

11

Autologous Mesenchymal Stem Cells for Post-Ischemic Myocardial Repair

Yao Liang Tang

Summary

Cell transplantation is a novel therapy for patients with postinfarction ventricular dysfunction and congestive heart failure. The potential of mesenchymal stem cells (MSCs) to be used in the injured myocardium is unlimited because of their ability to self-renew and differentiate into cardiomyocytes in vitro and in vivo. In addition, MSCs are easy to harvest and have a high proliferation capability. Finally, autologous MSCs can survive permanently and integrate with healthy host tissue to form new myocardium after implantation in vivo. We have used autologous cultured MSCs grafts for mouse and rat myocardial infarction in more than 500 cases. From these grafting experiments, it has been shown that cultured autologous MSCs grafting is a useful approach in the treatment of ischemic heart failure. This chapter offers a step-by-step guide for successful research on cultured MSCs for the treatment of myocardial infarction, as well as a set of techniques for evaluating postimplantation myocardial repair.

Key Words: Mesenchymal stem cells; cell transplantation; myocardial infarction.

1. Introduction

Cell transplantation is a novel therapy for patients with postinfarction ventricular dysfunction and congestive heart failure. Mesenchymal stem cells (MSCs) derived from bone marrow contain multipotent adult stem cells that have many advantages for clinical use in cellular cardiomyoplasty, as an autologous cell source with high proliferative capability and easy harvesting. Moreover, MSCs are capable of self-renewal, as well as differentiation into

From: *Methods in Molecular Medicine, vol. 112: Molecular Cardiology: Methods and Protocols*
Edited by: Z. Sun © Humana Press Inc., Totowa, NJ

many mesenchymally derived tissues *(1)*. MSCs have the ability to differentiate into cardiomyocytes and endothelial cells when they are exposed to the appropriate stimuli in vitro *(2)*. The cardiac host microenvironment is sufficient to permit MSC differentiation into a highly specific cell lineage, the cardiac ventricular myocytes *(3)*. This procedure may be induced by expression of related growth and differentiation factors in sequence *(4)*. New myocardium forms when MSCs integrate into healthy host tissue after implantation in vivo. This chapter discusses the methodology for MSC isolation, culture, and implantation. Specific protocols are given for techniques that have been shown to be effective in studying postimplantation myocardial repair. First, methods involved in the separation of MSCs from bone marrow are discussed, followed by a protocol for expansion and labeling of MSCs. Second, methods used for establishing a myocardial infarction model and topical MSC implantation into the damaged heart are described. Finally, the effects of implantation are assessed from myocardial regeneration and angiogenesis as well as left ventricular function.

2. Materials

1. Male Lewis rats (inbred) (Harlan, Indianapolis, IN).
2. Dulbecco's modified Eagle's medium (DMEM) (Gibco, Grand Island, NY).
3. Complete medium: DMEM supplemented with 20% fetal bovine serum (FBS) and 100 U/mL penicillin G and 100 μg/mg streptomycin.
4. 25- and 31-Gage needle (Becton Dickinson, Franklin Lakes, NJ).
5. D-Hanks', Hanks' balanced salt solutions (Gibco).
6. 0.25% Trypsin/1 mM EDTA solution (Gibco).
7. 4,6-diamidino-2-phenylindole (DAPI) (Sigma, St. Louis, MO).
8. Harvard Inspira advanced safety ventrilator (Harvard Apparatus, Boston, MA).
9. 18-Gage catheter (Abbott Ireland, Sligo, Rep. of Ireland).
10. Microcoagulator (Aaron Medical Industries, St. Petersburg, FL).
11. 30-μm nylon net filter (Millipore, Billerica, MA).
12. 5-0 and 6-0 Polyester fiber suture (Ethicon, Somerville, NJ).
13. Hemocytometer.
14. Krebs Henseleit buffer: 118 mM NaCl, 4.7 mM KCl, 1.2 mM KH$_2$PO$_4$, 2.5 mM CaCl$_2$, 1.2 mM MgSO$_4$, 25 mM NaHCO$_3$, 11 mM glucose, pH 7.4.
15. Langendorff apparatus and Latex balloon (Harvard Apparatus).
16. Weigert's iron hematoxylin, Accustain trichrome stain kit, and Bouin's solution (Sigma).
17. Radionuclide-labeled microspheres (New England Nuclear Company, D = 15 μm).
18. γ-Counter.
19. 4% Phosphate-buffered formalin solution.
20. Tissue-Tek® O.C.T. (Sakura Finetek U.S.A., Torrance, CA).
21. Mouse anti-α-actin (sarcomeric) clone EA-53 (Sigma, St. Louis, MO).
22. Mouse anti-Desmin IgG (BD Transduction Laboratories).

23. TRITC-conjugated goat antimouse lgG (Sigma).
24. Mouse monoclonal antibody to connexin-43 (BD Transduction Laboratories).
25. Fluorescent Mounting Medium (Dako, Carpinteria, CA).
26. Zeiss Axioplan 2 microscope.
27. Spot Software (Diagnostic Instruments).
28. TUNEL Apoptosis Detection Kit (Upstate Technology, Lake Placid, NY).
29. Bio-Rad 1024 ES confocal microscope.

3. Methods

The methods described below cover various aspects of bone marrow MSCs implantation for repairing ischemic myocardium: (1) the culture and expansion of MSCs, (2) a myocardial infarction model and MSCs implantation, (3) Langendorff preparation assessment of heart function, (4) examination of the angiogenesis and apoptosis of myocardium and myocardial differentiation of grafted MSCs.

3.1. Culture of Rat MSCs

The culture of rat mesenchymal stem cells is described in **Subheading 3.11.** and **3.12.** This includes (1) a description of bone marrow harvesting, and (2) a description of MSC isolation and expansion.

3.1.1. Marrow Harvest

1. Euthanize rats using an overdose of pentobarbital (80 mg/kg) injected ip.
2. Sink rats in 70% alcohol for 8 min.
3. Dissect the remaining muscle from the tibia and femoral bones using forceps and scissors; cut both ends of the long bones away from the diaphyses.
4. Insert the needle into both ends of the bone, and flush the bone marrow from the medullary cavity of the femur and tibia using a 25-gage needle attached to a 5-mL syringe with DMEM containing antibiotics (100 U/mL penicillin G, 100 µg/mL streptomycin), Flush each side twice to ensure removal of bone marrow completely from the medullary cavity.
5. Collect the marrow plug, and gently aspirate it several times with a 25-gage needle to disrupt cellular clumps.
6. Centrifuge the cells at 900g for 5 min, resuspend the cell pellet in complete medium, and adjust cell concentration to 5×10^7 nucleated cells per ml.
7. Plate cells into a 25-cm^2 Corning flask, and incubate it with 95% air and 5% CO_2 at 37°C.

3.1.2. MSC Isolation and Expansion

1. Change the medium every 4 d; retain the adherent cells, and discard nonadherent hematopoietic cells (*see* **Fig. 1A** and **Note 1**). Colonies of MSCs appear on average 7–9 d after plating.
2. When MSCs grow to approx 70% confluence (about 12 d), remove the medium

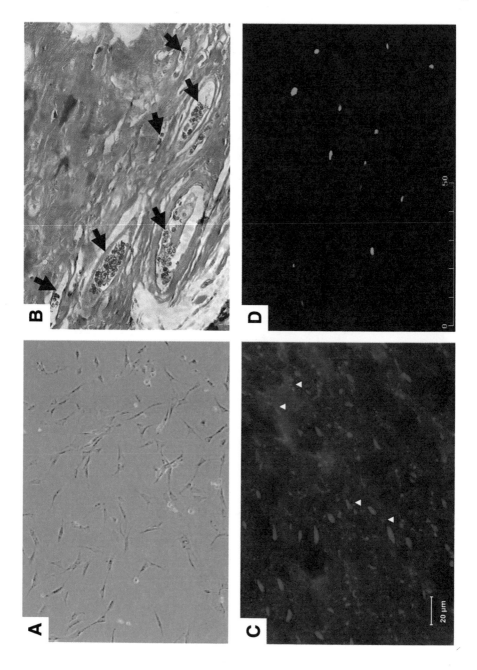

from the dish, wash the dishes twice with D-Hanks' solution to remove any trace of serum, and then incubate with 0.25% trypsin/1 mM EDTA for between 3 and 5 min at 37°C. Check cells until most of the cells are detached. Inhibit trypsin with complete medium, and centrifuge cells at 900g for 5 min. Replate at a 1:2 dilution.

3. In a series of passages, use homogeneous MSCs that were devoid of hematopoietic cells for cell expansion.

4. Keep nondifferentiated MSCs in long-term culture. MSCs have the potential to differentiate to multiple-cell types so that passaging before confluence is critical to avoid autodifferentiation in vitro (*see* **Note 2**).

3.2. Graft MSC Preparation (see Note 3)

1. Expand purified MSCs further in culture until the day before implantation.
2. To identify the graft cells, label MSCs with DAPI at a concentration of 10 μg/mL in the culture medium overnight. (DAPI is a fluorescent DNA-intercalating dye.)
3. Aspirate the medium; quickly wash the cells with Hanks' five times to remove unincorporated DAPI, and keep at 4°C.
4. Detect DAPI incorporation: the presence of DAPI-labeled nuclei is confirmed under the fluorescence microscope using the DAPI filter to focus on the cell nuclei.
5. Detach the labeled MSCs from the bottom of the flasks with 0.25% trypsin/1 mM EDTA, when most of the MSCs are in suspension, stop the enzymatic digestion by addition of the same amount of complete medium. Pellet the cells by centrifugation at 900g for 5 min, count the MSCs in a hemocytometer, and resuspend the cells in serum-free DMEM to adjust the cell concentration to 5×10^7/mL.

3.3. Myocardial Infarction Model

1. Anesthetize rats with sodium pentobarbital (40 mg/kg ip).
2. After anesthesia, place the rat in a supine position and tape all four paws on their respective sides
3. Intubate rats with an 18-gage intravenous catheter with a tapered tip via the oral cavity or a tracheotomy. Close a cooling blade to the catheter; vapor should appear on it if the catheter enters the trachea, and no vapor should appear if the

---

Fig. 1. (A) Phase contrast photomicrograph of rat mesenchymal stem cells (MSCs) in culture. MSCs appear spindle-shaped and mononucleard (original magnification ×10). **(B)** Section of a heart implanted with MSCs stained with Masson trichrome staining. Arrows indicate blood vessels in the transplanted scar (original magnification ×20). **(C)** Evidence for gap junction differentiation of engrafted cells. This section was stained with anti-connexin 43.TRITC-conjugated second antibody was used. One month after transplantation, DAPI-positive cells (blue) expressing connexin 43 (red, triangles). **(D)** TUNEL staining of ischemic myocardium implanted with MSCs demonstrates apoptotic nuclei.

catheter enters the esophagus. Rats are mechanically ventilated on a rodent ventilator with room air. (A respiratory rate of 110/min, a tidal volume of 1.5 mL, and a ventilator rate of 110/min were found to produce optimal values of pO_2, pCO_2, and pH.)

4. Open the chest through a left thoracotomy in the fourth intercostal space using a microcoagulator. Extend the medial aspect of the incision cranially to form a flap that is retracted to expose the heart.

5. Make a small opening in the pericardium using forceps and scissors. Pass a 6-0 nylon suture through the superficial myocardium of the left anterior descending coronary artery about 2–3 mm from the tip of the left auricle. Ligate the suture to induce coronary occlusion. Successful performance of coronary occlusion is verified by observation of the development of a pale color in the distal myocardium after ligation.

6. Close the chest in layers by using a 5-0 polyester fiber suture after the coronary occlusion is completed: close the muscle with a polypropylene suture, and close the skin with stainless steel wound clips that will be removed 10 d postoperatively.

7. Wean the rats from the ventilator when the animals wake, warm them with a heated water blanket, and give 100% oxygen via nasal cone.

3.4. MSC Implantation by Direct Intramyocardial Injection

1. Two weeks after production of a myocardial infarction, return the rats to the operating room for a second procedure. Anesthetize, intubate, and ventilate the rats as described in **Subheading 3.3.** Reexpose the heart via a midline sternotomy.

2. Under direct visualization, inject the suspension of MSCs (0.2 mL, 1×10^7 cells) into the periphery of the scar tissue at four sites (up, down, anterior, and posterior, 50 µL/site) using a 31-gage needle to facilitate the survival of transplant cells and potential connection with host cardiomyocytes. Inject the same volume of medium at corresponding sites in the control group (*see* **Note 4**).

3. Close the chest, muscle, and skin as described in Subheading 3.3., and allow the rats to recover.

3.5. Evaluation of Left Ventricular Function With Langendorff Preparation

1. Euthanize rats using an overdose of pentobarbital (80 mg/kg) 4 wk after cell transplantation. Isolate and perfuse hearts via the aorta in a Langendorff apparatus with oxygenated Krebs Henseleit buffer equilibrated with 5% CO_2 and 95% O_2 at 37°C.

2. Insert a latex balloon (filled with water and connected to the pressure transducer) into the left ventricle through the mitral valve, to connect to a pressure transducer, a transducer amplifier, and a differentiator amplifier.

3. After 30 min of stabilization at 37°C, measure coronary flow by taking the mean value of a 2-min timed collection in an empty beating state.

4. Increase the balloon volume gradually by stepwise addition of saline solution. Record the left ventricular systolic and diastolic pressure (LVSP and LVEDP), the maximal rate of myocardial contraction, and the maximal rate of myocardial relaxation (maximum dP/dt and minimum dP/dt) at each balloon volume. Increase

the balloon size by addition of water in 20-μL increments from 50 μL until the LVEDP reaches 30 mmHg. Calculate the developed pressure as the difference between peak systolic pressure and end-diastolic pressure.

5. After measurements are completed, inject 10 mL of a 20% solution of KCl into the aortic root to arrest the heart.

3.6. Assessment of Angiogenesis After MSC Implantation

This step is described in **Subheadings 3.6.1.** and **3.6.2.**, including (1) evaluation of myocardial blood flow using radioactive microsphere, and (2) measurement of vascular density using Masson trichrome.

3.6.1. Evaluation of Myocardial Blood Flow Using Radioactive Microsphere

1. Four weeks after transplantation, blood flow to the normal, border and infarct myocardium is measured with radionuclide-labeled microspheres.
2. A suspension of ^{99m}Tc-labeled microspheres (0.15 mL, 3×10^5 beads) is infused into the left atrium with aorta occlusion of 30 s.
3. The left ventricle is incised into normal tissue, border zone, and scar zone.
4. Each section is weighed, and the radioactivity in each fraction is measured with a γ-counter. The ratio of counts per milligram in the scar and border to the normal zone is characterized as relative myocardial blood flow (*see* **Note 5**).

3.6.2. Measurement of Vascular Density Using Masson Trichrome

The sections were stained with Masson trichrome, as follows:

1. Rinse in Bouin's solution overnight, then wash in water for 5 min the next day. Stain in Weigert's iron hematoxylin for 10 min.
2. Wash in ddH$_2$O, and stain in Biebrich scarlet-acid fuchsin solution for 15 min.
3. Wash in ddH$_2$O, and place the slides in phosphomolybdic-phosphotungstic acid solution for 15 min.
4. Stain sections in aniline blue solution for 10 min.
5. Wash in ddH$_2$O, and place slides in 1% acetic water for 5 min.
6. Following dehydrating and mounting, process the slides for morphometry using a computerized image analysis for quantitative assessment of vascular density in the myocardium.
7. In the images, red cells in blood vessels were stained red, and collagen in the infarct zone stained blue. Count the number of blood vessels in 10 random fields (magnification ×20). Calculate the average of the 10 high-power fields (hpf), and define the vascular density as blood vessels/hpf (**Fig. 1B**).

3.7. Myocardial Differentiation of Grafted MSCs by Immunohistochemistry

This step is described in **Subheadings 3.7.1.–3.7.4.**, including (1) tissue preparation, (2) identification of DAPI-positive cells to evaluate the survival

MSCs, (3) assessment of the myocardial differentiation of graft MSCs, and (4) analysis of graft–host myocardial gap junctions.

3.7.1. Tissue Preparation

1. After arrest of the heart, distend the ventricular volume to a balloon pressure of 30 mmHg.
2. Fix the heart with 4% phosphate-buffered formalin solution in the distended state.
3. One hour after fixation, remove the balloon, and remove the atria and great arteries at their origin. Embed the heart in Tissue-Tek O.C.T. compound, and then freeze it in dry ice. Section the heart into 8-μm slices, and process it for histological and immunohistochemical examination.

3.7.2. Celluar Identification of DAPI-Positive Cells

The survival of implanted MSCs is examined in rats by measuring the DAPI positive cells in sections harvested from ischemic myocardium as described in **Subheadings 3.7.3.** and **3.7.4.** Briefly, heart sections harvested from the left ventricle are embedded in Tissue-Tek O.C.T compound, and the specimens are frozen in dry ice and stored at –70°C until use. Frozen sections are quantified for DAPI fluorescence-positive MSCs nuclei.

3.7.3. Regeneration of Myocardial Tissue

1. The same section is selected for immunofluorescent staining.
2. The following cardiac markers are tested using primary mouse monoclonal antibodies: α-actin and desmin.
3. After blocking in normal serum, sections are treated with the appropriate monoclonal antibodies (1:50) for 30 min at 37°C and then incubated with secondary TRITC-conjugated goat antimouse IgG (1:200) for 30 min at 37°C.
4. Cells derived from MSCs are identified by their blue nuclei under the Zeiss Axioplan 2 microscope.
5. Digital images are transferred to a computer equipped with Spot Software for assessment.

3.7.4. Analysis of Graft–Host Myocardium Gap Junctions

1. The cardiac muscle-specific intercalated disk is examined using primary mouse monoclonal antibody to connexin 43 by the immunofluorescent staining protocol as described in **Subheading 3.7.3.** Sections are treated with the first antibodies (1:50) for 30 min at 37°C and then incubated with secondary TRITC-conjugated goat antimouse IgG (1:200) for 30 min at 37°C (**Fig. 1C**).

3.8. Determination of Peri-Infarct Cardiomyocyte Apoptosis Using TUNEL Assay

1. The cryosections from the midcavity of rat heart were stained with fluorescent TUNEL using a commercially available kit, as described in **Subheading 2.**

2. Thin myocardial sections are first treated with proteinase K (250 µL) and then incubated with biotin-dUTP, TdT.
3. Slides are finally treated with avidin-FITC.
4. Apoptosis cells are visualized and acquired by the Bio-Rad 1024 ES confocal microscope. Apoptotic nuclei show strong but diffuse FITC fluorescence.
5. The TUNEL-positive cells are counted in peri-infarct regions. For each heart, the numbers of TUNEL-positive myocyte nuclei are scored per unit field. Images are taken at high magnification (×100) (**Fig. 1D**).

4. Notes

1. An alternative for removing contaminating hematopoietic cells prior to plating is density gradient *(5,6)*. Briefly, load the bone marrow aspirate on a 20 to 60% Percoll gradient and centrifuge at 2000*g* for 30 min; then transfer the interface cell layer to a tube with PBS and centrifuge at 900*g* for 5 min twice to remove the Percoll. After that step, the pellets contain the mononuclear cells for MSC culture. According to our experience, density gradient is not necessary because MSCs can be isolated from hematopoietic cells by its adherent characterization. This additional step can compromise the activity and proliferative potential of MSCs.
2. Purification of MSCs: MSCs have been shown to contain a heterogenous population of cells, most of which are nondifferentiating cells. However, when they are subcloned, special subsets of progenitor cells can be isolated for further research.
3. To trace the fate of grafted MSCs, bromodeoxyuridine (BrdU) and DAPI are common reagents for cell labeling. DAPI, a fluorescent dye labeling the nucleus of cells, is nontoxic to living cells *(7)*. As for slow loss of fluorescence, in vivo DAPI-labeled MSC trafficking can be observed for about 1 mo, suggesting that DAPI will be useful for short-term in vivo tracking studies. Compared with DAPI, BrdU is suitable for long-term investigation because BrdU can incorporate stably into DNA. Intensively positive grafted cells in myocardium staining can be identified when cells are incubated with high levels of BrdU (0.1 mg BrdU/mL culture medium) for 2 d before transplantation *(8)*. BrdU can also appear in cytoplasm in immunohistochemical staining for low-level unincorporated BrdU in plasma.
4. An alternative method to administer the cells in small animals is nonselective coronary delivery *(9)*, which can improve the region of distribution *(10)*. Briefly, the ascending aorta is exposed through a parasternotomy and looped after dissection. An MSC suspension is infused into the left ventricular chamber with an insulin syringe while ascending aorta was temporarily occluded for 20 s. When the needle reaches the high-pressure left ventricular chamber, a rush of blood will enter the syringe. After the infusion, the MSCs were trapped within the coronary capillaries in the noninfarct area. MSCs have the ability to migrate to the infarct zone thereafter. Our data show that grafted MSCs no longer stay in the coronary capillaries but appear to be integrated into the myocardium interstitium at 1 wk after intracoronary infusion. The apparent risk of intracoronary trans-

plantation is coronary embolism, that will develop into a large-scale infarction. According to our experience, controlling the number of graft cells (less than 1×10^6) and filtering the cells through a 30-μm nylon mesh is crucial for success in intracoronary infusion. Cell clumps can be avoided by filtering before infusion *(11)*.

5. For measuring myocardial blood flow, we developed an in vivo technique of microsphere injection to avoid leakage to the systemic circulation. Injection of microspheres into the left atrium in vivo may cause most of the microspheres to be dispersed into cardiac capillaries when the ascending aorta is temporarily occluded. Although ex vivo microsphere injection in an isolated heart can deliver most of the microspheres into the myocardium, it is not in a physiologic condition because the left atrium plays an important role in mixing microspheres with blood.

References

1. Krause, D. S. (2002) Plasticity of marrow-derived stem cells. *Gene Ther.* **9**, 754–758.
2. Makino, S., Fukuda, K., Miyoshi, S. et al. (1999) Cardiomyocytes can be generated from marrow stromal cells in vitro. *J. Clin. Invest.* **103**, 697–705.
3. Toma, C., Pittenger, M. F., Cahill, K. S., et al. (2002) Human mesenchymal stem cells differentiate to a cardiomyocyte phenotype in the adult murine heart. *Circulation* **105**, 93–98.
4. Wang, J. S., Shum-Tim, D., Galipeau, J., et al. (2000) Marrow stromal cells for cellular cardiomyoplasty: feasibility and potential clinical advantages. *J. Thorac. Cardiovasc. Surg.* **120**, 999–1005.
5. Tomita, S., Li, R. K., Weisel, R. D., et al. (1999) Autologous transplantation of bone marrow cells improves damaged heart function. *Circulation* **100**, II247–II256.
6. Shake, J. G., Gruber, P. J., Baumgartner, W. A., et al. (2002) Mesenchymal stem cell implantation in a swine myocardial infarct model: engraftment and functional effects. *Ann. Thorac. Surg.* **73**, 1919–1925.
7. Dorfman, J., Duong, M., Zibaitis, A., et al. (1998) Myocardial tissue engineering with autologous myoblast implantation. *J. Thorac. Cardiovasc. Surg.* **116**, 744–751.
8. Kim, E. J., Li, R. K., Weisel, R. D., et al. (2001) Angiogenesis by endothelial cell transplantation. *J. Thorac. Cardiovasc. Surg.* **122**, 963–971.
9. Wang, J. S., Shum-Tim, D., Chedrawy, E., and Chiu, R. C. (2001) The coronary delivery of marrow stromal cells for myocardial regeneration: pathophysiologic and therapeutic implications. *J. Thorac. Cardiovasc. Surg.* **122**, 699–705.
10. Kessler, P. D. and Byrne, B. J. (1999) Myoblast cell grafting into heart muscle: cellular biology and potential applications. *Annu. Rev. Physiol.* **61**, 219–242.
11. Suzuki, K., Brand, N. J., Smolenski, R. T., et al. (2000) Development of a novel method for cell transplantation through the coronary artery. *Circulation* **102**, III359–III364.

12

Cellular Therapy With Autologous Skeletal Myoblasts for Ischemic Heart Disease and Heart Failure

Yao Liang Tang

Summary

Cardiomyocytes are final differentiated cells that lose the ability to regenerate. Autologous cellular transplantation for cardiac repair has recently emerged as a promising new approach for end-stage heart failure that avoids the risk of immune rejection and ethical problems. Skeletal myoblasts (or satellite cells) are committed progenitor cells located under the basal lamina of adult skeletal muscle; they are committed to multiply after injury. They are highly resistant to ischemia and possess a considerable potential for division in culture. The cardiac milieu might alter the developmental program of grafted myoblast and facilitate their conversion to the slow-twitch phenotype, which is capable of performing cardiac work. We have used autologous cultured myoblast grafts for mouse and rat myocardial infarction in more than 200 cases. From these grafting experiments, it has been shown that cultured autologous myoblast grafting is a useful technique in the treatment of ischemic heart failure. This chapter offers a step-by-step guide to a successful research project on cultured myoblasts for the treatment of myocardial infarction, as well as a set of special techniques for yielding large numbers of skeletal myoblasts and studying postimplantation myocardial repair.

Key Words: Myoblast; cell transplantation; myocardial infarction.

1. Introduction

Cardiac muscle is composed of terminally differentiated cell that have lost the ability to regenerate. Autologous cellular transplantation for cardiac repair

From: *Methods in Molecular Medicine, vol. 112: Molecular Cardiology: Methods and Protocols*
Edited by: Z. Sun © Humana Press Inc., Totowa, NJ

has recently emerged as a promising new approach for end-stage heart failure that avoids the risk of immune rejection and ethical problems. Skeletal myoblasts (or satellite cells) are committed progenitor cells located under the basal lamina of adult skeletal muscle *(1)*; they are committed to multiply after injury *(2)*. They are highly resistant to ischemia and possess a considerable potential for division in culture. The cardiac milieu contains specific signal molecules and growth factors that might alter the developmental program of grafted myoblasts and facilitate their conversion to a slow-twitch phenotype capable of performing cardiac work *(3)*. This procedure may be induced by expression of related development genes in sequence. New myocardium forms when myoblasts integrate into healthy host tissue after implantation in vivo. This chapter discusses approaches to myoblast isolation, culture, and cell implantation. Specific protocols are given for techniques that have been shown to be effective in yielding large numbers of skeletal myoblasts and studying postimplantation myocardial repair. First, two methods for separation of myoblasts from skeletal muscle are given, followed by techniques for myoblast expansion and labeling. Second, methods used for establishing myocardial infarction model and delivery of a myoblasts into the damaged heart are described. Finally, the therapeutic effect of implantation is assessed through myocardial regeneration and left ventricular function.

2. Materials

1. Male (inbred) Lewis rats (Harlan, Indianapolis, IN).
2. Dulbecco's modified Eagle's medium (DMEM; Gibco, Grand Island, NY).
3. Collagenase IA and hyaluronidase I (Worthington, Lakewood, NJ).
4. Sterile gauze pads (Tyco Healthcare Group, Mansfield, MA).
5. Scalpel, blade, small forceps, and dissecting scissors (F.S.T., North Vancouver, BC, Canada).
6. 0.25% Trypsin/1 mM EDTA (Gibco).
7. 25 cm^2 Flask (Corning, Corning, NY).
8. Matrigel (Universal Biologicals, London, UK).
9. Complete medium: 20% fetal bovine serum (FBS), 10% horse serum, and 0.5% chicken embryo extract in DMEM.
10. Sterile cloning cylinders (Bel-Art Products, Pequannock, NJ).
11. 4,6-Diamino-2-phenylindole (DAPI; Sigma, St. Louis, MO).
12. 18-Gage catheter (Abbott Ireland, Sligo, Rep. of Ireland).
13. 6-0 polypropylene thread (Ethilon, Somerville, NJ).
14. 31-Gage needle (Becton Dickinson, Franklin Lakes, NJ).
15. 30-μm Nylon net filter (Millipore, Billerica, MA).
16. Harvard Inspira advanced safety ventilator (Harvard Apparatus, Boston, MA).
17. Langendorff apparatus (Harvard Apparatus).
18. Echocardiograms (Hewlett-Packard Sonos 5500).

19. Tissue-Tek® O.C.T (Sakura Finetek U.S.A., Torrance, CA).
20. Weigert's iron hematoxylin, Accustain trichrome stain kit, and Boulin's solution (Sigma).
21. Mouse antihuman Desmin monoclonal antibody (BD Transduction Laboratories).
22. Mouse monoclonal antibody to connexin-43 (BD Transduction Laboratories).
23. TRITC-conjugated goat antimouse IgG (Sigma).
24. Fluorescent Mounting Medium (DAKO, Carpinteria, CA).
25. Zeiss Axioplan 2 Microscope.
26. Spot Software (Diagnostic Instruments).

3. Methods

The methods described below cover various aspects of skeletal myoblast implantation for improving heart function: (1) culture of skeletal myoblasts, (2) purification and evaluation of myoblasts, (3) myocardial infarction model and myoblast implantation, (4) echocardiographical assessment of heart function, and (5) examination of the myocardial differentiation of grafted myoblasts.

3.1. Skeletal Myoblast Cultures

Myoblasts may be cultured by a variety of methods. Two commonly used approaches are described here. The standard method provides an effective means of producing large quantities of myoblasts, whereas the single myoblast isolation method yields highly purified myoblasts.

3.1.1. Standard Methods (4)

1. Euthanize rats using an overdose of pentobarbital (80 mg/kg) injected ip.
2. Sink rats in 70% alcohol for 8 min.
3. Incise the skin in the hindlimb, excise the right and left tibialis anterior, soleus, gastrocnemius, quadriceps, and extensor digitorum longus, and put them in a dish containing Tyrode solution.
4. Carefully remove the tendon and the aponeurotic tissue from the muscle tissue with a scissor.
5. Mince the muscles in 2% FBS/Hanks' solution with a scalpel.
6. Digest the muscle tissue at 37°C with 2 mg/mL collagenase I and 0.2% hyaluronidase/DMEM for 1 h in a shaker at 37°C.
7. Enzymatically dissociate with 0.25% trypsin/1 mM EDTA for 20 min at 37°C.
8. Pass samples through a sterile gauze pad.
9. Collect the cells by centrifugation at 900g for 7 min.
10. Resuspend the cells in full DMEM medium, and count the cells with a hematocytometer to adjust the concentration of 5×10^5 cells/mL.
11. Assess the viability by the trypan blue exclusion test.
12. Plate the cells in a 25-cm^2 Corning flask in full DMEM. Incubate the cells with 95% air and 5% CO_2 at 37°C.

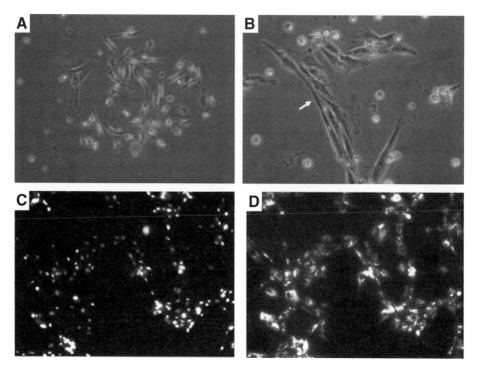

Fig. 1. (A) Primary skeletal myoblasts in culture. **(B)** The myoblasts fused (arrow) when cultured in low serum medium. **(C)** and **(D)** In vitro characterization of myoblasts using immunofluorescence staining with anti-desmin antibody. Nuclei were counterstained blue with DAPI, in the same field, Note that some myoblasts fused and differentiated into multinucleated myotubes (original magnification ×20).

13. One day later, wash the cells and change the growth medium.
14. At 70% confluence, split the cells into two flasks to avoid fusion. The first passage is carried out on d 4 and is followed by subsequent passage every 48–72 h (*see* **Note 1** and **Fig. 1A,B**).

3.1.2. Single Myofiber Isolation Method

This method was developed by Rosemblatt *(5)* to obtain highly purified myoblasts.

1. Dissect the extensor digitorum longus carefully away from the surrounding musculature in rat.
2. Digest muscles for 90 min at 37°C in 0.2% (w/v) type 1 collagenase in DMEM, supplemented with 2 m*M* L-glutamine (Sigma) and 1% penicillin/streptomycin solution.
3. Transfer the digested muscle to a plastic Petri dish containing 8 mL DMEM with a Pasteur pipet.

4. Separate muscle fibers from the whole muscle by repeated pipeting with a wide-mouth Pasteur pipet until most of the muscle fibers are liberated from the muscle surface under a dissecting microscope.
5. Place single, intact muscle fibers into each well of a 24-well culture plate.
6. Prior to plating, coat flask with 0.1% Matrigel, a solubilized basement membrane to which muscle fibers adhere and on which differentiation of myogenic cells is enhanced.
7. Bathe the fibers in 0.5 mL of medium comprising 20% FBS, 10% horse serum, and 5 ng/mL recombinant basic fibroblast growth factor (rbFGF) in DMEM after fibers attach to the dish. Incubate in a water-saturated environment at 5% CO_2 and 37°C for 3 d. In these culture conditions, skeletal myoblasts emigrate from the fiber and divide.
8. Remove the muscle fiber from culture at 90 h to prevent it from contributing further to the surrounding cell population (optional), and feed the myoblasts with complete medium (*see* **Note 2**).
9. Passage cells using 0.25% trypsin before cells reach 75% confluence to maintain the undifferentiated state.

Rosenblatt's method can yield myoblasts of higher purity than traditional methods. With one to two passages, each muscle fiber can generate 3×10^4 to 5×10^5 myoblast. The intact muscle is critical for harvesting highly purified myoblasts (*see* **Note 3**).

3.2. Purification of Myoblast and Purity Evaluation

The steps are described in **Subheading s3.2.1.–3.2.3.**, including (1) purification of myoblasts by cloning ring or different adhesion procedures and (2) evaluation of purity by fluorescent immunocytochemical method.

3.2.1. Cloning of Myoblasts Using Cloning Cylinders

1. Dilute cells at a concentration of 100 cells/mL, and seed diluted cells into a 60-mm² Petri dishes. Incubate the cells at 37°C in a humidified chamber equilibrated with 5% CO_2 for 10 d.
2. Inspect the dish with the aid of a microscope, and mark the desired colonies that have the myoblast phenotype on the bottom of the dish.
3. Remove the growth medium from dish, and wash twice with 5 mL D-Hank's solution to remove any trace of serum.
4. Dip the thicker edge of the cloning cylinder into sterile silicone, and apply it around the selected colony by lightly pressing against the Petri dish.
5. Add 75 µL of 0.25% trypsin/1 m*M* EDTA solution to the center of the cylinder. Incubate at 37°C for 5 min, and check the colony under the microscope to ensure that the cells have rounded up and detached.
6. Collect the cells with a pipet, and transfer to a centrifuge tube.
7. Add complete medium to neutralize the trypsin, and incubate at 37°C in a humidified chamber equilibrated with 5% CO_2.

3.2.2. Purification of Myoblasts From Fibroblasts by Adhesive Difference

Remove fibroblasts from the cultures by repeated differential adhesion steps whereby the supernatant containing the slowly adhering myoblasts is removed and transferred to a fresh flask, and the fibroblasts are discarded. Repeat this isolation step three times.

3.2.3. Evaluation of the Purity of the Cells for Presence of Desmin

1. Culture cells on chamber slides, incubated to about 75% confluence.
2. Wash the cells in three changes of phosphate-buffered saline solution (PBS).
3. Aspirate the last change of PBS. Fixed the cells with –20°C methanol for 5 min.
4. Wash three times in PBS. Leave the third wash in contact with the slide.
5. Incubate cells with 100 μL 5% horse serum in PBS at room temperature for 30 min.
6. Place 100 μL 1:50 dilution of mouse antihuman desmin monoclonal antibody, and incubate for 30 min at 37 °C.
7. Wash three times in PBS.
8. Incubate slide with 100 μL 1:200 dilution TRITC-conjugated antimouse IgG for 30 min at 37°C in the darkness.
9. Wash the cover slip three times in PBS as above.
10. Counterstain nuclei with DAPI.
11. Place a drop of DAKO Flu-mountant onto a clean glass slide, and place the cover slip face down onto the mountant.
12. View under a fluorescent microscope using a Texas Red filter to focus on the cell plasma, followed by a DAPI filter to focus on the nuclei (**Fig. 1C,D**).
13. Calculate the proportion of myoblasts by dividing the number of desmin-positive cells by the total number of DAPI-positive cells in random fields.

3.3. Cell Preparation for Implantation

1. Expand purified myoblasts further in culture until the day of implantation.
2. To identify the graft cells, label myoblasts with DAPI at a concentration of 10 μg/mL in the culture medium overnight. (DAPI is a fluorescent DNA-intercalating dye.)
3. Aspirate the medium. Quick wash the cells in five changes of Hanks' solution to get rid of uncombined DAPI.
4. Harvest the cells with trypsinization, and assess the viability with 0.4% trypan blue. Keep the cells at 4°C before implantation.
5. Detection of DAPI incorporation: view the flask under the fluorescent microscope using the DAPI filter to focus on the cell nuclei.
6. Transfer cells to 1-mL syringes, and warm them to room temperature before implantation.

3.4. Myocardial Infarction Model

1. Anesthetize rats with sodium pentobarbital (40 mg/kg, ip).
2. After anesthesia, place the rat in a supine position and tape all four paws on their respective sides.

3. Intubate rats with an 18-gage intravenous catheter with a tapered tip via the oral cavity or a tracheotomy. Close a cooling blade to the catheter. Vapor should appear on it if the catheter enters the trachea; no vapor will appear on it if the catheter enters the esophagus. Rats will be mechanically ventilated on a rodent ventilator with room air. (A respiratory rate of 110/min, a tidal volume of 1.5 mL, and a ventilator rate of 110/min was found to produce optimal values of pO_2, pCO_2, and pH.)

4. Open the chest through a left thoracotomy in the fourth intercostal space using a microcoagulator. Extend the medial aspect of the incision cranially to form a flap that is retracted to expose the heart.

5. Make a small opening in the pericardium using forceps and scissors. Pass a 6-0 nylon suture through the superficial myocardium of the left anterior descending coronary artery about 2–3 mm from the tip of the left auricle. Ligate the suture to induce coronary occlusion. Verify successful performance of coronary occlusion by observation of the development of a pale color in the distal myocardium after ligation

6. Close the chest in layers using a 5-0 polyester fiber suture after the coronary occlusion is completed, close the muscle with a polypropylene suture, and close the skin with a stainless steel wound clip, which will be removed 10 d postoperatively.

7. Remove rats from the respirator, keep warm using a heated water blanket, and give 100% oxygen via a nasal cone.

3.5. Myoblast Implantation

Successful delivery of myoblasts in the myocardium can be achieved by intramyocardial injection and intracoronary infusion.

1. Intramyocardial injection is relative simple. Briefly, under direct vision, inject 0.2 mL (1×10^7) of DAPI labeled myoblast into the border zone of infarction at four sites (up, down, anterior, and posterior, 50 μL/site) using a 31-gage needle to facilitate the survival of transplant cells. Inject control groups with the same volume of cell-free DMEM at corresponding sites (*see* **Note 4**). The site appears edemic after successful injection.

2. Intracoronary infusion is achieved through a trans-left ventricular chamber infusion in rats or by selective coronary infusion in larger animal. In brief, expose the ascending aorta through a parasternotomy and loop after dissection. Infuse the myoblast suspension into the left ventricular chamber while occluding the ascending aorta temporarily for 20 s. After the infusion, the myoblasts are trapped within the coronary capillaries in the noninfarct area and have the ability to migrate to the infarct zone thereafter (*see* **Note 5**).

3.6. Left Ventricular Functional Assessment

Left ventricular function can be analyzed by a Langendorff preparation (**Subheading 3.6.1.**) or echocardiography (**Subheading 3.6.2.**).

3.6.1. Functional Assessment of the Heart in a Langendorff Perfusion System

1. Euthanize rats using an overdose of pentobarbital (80 mg/kg) 4 wk after cell transplantation. Isolate and perfuse hearts via the aorta in a Langendorff apparatus with oxygenated Krebs Henseleit buffer equilibrated with 5% CO_2 and 95% O_2 at 37°C.
2. Insert a latex balloon (filled with water and connected to the pressure transducer) into the left ventricle through the mitral valve to connect to a pressure transducer, a transducer amplifier, and a differentiator amplifier.
3. After 30 min of stabilization at 37°C, measure coronary flow by taking the mean value of 2-min timed collection in an empty beating state.
4. Increase the balloon volume gradually by stepwise addition of saline solution. Record the left ventricular systolic and diastolic pressure (LVSP and LVEDP), the maximal rate of myocardial contraction and the maximal rate of myocardial relaxation (maximum dP/dt and minimum dP/dt) at each balloon volume. the balloon size was increased by the addition of water in 20-µL increments from 50 µL until the LVEDP reaches 30 mmHg. Calculate the developed pressure as the difference between peak systolic pressure and end-diastolic pressure.
5. After the measurement is completed, inject 10 mL of a 20% KCl solution into the aortic root to arrest the heart.

3.6.2. Left Ventricular Function Can Be Assessed by 2D Echocardiography (see *Fig. 2*)

1. Under general anesthesia with pentobarbital (40 mg/kg), shave the rat's chest, and apply a layer of acoustic coupling gel to minimize imaging artifacts.
2. Perform B- and M-mode measurements with a commercially available 15 MHz transducer system. Place the rats in the supine position.
3. Record echocardiograms through parasternal long-axis views followed by parasternal short-axis views, making the mitral valve, aortic valve, and the papillary muscle visible.
4. Take measurements of the left ventricular end-diastolic volume (LVEDV) and the left ventricular end-systolic volume (LVESV). Then calculate the left ventricular ejection fractions (LVEF %) (LVEF = (LVEDV – LVESV)/LVEDV) (*6*).

3.7. Pathologic Assessment

The pathologic assessment is described in **Subheadings 3.7.1.–3.7.5.**, including (1) tissue preparation, (2) assessment of left ventricular remodeling, (3) survival of grafted cells, (4) regeneration of myocardial tissue, and (5) gap junction between grafted cells and host myocardium.

3.7.1. Heart Preparation

1. After the last echocardiography evaluation, euthanize rats with an overdose of pentobarbital. Remove the heart and rapidly rinse into PBS.

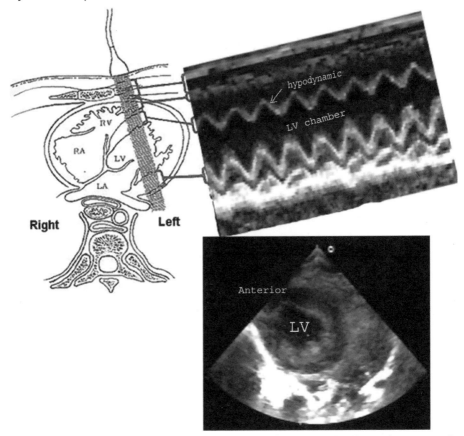

Fig. 2. Functional assessment with echocardiography. Left: the probe was positioned for a parasternal short-axis view, obtaining a good image quality at the midpapillary muscle level of the left ventricle (LV) in 2D echocardiography. Right bottom: 2D measurement of LV anterior and posterior wall movement. Right top: M-mode was acquired for measurement of LV dimension at end-diastole and end-systole in the cardiac cycle. LA, left atrium; RA, right atrium; RV, right ventricle.

2. Embed the left ventricle in Tissue-Tek O.C.T compound, freeze the specimen in dry ice, and store it at –80°C until use.
3. Section heart tissue to yield 8-μm-thick slices with a cryostat.
4. The heart sections were processed for morphometry (Masson trichrome staining) and immunohistochemical examination (cardiac α-actin, connexin 43).

3.7.2. Assessment of Left Ventricular Remodeling Using Masson Trichrome

The sections were stained with Masson trichrome:

1. Rinse in Bovin's solution overnight, then wash in water for 5 min the next day. Stain in Weigert's iron hematoxylin for 10 min.

2. Wash in ddH$_2$O, and stain in Biebrich scarlet-acid fuchsin solution for 15 min.
3. Wash in ddH$_2$O, and place the slides in phosphomolybdic-phosphotungstic acid solution for 15 min.
4. Stain sections in aniline blue solution for 10 min.
5. Wash in ddH$_2$O, and place slides in 1% acetic water for 5 min.
6. Following dehydration and mounting, process slides to morphometry using a computerized image analysis for quantitative assessment of left ventricular re-modeling.
7. In the images, nuclei display black, muscle fibers display red, and collagen displays blue. Measure the ratio of scar length to the left ventricular circumference of the endocardium and epicardium as a percentage to define the infarct index *(7)*.

3.7.3. Celluar Identification of DAPI-Positive Cells

, The survival of implanted myoblasts was examined in rats by measuring the DAPI positive cells in sections harvested from ischemic myocardium as described below in **Subheading 3.7.4.** Frozen sections were quantified for DAPI fluorescence-positive myoblast nuclei.

3.7.4. Regeneration of Myocardial Tissue

The same section was selected for immunofluorescent staining. The following cardiac markers were tested using primary mouse monoclonal antibodies: cardiac α-actin and connexin 43.

1. Block with 5% horse serum in PBS for 10 min.
2. Treat sections with the mouse monoclonal anticardiac α-actin 1:50 for 30 min at 37°C.
3. Wash three times in PBS, and incubate sections with secondary TRITC-conjugated goat antimouse IgG 1:200 for 30 min at 37°C.
4. After several washes, mount the sections with Fluorescent Mounting Medium.
5. Identify myoblasts by their blue nuclei under the Zeiss Axioplan 2 Microscope. Transfer digital images to a computer equipped with Spot Software.

3.7.5. Analysis of Graft–Host Myocardium Gap Junction

The cardiac muscle-specific intercalated disks were evaluated using primary mouse monoclonal antibody to connexin 43. The immunofluorescent method is in **Subheading 3.7.4.** Sections were treated with the first antibodies (1:50) for 30 min at 37°C and then incubated with secondary TRITC-conjugated goat antimouse IgG (1:200) for 30 min at 37°C (*see* **Note 6**).

4. Notes

1. To prevent myoblasts from premature differentiation and fusion in vitro, keeping high-serum medium and passaging the myoblast cultures every 4 d before 75% confluence are critical because the terminal differentiation will happen in low-

level serum (2% horse serum, 2 mmol/L glutamine in DMEM) or when myoblasts reach confluence *(8)*. Keeping myoblast in low-serum medium for 5 d facilitates formation of myotubes.

2. bFGF can be added to the medium to increase in vitro myoblast expansion. The recommended concentration of bFGF is 5 ng/mL. We suggest using bFGF only after the myoblast purification procedure *(9)*.

3. The standard method has the attractive feature of simplicity. Cultured myoblasts are composed of about 80% myoblasts and 20% fibroblasts. The fibroblasts have a higher proliferation capacity than myoblast. It will outgrow myoblasts and cause detrimental effects in implantation by facilitating scar expansion. Although the single myofiber isolation method is complicated to handle, it has the advantage of ensuring purification of myoblasts from the first step. Despite the larger total number of cells produced by the standard method, the intact myoblasts that maintain normal morphology and function obtained by the standard method are less than 0.01% of what can be recovered by the single myofiber isolation method *(5)*. The cloning cylinder technique can be used for selecting myoblasts with superior characteristics and propagating them for implantation. It is a feasible way to free myoblasts from fibroblast contamination.

4. As for the site of cell grafting, implanting myoblasts in the peri-infarct zone is more ideal than at the center of the infarct region for two reasons: (1) grafted cells need a blood supply for survival, whereas the infarct zone is severely ischemic; and (2) it is important to salvage hibernating myocardium in the border zone to recover LV contract function though contacting with host myocardium *(7)*.

5. The intracoronary infusion method, aimed at wide dissemination of donor myoblasts, has the apparent risk of coronary embolism *(10)* that could develop into a large-scale infarction *(11)*. However, it has been shown that myoblasts are able to cross the endothelium into the muscle interstitium. According to our experience, controlling the graft cell number (less than 1×10^6) and filtering the cells through 30-μm nylon mesh are two crucial measures for successful prevention of coronary embolism. Myoblast fusion need be controlled in cell culture and can be avoid by pregrafting.

6. It remains controversial whether grafted myoblasts could form excitation–contraction coupling with native cardiomyocytes *(12)*. Some reports identified gap junction (Connexin 43 expression) at the interfaces between grafted myoblasts and native cardiomyocytes, whereas some coupling exists between two adjacent myoblast-derived structures.

References

1. Hughes, S. (2002) Cardiac stem cells. *J Pathol.* **197,** 468–478.
2. Ghostine, S., Carrion, C., Souza, L. C., et al. (2002) Long-term efficacy of myoblast transplantation on regional structure and function after myocardial infarction. *Circulation* **106,** I131–I136.
3. Kessler, P. D. and Byrne, B. J. (1999) Myoblast cell grafting into heart muscle: cellular biology and potential applications. *Annu. Rev. Physiol.* **61,** 219–242.

4. Dorfman, J., Duong, M., Zibaitis, A., et al. (1998) Myocardial tissue engineering with autologous myoblast implantation. *J. Thorac. Cardiovasc. Surg.* **116,** 744–751.

5. Bockhold, K. J., Rosenblatt, J. D., and Partridge, T. A. (1998) Aging normal and dystrophic mouse muscle: analysis of myogenicity in cultures of living single fibers. *Muscle Nerve* **21,** 173–183.

6. Scorsin, M., Hagege, A., Vilquin, J. T., et al. (2000) Comparison of the effects of fetal cardiomyocyte and skeletal myoblast transplantation on postinfarction left ventricular function. *J. Thorac. Cardiovasc. Surg.* **119,** 1169–1175.

7. Suzuki, K., Murtuza, B., Smolenski, R. T., et al. (2001) Cell transplantation for the treatment of acute myocardial infarction using vascular endothelial growth factor-expressing skeletal myoblasts. *Circulation* **104,** I207–I212.

8. Lawson, M. A. and Purslow, P. P. (2000) Differentiation of myoblasts in serum-free media: effects of modified media are cell line-specific. *Cells Tissues Organs* **167,** 130–137.

9. Pouzet, B., Vilquin, J. T., Hagege, A. A., et al. (2000) Intramyocardial transplantation of autologous myoblasts: can tissue processing be optimized? *Circulation* **102,** III210–III215.

10. Suzuki, K., Murtuza, B., Suzuki, N., et al. (2001) Intracoronary infusion of skeletal myoblasts improves cardiac function in doxorubicin-induced heart failure. *Circulation* **104,** I213–I217.

11. Suzuki, K., Brand, N. J., Smolenski, R. T., et al. (2000) Development of a novel method for cell transplantation through the coronary artery. *Circulation* **102,** III359–III364.

12. Pouzet, B., Vilquin, J. T., Hagege, A. A., et al. (2001) Factors affecting functional outcome after autologous skeletal myoblast transplantation. *Ann. Thorac. Surg.* **71,** 844–850.

13

Protocols for Myocardial Infarction Repair Using Fetal Cardiac Myocytes

Sharon Etzion, Radka Holbova, Liron Miller, and Jonathan Leor

Summary

We review an experimental protocol for investigating concepts and methods for myocardial repair using fetal cardiomyocyte transplantation. We describe methods of cell isolation, culture, labeling, and assessment of the influence of the engrafted cells on left ventricular remodeling and function.

Key Words: Cardiomyocyte; cell; gene; heart failure; myocardium; transplantation.

1. Introduction

Efforts to reduce the extent of muscle damage from acute myocardial infarction (MI) have been successful in many ways, but the problems of postinfarction scarring, remodeling, dilatation, and consequent heart failure persist. Consequently, researchers are intensively developing new strategies aimed at replacing infarcted myocardium with new viable tissue (1). Recent animal studies have shown that transplantation of fetal or neonatal cardiac myocytes, skeletal myoblasts, and smooth muscle cells into the infarcted myocardium has been associated with improved remodeling and contractility of infarcted myocardium. Other animal research has evaluated the implantation of bone marrow stem cells into myocardium.

Fetal cardiomyocytes are the gold standard cell for investigating and testing concepts and strategies for myocardial repair. These cells are committed to develop into mature, functional cardiomyocytes. Most of the pioneering experiments on cardiac cell transplantation used fetal cardiomyocytes as the donor cells for myocardial repair (2–6). In animal studies, transplantation of fetal or neonatal cardiomyocytes within an infarcted myocardium limited

From: *Methods in Molecular Medicine, vol. 112: Molecular Cardiology: Methods and Protocols*
Edited by: Z. Sun © Humana Press Inc., Totowa, NJ

postinfarction remodeling and ejection fraction deterioration *(2,4–6)*. Some evidence suggests that the engrafted cells integrate structurally and display characteristic physiological functions *(7,8)*.

Promising reports on creating embryonic stem (ES) cell lines *(9)*, ES-derived cardiomyocytes *(10)*, and nuclear transfer *(11)* have raised hope that ES-derived cardiomyocytes will some day be available as "autologous" cells for transplantation.

The purpose of this chapter is to review the experimental protocol for testing and investigating strategies for myocardial repair using fetal cardiomyocyte transplantation. This model is feasible and useful for testing various techniques to enhance survival and function of the graft. Strategies such as genetic engineering, therapeutic angiogenesis, anti-apoptotic proteins and immune tolerance, are all relevant to the success of cardiac cell therapy *(1)*.

2. Materials
2.1. MI Model

1. Surgical equipment.
2. Ketamine and xylazine.
3. Polypropylene 6-0 suture (Johnson-Johnson Int., Brussels, Belgium), 4-0 absorbable vicryl suture (Ethicon, Edinburgh, UK).
4. Echocardiography system equipped with 12.5-MHz phased-array transducer.
5. Standard ECG system.

2.2. Cardiomyocyte Tissue Culture
2.2.1. Fetal Cardiomyocyte Culture Based on Trypsin-DNase I

1. Full M-199 culture medium (Biological Industries, Kibbutz Beit Haemek, Israel): M-199 medium supplement with 0.12 μM $CuSO_4$ (Sigma), 0.1 μM $ZnSO_4$ (Sigma), 15 μM vitamin B_{12} (Sigma), 1% penicillin/streptomycin, 5% fetal calf serum (FCS, Biological Industries), pH 7.5.
2. Dissociation buffer: 137 mM NaCl, 5.4 mM KCl, 0.8 mM $MgSO_4$, 5.6 mM dextrose, 0.4 mM KH_2PO_4, 0.3 mM Na_2HPO_4, 20 mM HEPES, 500 U/mL penicillin, 100 mg/mL streptomycin, pH 7.5.
3. 0.002% DNase I (Sigma): dissolve each vial of DNase I in 150 μL 1 M NaCl + 850 μL H_2O.
4. 0.1% Trypsin (CalBiochem).

2.2.2. Fetal Cardiomyocyte Culture Based on RDB

1. RDB proteolytic enzyme (Biological Institute, Ness-Ziona, Israel).
2. Full DMEM culture medium: Dulbecco's modified Eagle's medium (4500 mg/L glucose) supplemented with 10% inactivated horse serum, 2% chicken embryos extract, 1% L-glutamine, and 1% penicillin/streptomycin (all from Biological Industries).

3. Collagen–gelatin: collagen (CalBiochem) 50 mg/100 mL DDW, gelatin (Sigma) 0.1 g/100 mL DDW in a proportion of 1:1 (v/v). Store separately and mix before use. Cover the dishes at least 24 h before plating the cells.
   a. PBS I: 8 mM NaCl, 0.2 mM KCl, 0.2 mM KH$_2$PO$_4$, 1.15 mM Na$_2$HPO$_4$, 2.5 mM dextrose, pH 7.5.
   b. PBS II: 8 mM NaCl, 0.2 mM KCl, 0.2 mM KH$_2$PO$_4$, 1.15 mM Na$_2$HPO$_4$, 0.1 mM CaCl$_2$, 0.1 mM MgCl$_2$, pH 7.5.

2.2.3. Fetal Cardiomyocyte Culture Based on Collagenase–Pancreatin

1. Buffer: 116.4 mM NaCl, 5.4 mM KCl, 1 mM Na$_2$HPO$_4$, 20 mM HEPES, 5.5 mM glucose, 0.8 mM MgSO$_4$, pH 7.4.
2. DMEM/M-199 medium: DMEM and M-199 (1:4) supplemented with 10% horse serum, 50% fetal bovine serum (FBS), 100 U/mL penicillin G, 100 µg/mL streptomycin, and 0.25 µg/mL amphotericin B.
3. 0.1 mM Bromodeoxyuridine (BrdU; Sigma).
4. 0.25% Trypsin–EDTA (Biological Industries).

3. Methods

The methods describe below outline (1) two possibilities for myocardial injury model, (2) three methods for cardiomyocyte tissue culture, (3) method for cell labeling and transplantation into the infarct or border zone, and (4) measurements to evaluate remodeling and function following infarction and transplantation.

3.1. Myocardial Infarction Model

3.1.1. Acute Myocardial Infarction Model in Rat (4,12) (see Notes 1 and 2)

The standard model used for MI studies of is left anterior descending coronary artery ligation through left anterolateral thoracotomy. Syngeneic Fischer 344, Lewis, or Sprague-Dawley rats weighing 200–250 g are used.

1. Anesthetize rats with 90 mg/kg ketamine and 10 mg/kg xylazine im. Shave the chest, and place the rats in the supine position. If using athymic nude rats, half of the dose should be injected carefully, as they are more sensitive to anesthesia (*see* Note 2).
2. Monitor lead I of the ECG throughout the operation.
3. Intubate the anesthetized rat with an 18-gage intravenous catheter, connected to the rodent ventilator (Harvard Apparatus), and ventilate with room air, volume 2 mL, respiratory rate 70 breaths/min.
4. Perform a left anterolateral thoracotomy through fourth intercostal space and expose the beating heart.
5. Remove the pericardium, pass 6-0 polypropylene suture under the left coronary artery, and tie. You may visually confirm formation of acute MI by a pale

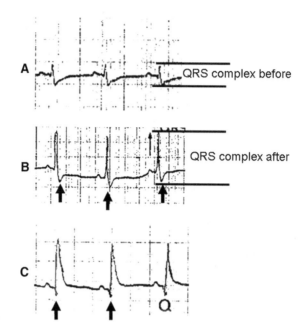

Fig. 1. ECG. (**A**) Lead I before coronary artery occlusion. (**B**) After LAD coronary artery occlusion, there is a significant increase in QRS complex amplitude and width, accompanied by typical ST-segment deviation (arrow). (**C**) After 2–3 h, the ECG tracing discloses development of Q wave (arrow).

    nonbeating or dyskinetic area of the left ventricle and by typical ST-segment deviation and tachyarrhythmias on the ECG (*see* **Fig. 1** and **Note 1**).

6. Expel the air from the chest by gentle compression, and close the skin with 4-0 absorbable vicryl or silk suture. Animals should be allowed to recover under the heat lamp and then returned to their cages.

3.1.2. Myocardial Cryoinjury (13)

    An alternative and possibly easier method for myocardial scar formation is cryoinjury.

1. Repeat preparation procedures as in the MI model (**Subheading 3.1.1., steps 1–4**).
2. Place a 5-mm-diameter metal probe cooled to –190°C for 2 min on the apex of the heart for 2 seconds. Repeat this procedure eight times.
3. Expel the air from the chest by gentle compression, and close the skin with 4-0 absorbable vicryl or silk suture. Animals are allowed to recover under the heat lamp and returned to their cages.

3.1.3. Myocardial Infarction by LAD Ligation: Mouse Model

This model is useful for protocols requiring transgenic, SCID, or nude mice.

1. Anesthetize the mouse (weight range 20–30 g) using a mixture of 200 mg/kg ketamine and 10 mg/kg xylazine in a single ip injection.
2. Shave the chest, and place the animal in the supine position on the heating pad (37°C).
3. Intubate the mouse with a 20-gage intravenous catheter, and ventilate with room air, using a Minivent ventilator (Harvard Apparatus). The stroke volume is 0.2 mL and the respiratory rate is 150 breaths/min.
4. After left anterior thoracotomy is performed, expose the heart and identify the left coronary artery on the surface of the left ventricular (LV) anterior wall.
5. Place a 7-0 or 6-0 nylon suture (Prolene) around the left anterior descending (LAD) coronary artery. Occlusion of the LAD is confirmed immediately by change in the color of the LV free wall and by echocardiography performed the day after the occlusion.
6. Place the animal into a heated cage with 95% oxygen supply until full recovery from the anesthesia. After recovery, place the mouse in the cage and give standard mouse chow and water *ad libitum* (*see* **Note 3**).

3.2. Fetal Cardiomyocytes Isolation (see Notes 4–6)

Primary cardiomyocyte tissue culture can be performed by three different methods, based on various dissociation enzymes. Cardiomyocyte tissue culture is usually one-passage culture.

3.2.1. Fetal Cardiomyocyte Culture Based on Trypsin-DNase I (12,14)

1. Anesthetize female rats carrying 14–15-d-old embryos with sodium pentobarbital.
2. Under sterile conditions, remove the embryos and their hearts, dissect the heart under the dissecting microscope, and place the ventricles in cold dissociation buffer.
3. Cut the ventricles into 1–2-mm cubes, and dissociate them at 24°C in 10 cycles using the following treatments:
    a. Add 15 mL of 0.1% trypsin + 0.002% DNase I in dissociation buffer to the tissue cubes in the test tube for 5 min and mix gently. Remove the buffer and place in a clean test tube.
    b. Add 15 mL of 2% FCS in dissociation buffer to the ventricles for 5 min with gentle pipeting, and insert the buffer into the test tube from **step a**.
    c. Centrifuge the buffer from **steps a** and **b** (30 mL) at room temperature for 10 min at 500*g*.
    d. Resuspend the sediment cells in cold M-199 culture medium (5–6 mL) containing 0.5% calf serum and 0.002% DNase and keep on ice.
4. Repeat this cycle until all tissue dissociates (about 10 times). Cells from the first two cycles will be discarded.

5. At the end of the cycles, collect the M-199 medium from all test tubes (cycles 3–10) and centrifuge (0°C, 10 min, 500g).
6. Wash the sediment in full M-199 culture medium, and incubate in a 100-mm dish for 15–20 min at 37°C in humidified air with 5% CO_2 for preplating. Collect the nonattached cells (*see* **Note 7**).
7. Place an aliquot of the nonattached cells on the hemocytometer, add 0.4% trypan blue to identify dead cells, and count in quadruplicate.
8. Plate 1.5 mL of culture medium (1 × 10^6 cells/mL) containing 5% FCS in prewetted 35-mm culture dishes (Costar). If the cell concentration is low, you can centrifuge again at 25°C, 10 min, 500g.
9. After 24 h, wash the cells with phosphate-buffered saline (PBS) containing 5.5 mM glucose, and renew the culture medium at this time and every third day thereafter (*see* **Note 8**).

3.2.2. Fetal Cardiomyocyte Culture Based on RDB

This method is based on the proteolytic enzyme RDB (Biological Institute, Ness-Ziona), prepared from fig tree extract *(15)*. Compared with other methods, this method is simpler and quicker. Theoretically, this method should reduce the immunogenicity and damage associated with trypsin or collagenase.

1. Anesthetize female rats carrying 14–15-d-old embryos with sodium pentobarbital.
2. Remove the embryos and their hearts, and place the hearts in DMEM medium. Cut into 1–2-mm pieces.
3. Wash the pieces in a test tube with PBS I for 10 min and mix gently.
4. Dilute the RDB 1:200 in PBS I, and dissociate the ventricles in a test tube with 20 mL RDB solution for 10 min, mixing gently.
5. Collect the supernatant, centrifuge (500g, 10 min, room temperature), and resuspend the cells in 5 mL full DMEM culture medium.
6. Repeat this sequence (**steps 4** and **5**) until all tissue dissociates (about 10 times). Pool the medium from all test tubes except for the first two cycles.
7. Preplate the cells in a 60- or 100-mm dish for 15–20 min at 37°C in full DMEM culture medium (*see* **Note 7**).
8. Count (by a hemacytometer), in quadruplicate, an aliquot of the nonattached cells with 0.4% trypan blue.
9. Plate 1.5 mL of culture medium (1 × 10^6 cells/mL) in collagen–gelatin-coated 35-mm culture dishes (Costar) (*see* **Subheading 2.2.2.**).
10. After 24 h, wash the cultures with PBS II, and incubate with full DMEM at 37°C humidity air chamber, 5% CO_2. Renew the culture medium every third day thereafter. Cardiomyocyte contraction begins approx 48 h after seeding (*see* **Note 8**).

3.2.3. Fetal Cardiomyocyte Culture Based on Collagenase–Pancreatin **(16)**

1. Anesthetize female rats carrying 14- to 15-d-old embryos with sodium pentobarbital.

2. Remove the embryos and their hearts, and place the hearts in DMEM medium. Cut into 1–2-mm pieces, and wash the pieces in ice-cold buffer
3. Incubate the ventricles at 37°C for 25 min repeatedly (five to six times) in buffer supplemented with 95 U/mL collagenase type II and 0.6 mg/mL pancreatin.
4. After each round of digestion, centrifuge the supernatant (600g, 5 min), and resuspend the resulting cell pellet in DMEM/M-199 medium.
5. After preplating for 30 min, pool the cells, count them, and incubate at 37°C in 5% CO_2 (*see* **Notes 7** and **8**).

3.3. Labeling of Cells Before Transplantation (12)

Identification of the engrafted cells in the infarcted myocardium can be obtained by labeling the cells while they are in tissue culture, before transplanting them into the infarcted zone. Several labeling methods can be used.

3.3.1. Recombinant Adenovirus Encoding the LacZ Reporter Gene

In our studies, samples of cultured cells are genetically labeled by transfection with recombinant E1a deleted adenovirus-5 carrying the nuclear *LacZ* reporter gene under the cytomegalovirus (CMV) promoter.

1. Wash cardiomyocyte tissue culture once with serum-free medium, and then incubate with 10 µL of adenovirus in 1 mL of serum-free medium (1 × 10^{11} viral particles/mL) for 60 min at 37°C.
2. Wash the cells three times with serum-free medium to remove any remaining virus, and incubate for 24 h in medium containing 10% FCS.
3. Prepare the cells for transplantation (*see* **Subheading 3.4.** and **Note 9**) or stain representative sample of the cells in vitro (*see* **Subheading 3.6.**). Labeling efficacy is approx 90% (**Fig. 2A**).

3.3.2. Labeling Cells With BrdU

1. Wash the cells once with PBS and incubate with 1 mL of 1% BrdU solution from 2 h to overnight at 37°C (thymidine analog BrdU, dilution 1:100 with complete culture medium; Zymed). The solution must be sterilized (by filtration) and warmed to 37°C before use.
2. Remove labeling medium from cells, and wash gently with PBS.
3. Prepare the labeled cells for transplantation (*see* **Subheading 3.4.**), and after sacrificing the rats prepare paraffin sections for staining with the BrdU kit (Zymed, BrdU staining kit, streptavidin–Biotin system for BrdU staining).
4. For in vitro staining: fix cells with 70 to 80% alcohol for 20–30 min, and wash with PBS (three times, 2 min each). Incubate with biotinylated Ms anti-BrdU antibody as described in the BrdU staining kit. Labeling efficacy is approx 50% (**Fig. 2B**).

3.3.3. Labeling Cells With Fluorescent Dye

1. Remove the culture medium, and rinse the cells with serum-free medium.

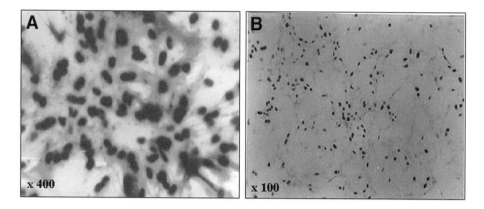

Fig. 2. Cell labeling before transplantation. (**A**) Cultured fetal cardiomyocytes 24 h after transfection with recombinant adenovirus carrying the reporter gene *LacZ*. Approximately all cultured cells stained positive with X-gal, as demonstrated by nuclear dark color. (**B**) Cultured fetal cardiomyocytes 24 h after incubation with BrdU. Roughly 50 to 60% of the cells showed positive staining in vitro using anti-BrdU immunostaining.

2. Mix the dye PKH2-GL 1:10 with the diluent supplied with the product (PKH2 Green Fluorescent General Cell Linker Kit, Sigma). Make sufficient solution to immerse all cell culture completely.
3. Incubate the cells in the dye for 5–10 min at 37°C with mild agitation.
4. Add pure serum in equal amounts to the dye solution, and incubate further for 1 min. Add an equal amount of full medium.
5. Remove the dye solution, and replace with full medium. Repeat and return the cells to the culture medium to await examination under the fluorescent microscope, or prepare cells for transplantation (*see* **Subheading 3.4.** and **Note 10**).

3.4. Cell Transplantation

In most experiments, cell transplantations are performed 10–14 d after myocardial infarction, and viable beating cardiomyocytes are selected microscopically after 3–4 d in culture. Alternatively, fresh cells can be transplanted immediately after the preplating stage.

1. Wash the cells once in serum free-DMEM, and prepare the cells for transplantation by trypsinization with 0.4 mL of 0.25% trypsin/EDTA for 1–2 min at 37°C.
2. Stop the reaction by adding 2 mL culture medium supplemented with 10% serum. Collect the medium in a test tube.
3. Centrifuge at 1000 rpm for 10 min, at room temperature, and resuspend the cells in small volume (100 µL for each rat) of serum-free M-199 medium or DMEM.

4. Anesthetize the rats, and under sterile technique open the chest. The infarcted area can be identified visually on the basis of surface scarring and wall motion akinesis.

5. Select rats either for injection of $1.5–2 \times 10^6$ fetal/neonatal cardiomyocytes by two injections of 50 mL using an insulin syringe with a 27-gage needle or for injection of serum-free culture medium as control (*see* **Note 11**).

6. After injections into the scar, close the surgical incision by sutures as described in **Subheading 3.1.1.**

3.5. Echocardiography to Evaluate Remodeling and Contractility (5,12,17)

1. Anesthetize the rats with a combination of 40 mg/kg ketamine and 10 mg/kg xylazine.

2. Shave the chest, and place the rats on their backs.

3. A conventional echocardiography paste is used. Place the transducer against the chest on the left anterior side of the chest.

4. In our experiments, echocardiograms are performed with a commercially available echocardiography system equipped with 12.5-MHz phased-array pediatric transducer (Hewlett Packard). Transthoracic echocardiography is performed on all animals after MI, before transplantation (baseline echocardiogram), and 4 and 8 wk after cell transplantation.

5. The heart is first imaged in the 2D mode in the parasternal long- and short-axis views of the LV (**Fig. 3A,B**).

6. M-mode images are obtained at the level below the tip of the mitral valve leaflets at the level of the papillary muscles (**Fig. 3C,D**).

7. The following measurements should be taken:
   a. Maximal LV end-diastolic dimension, minimal LV end-systolic dimension, and fractional shortening (FS) as a measure of systolic function, calculated as FS (%) = [(LVIDd – LVIDs)/LVIDd] × 100, where LVID indicates LV internal dimension, s is systole, and d is diastole.
   b. Index of change in LV area (%) is calculated as [(EDA – ESA)/EDA] × 100 where EDA indicates LV end diastolic area and ESA indicates LV end-systolic area.
   c. Cardiac output and stroke volume are calculated using pulmonary artery Doppler flow and diameter, measured on a 2D short-axis view taken at the base to allow adequate visualization of the pulmonary artery trunk and correct alignment of pulsed-wave Doppler along the pulmonary flow.

3.6. Histology to Identify the Donor Cells

Histological identification should be performed in representative samples, sectioned and either frozen or paraffin-embedded.

3.6.1. Staining of Ad-LacZ-Transfected Cardiac Myocytes In Vitro

1. Twenty-four hours after transfection, wash the cells once with PBS, and fix the cells in culture with 0.05% glutaraldehyde in PBS for 10 min at room temperature.

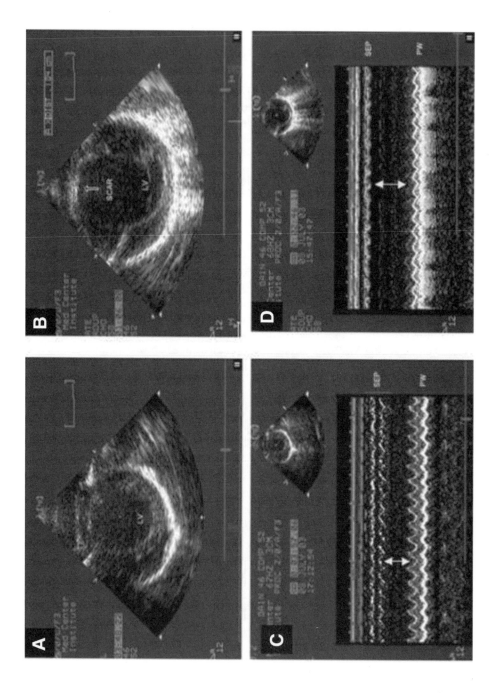

2. Wash twice with PBS, 5 min each.
3. Incubate the cells with X-gal staining solution 30 min to overnight, depending on cells.
   a. Fe solution: 5 mM potassium ferricyanide ($K_3Fe[CN]_6$), 5 mM potassium ferrocyanide ($K_4Fe[CN]_4$), 2 mM $MgCl_2$ in PBS. (Can be stored in dark at 4°C for up to 1 yr).
   b. X-gal solution: 1 mg X-gal (5-bromo-4-chloro-3-indolyl-D-galactosyranosid) in 10 μL dimethyl sulfoxide (DMSO). Add the 10 μL of X-gal (in DMSO) to 1 mL Fe solution (room temperature). The final concentration is 1 mg/mL X-gal (freshly prepared).
4. Cells that express the marker gene *LacZ* are stained dark blue (**Fig. 2A**).

3.6.2. Staining Heart Tissue for the Marker Gene LacZ

To identify *LacZ* activity in the infarcted tissue and engrafted cardiomyocytes, the hearts will be harvested after 1–3 wk.

1. Sacrifice the rats with an overdose of pentobarbital. Arrest the heart by intravenous injection of KCl, while the rats are under deep anesthesia.
2. After the heart is excised, wash it with ice-cold saline or PBS, cut into four transverse slices, and immediately frozen-section.
3. Cut adjacent serial sections of 5 μm thickness. Fix the slides with 0.05% glutaraldehyde for 10 min, and wash the slides twice with PBS, 5 min each.
4. Stain with the X-gal solution as described above in **Subheading 3.6.1.** Wash once in PBS. Blue nuclear stain will mark the engrafted cells (**Fig. 4A,B**).
5. Counterstain representative samples with hematoxylin and eosin (H&E).

3.6.3. Identification of Transplanted Cardiomyocytes by Specific Antibodies

Several protein isoforms are expressed in the fetal hearts but not in the adult, normal myocardium. The α-smooth muscle actin (α-SMA) and slow-myosin heavy chain (slow-MHC) isoforms are present in embryonic cardiomyocytes, whereas α-sarcomeric actin, cardiac actin, or fast-MHC isoforms are found in the adult myocardium. Immunostaining with the specific fetal antibodies allows one to identify the grafted fetal cardiomyocytes in the host myocardium.

1. Sacrifice rats with an overdose of pentobarbital. Arrest the heart by intravenous injection of KCl, while the rats are under deep anesthesia.
2. After the heart is excised, wash it with ice-cold saline or PBS, cut into four transverse slices, and incubate in 4% formaldehyde for paraffin embedding.

Fig. 3. *(opposite page)* Echocardiography before and 2 mo after MI. Two-dimensional mode in short-axis views of the left ventricle before MI formation (**A**) and 2 mo after coronary artery occlusion (**B**), demonstrating LV dilatation and scar formation. M-mode images before coronary artery occlusion (**C**) and 2 mo after MI (**D**) demonstrate anterior wall akinesis. Arrows designate LV cavity.

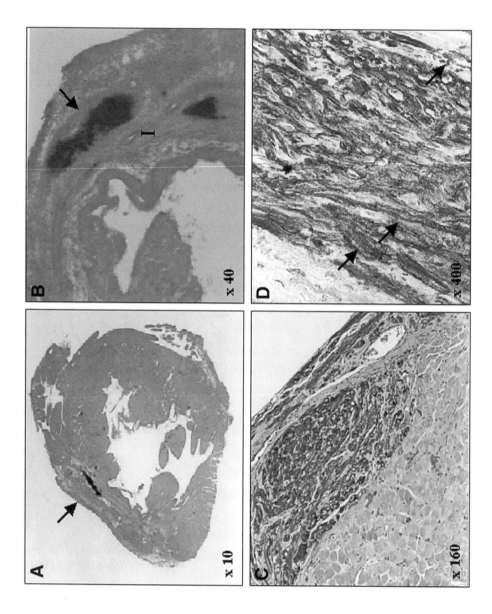

3. Cut adjacent serial sections of 5 μm thickness.
4. Stain with specific antibodies according to the staining kit instructions (**Fig. 4C,D**).
5. Counterstain representative samples with (H&E).

3.7. Histology, Immunohistochemistry, and Morphometric Analysis (12,18)

1. After the heart is excised, cannulate the LV via the aorta, and suspend the heart from a cylinder containing 10% formalin subjected to pressure fixation at 15 mmHg for 30 min.
2. After LV volume measurements, cut the heart into four transverse slices, and process for histology. Cut serial sections of 5 μm thickness, and stain with H&E.
3. To determine infarct size, thickness of the LV free wall and noninfarcted region, and expansion index, we photograph H&E slides, obtained by pressure fixation (**Fig. 5**). Measurements are made using Scion Image software (version 4.0.2).
4. The following measurements should be taken:
   a. LV maximal diameter (mm; maximal diameter is defined as the longest diameter perpendicular to a line connecting the insertions of the septum to the ventricular wall).
   b. Average wall thickness (mm; averaged from three measurements of septum thickness).
   c. Average scar thickness (mm; averaged from three measurements of scar thickness).
   d. Relative scar thickness (average scar thickness/average wall thickness).
   e. Muscle area (mm^2; including the septum).
   f. Scar area (mm^2).
   g. Relative scar area (scar area/muscle area).
   h. LV cavity area (mm^2).
   i. Whole LV area (mm^2).
   j. Expansion index [(LV cavity area/whole LV area)/relative scar thickness].
   k. Epicardial scar length (mm).

Fig. 4. *(opposite page)* Labeled cardiomyocytes following transplantation. (**A**) Macroscopic photograph of infarcted heart 14 d after myocardial infarction and 7 d after transplantation of genetically marked fetal cardiomyocytes. Examination of infarcted hearts revealed an island of dark staining reflecting strong β-galactosidase activity (arrow) in the mid-scar. (**B**) Microscopic view of genetically marked cells 1 wk after transplantation into the infarcted myocardium (I). Engrafted cardiomyocytes (blue nuclei, arrow) were located in the granulation tissue and were surrounded by inflammatory infiltrate. (**C**) Fetal cardiac cell implant 8 wk after transplantation and 9 wk after myocardial infarction. Tissue was stained with antibody to the α-SMA isoform, which is typical for fetal myocardium. Positive cells appear yellow-brown. (**D**) Positive staining cells are enlongated and exhibit the typical cross-striations of early sarcomere formation (arrows).

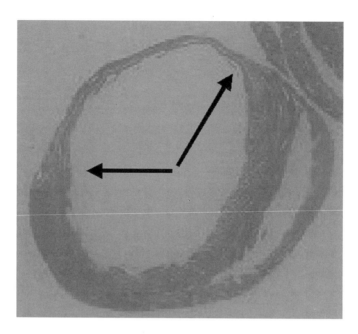

Fig. 5. Myocardial infarction and LV remodeling. With the acute myocardial infarction model, an anterior infarction was created in 20 to 50% of the left ventricle mass (arrows). Measurements of infarct size, thickness of the LV free wall and noninfarcted region, and expansion index were obtained by measurements of the photographed H&E slide, with by pressure fixation, 5 mm from the apex.

   l. Endocardial scar length (mm).
   m. Epicardial LV free wall length (including the septum; mm).
   n. Endocardial LV free wall length (including the septum; mm).
   o. Percentage of scar tissue out of the surface area [(epicardial scar length + endocardial scar length) × 100/(epicardial LV free wall length + endocardial LV free wall length)] *(18)*.
  5. Slices immunolabeled for α-actin are used to identify angiogenesis in the scar tissue (**Fig. 6**). We average the number of small blood vessels (arterioles, venules, and capillaries) per high power field (magnification ×200, true 22.5 μm × 30 μm) in nine random fields from the scar area in each heart and compare the groups using the unpaired Student's *t*-test (InStat, version 3.01, GraphPad Software).

4. Notes

  1. Using this model, it is possible to create an anterior infarct in 20 to 50% of the LV mass (**Fig. 5**). In the rat the infarct is large, partly owing to a lack of coronary collateral flow, an extensive area at risk, and a high metabolic demand of the

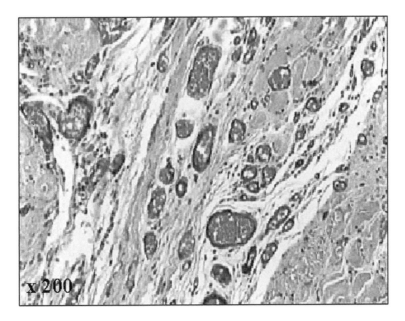

Fig. 6. Angiogenesis. Immunohistologic staining of representative slides with α-SMA antibody, to localize functional blood vessels. Nine consecutive adjacent fields were photographed, and the differences in the extent of neovascularization were obtained by counting the number of vessels and calculating vessel density in the infarcted zone of transplanted and control groups.

heart. Perioperative mortality ranges from 10 to 60%, depending on operator experience, infarct size, and animal strain. In the mouse model of chronic coronary artery occlusion, mortality is higher than 50%. Animal death results from ventricular tachy- or bradyarrhythmias or pump or respiratory failure. Some rats develop intractable ventricular flutter and shock and need resuscitation. Resuscitation is performed by a few gentle compressions of the chest until sinus rhythm is restored. In some rats, the suture misses the coronary artery, and no infarct develops. This can be immediately identified by visual inspection: absence of pale and akinetic region, absence of typical ECG signs of ischemia (**Fig. 1**) and later by wall motion contractility imaged by echocardiography (**Fig. 3**).

The infarcted wall gradually thins as the necrotic tissue reabsorbs. In large infarcts the necrotic tissue not only thins but also stretches, resulting in LV dilatation. The early phase of infarct thinning and stretching is termed infarct expansion (**Fig. 5**).

2. Athymic immunocompromised nude rats (~150 g) are used in experiments with human donor cells. Alternatively, 15 mg/kg cyclosporine-A, 20 mg/kg mycophenolate mofetil, or both should be administered daily *(4)*.

Nude rats require sterile cages, rodent chow, and sterile water throughout the experiment. They are very sensitive to nonsterile environments and easily develop infections; we advise injecting nude rats with antibiotics (20 mg/kg ampicillin) 5 d after surgery.

3. Mortality in the mouse model of chronic myocardial infarction is >50%. Careful postoperative care is essential to reduce mortality.

4. These three methods can also be used for neonatal cardiomyocytes. In this case, anesthetize 1- to 2-d-old neonatal rats with isoflurane (USP).

5. For neonatal culture 0.1 mM BrdU may be used in the culture medium to avoid domination of the proliferating fibroblasts in the culture. In early experiments use the BrdU continuously; in later studies omit it after d 3.

6. The purity of the cardiomyocytes in culture may be evaluated using specific monoclonal antibodies: Wash the cells in PBS and fix with 100% methanol at –20°C for 15min. Wash in PBS three times, and incubate with the specific antibody, such as sarcomeric actin, accordingly to the staining kit orders.

7. During the preplating phase, the proliferating nonmyocardial cells (mostly fibroblasts) are more rapidly attached to the dish surface, leaving the myocardial cells in suspension. This method allows reduction of myocyte culture contamination by the nonmyocyte cells.

8. The cell yield is approx 3×10^5 per fetal heart and approx 2×10^6 per neonatal heart. Preparation average approx 85 to 90% cardiomyocytes, as determined by specific antibodies.

9. Adenovector may compromise the viability and function of the engrafted cells, probably owing to immune response against viral antigens.

10. An alternative popular approach is the marker gene green fluorescent protein (GFP). Based on our experience, this marker gene is very useful in vitro but is toxic to the cells in vivo. In addition, because of the scar autofluorescence activity, the engrafted cells, transfected with GFP, are difficult to identify in the scar.

11. Zhang et al. *(19)* studied the optimal number of cells grafted into the injured heart. They injected neonatal cardiomyocytes of syngeneic rats immediately after cryoinjury. After 7 d, they found that graft sizes were small regardless of the number of cells ($5–20 \times 10^6$) implanted, ranging from 0.4% to 2.7% of the LV. There was no increase in graft size with increasing donor cell number.

References

1. Etzion, S., Kedes, L. H., Kloner, R. A., and Leor, J. (2001) Myocardial regeneration: present and future trends. *Am. J. Cardiovasc. Drugs* **1,** 233–244.

2. Li, R. K., Jia, Z. Q., Weisel, R. D., et al. (1996) Cardiomyocyte transplantation improves heart function. *Ann. Thorac. Surg.* **62,** 654–660; discussion 660,661.

3. Kim, K. K., Soonpaa, M. H., Daud, A. I., Koh, G. Y., Kim, J. S., and Field, L. J. (1994) Tumor suppressor gene expression during normal and pathologic myocardial growth. *J. Biol. Chem.* **269,** 22,607–22613.

4. Leor, J., Patterson, M., Quinones, M. J., Kedes, L. H., and Kloner, R. A. (1996) Transplantation of fetal myocardial tissue into the infarcted myocardium of rat. A potential method for repair of infarcted myocardium? *Circulation* **94,** II332–336.

5. Scorsin, M., Hagege, A. A., Marotte, F., et al. (1997) Does transplantation of cardiomyocytes improve function of infarcted myocardium? *Circulation* **96,** II-188–193.

6. Scorsin, M., Marotte, F., Sabri, A., et al. (1996) Can grafted cardiomyocytes colonize peri-infarct myocardial areas? *Circulation* **94,** II337–340.

7. Soonpaa, M. H., Koh, G. Y., Klug, M. G., and Field, L. J. (1994) Formation of nascent intercalated disks between grafted fetal cardiomyocytes and host myocardium [see comments]. *Science* **264,** 98–101.

8. Rubart, M., Pasumarthi, K. B., Nakajima, H., Soonpaa, M. H., Nakajima, H. O., and Field, L. J. (2003) Physiological coupling of donor and host cardiomyocytes after cellular transplantation. *Circ. Res.* **92,** 1217–1224.

9. Thomson, J. A., Itskovitz-Eldor, J., Shapiro, S. S., Waknitz, M. A., Swiergiel, J. J., Marshall, V. S., and Jones, J. M. (1998) Embryonic stem cell lines derived from human blastocysts. *Science* **282,** 1145–1147.

10. Kehat, I., Kenyagin-Karsenti, D., Snir, M., et al. (2001) Human embryonic stem cells can differentiate into myocytes with structural and functional properties of cardiomyocytes. *J. Clin. Invest.* **108,** 407–414.

11. Lanza, R. P., Cibelli, J. B., and West, M. D. (1999) Prospects for the use of nuclear transfer in human transplantation. *Nat. Biotechnol.* **17,** 1171–1174.

12. Etzion, S., Battler, A., Barbash, I. M., et al. (2001) Influence of embryonic cardiomyocyte transplantation on the progression of heart failure in a rat model of extensive myocardial infarction. *J. Mol. Cell. Cardiol.* **33,** 1321–1330.

13. Li, R. K., Mickle, D. A., Weisel, R. D., et al. (1997) Natural history of fetal rat cardiomyocytes transplanted into adult rat myocardial scar tissue. *Circulation* **96,** II-179–186; discussion 186,187.

14. Simpson, P. and Savion, S. (1982) Differentiation of rat myocytes in single cell cultures with and without proliferating nonmyocardial cells. Cross-striations, ultrastructure, and chronotropic response to isoproterenol. *Circ. Res.* **50,** 101–116.

15. Shneyvays, V., Nawrath, H., Jacobson, K. A., and Shainberg, A. (1998) Induction of apoptosis in cardiac myocytes by an A3 adenosine receptor agonist. *Exp. Cell. Res.* **243,** 383–397.

16. Reinecke, H., Zhang, M., Bartosek, T., and Murry, C. E. (1999) Survival, integration, and differentiation of cardiomyocyte grafts: a study in normal and injured rat hearts [In Process Citation]. *Circulation* **100,** 193–202.

17. Litwin, S. E., Katz, S. E., Morgan, J. P., and Douglas, P. S. (1994) Serial echocardiographic assessment of left ventricular geometry and function after large myocardial infarction in the rat. *Circulation* **89,** 345–354.

18. Mehta, P. M., Alker, K. J., and Kloner, R. A. (1988) Functional infarct expansion, left ventricular dilation and isovolumic relaxation time after coronary occlusion: a two-dimensional echocardiographic study. *J. Am. Coll. Cardiol.* **11,** 630–636.

19. Zhang, M., Methot, D., Poppa, V., Fujio, Y., Walsh, K., and Murry, C. E. (2001) Cardiomyocyte grafting for cardiac repair: graft cell death and anti-death strategies. *J. Mol. Cell. Cardiol.* **33,** 907–921.

14

Methods for Examining Stem Cells in Post-Ischemic and Transplanted Hearts

Nana Rezai, Hubert Walinski, Alexandra Kerjner, Lubos Bohunek, Fabio M. V. Rossi, Bruce M. McManus, and Thomas J. Podor

Summary

Currently, the tenet that heart muscle cells are terminally differentiated and incapable of self-repair is being challenged. Recent experimental observations suggest that both endogenous and exogenous stem cell populations have the potential to regenerate damaged areas within the heart. These findings hold promise for new therapeutic strategies to treat cardiovascular diseases, including common conditions like myocardial infarction and transplant vascular disease (TVD). In this chapter, we focus on the study of endogenous stem cells in the context of their role in modulation of cardiovascular diseases, including ischemic heart disease and TVD. Specific experimental models and methods used to study the phenomena of endogenous bone marrow-derived stem cell migration and potential differentiation are also described.

Key Words: Myocardial infarction; transplant vascular disease; stem cells; cardiomyocytes; endothelial cells; smooth muscle cells; confocal microscopy.

1. Introduction

Complex chronic heart ailments, such as ischemic heart disease and transplant vascular disease (TVD), levy a heavy burden on society. To date, the ability to repair or regenerate ischemic or damaged heart tissue has presented a major challenge, in part owing to the perceived terminal differentiation of cardiomyocytes. However, recent observations suggest that the body can recruit endogenous bone marrow stem cells to sites of myocardial damage and that these cells have the ability to engraft within the myocardium and may participate in the regeneration of heart function. Other work suggests a regenerative

From: *Methods in Molecular Medicine, vol. 112: Molecular Cardiology: Methods and Protocols*
Edited by: Z. Sun © Humana Press Inc., Totowa, NJ

role for resident cardiac stem cells. Consequently, the replacement of cells within the damaged myocardium and vasculature with endogenous stem cells, which may restore structural and physiological heart function, represents a tremendous opportunity for developing new therapeutic strategies.

1.1. Bone Marrow Stem Cells

The bone marrow is an important source of stem cells for possible transplantation into the heart. In contrast to embryonic stem cells, bone marrow stem cells can be collected from adults and used for transplantation without instigating ethical dilemmas or incurring immunogenicity issues related to tissue mismatches or rejection. Bone marrow stem cells retain the capacity for unlimited, undifferentiated proliferation and demonstrate the potential to develop into different cell types, including cardiomyocytes *(1–5)*. Hematopoietic stem cells (HSCs) are a population of stem cells found within the bone marrow that demonstrate the ability to provide permanent long-term reconstitution of the entire hematopoietic system by constantly replenishing the differentiated cells of the peripheral blood through a population of committed progenitors *(6)*. Recent experimental studies suggest that HSCs have the ability to differentiate into a variety of phenotypes, including skeletal muscle *(7,8)*, cardiomyocytes *(9–11)*, and endothelial cells *(9)*. Mesenchymal stem cells (MSCs) are another class of progenitors found in the bone marrow, as well as in other tissues, including fat, skin, and muscle *(1)*. The precise relationship between MSCs and HSCs is still unclear at this point; however, MSCs are thought to support HSCs by the production of crucial cytokines, such as interleukin-6 (IL-6); leukocyte inhibitory factor (LIF), and extracellular matrix, all of which aid in HSC function within the bone marrow microenvironment *(1)*. Recently, MSCs have demonstrated transdifferentiation properties or plasticity under appropriate stimuli and environmental conditions. In vivo and in vitro techniques have been developed to induce MSC differentiation into cells of mesenchymal lineage, including cartilage and bone *(4,12)*, as well as skeletal and cardiac muscle *(2,3,5)*, in an attempt to determine MSC potential for plasticity and directed transdifferentiation.

Human cardiomyocytes have tradionally been regarded as terminally differentiated, with permanent withdrawal of cardiomyocytes from the cell cycle along with a loss of capacity for renewal *(13,14)*. However, compelling evidence has emerged that challenges the long-standing perception of the adult human heart's limited capacity for regeneration. Evidence suggests that transplanted hearts harbor a population of primitive cells derived from the recipient *(15,16)*. Furthermore, there is compelling evidence from studies of adult hearts following myocardial infarction demonstrating the potential for stem cells to regenerate damaged areas of the heart by natural homing mechanisms following direct injection of isolated cells. In order to determine their potential for future clinical use, it will be necessary first to clarify a number of issues such as the sufficient numbers of cells required for therapeutic effect, methods to optimize stem cell recruitment to areas of myocardial damage, and the safety and efficacy of altered stem cell homing within the heart.

1.2. Transplant Vascular Disease

Heart transplantation is a life-saving procedure for surgical treatment of patients with end-stage congestive heart failure. Despite advances in the field of heart transplantation, rejection continues to limit survival and quality of life in heart transplant recipients. TVD is a rapidly progressive form of atherosclerosis that occurs in the vessels of solid organ transplants. Cardiac TVD is estimated to affect significantly affect more than 40% of recipients who survive beyond 4 yr after transplantation *(17,18)*.

The pathogenesis of TVD has a multifactorial basis and is believed to arise from a complicated interplay between immunological and nonimmunological factors. Together, these factors result in endothelial cell damage leading to the accumulation of a cellular infiltrate consisting of lymphocytes, macrophages, and modified smooth muscle cells (SMCs) in the arterial walls of the transplanted heart *(19)*. The events and environment convey repetitive vascular injury, thereby fostering the formation of concentric plaques with myointimal hyperplasia and extracellular matrix accumulation *(20)*. However, the precise pathogenesis of TVD is still undetermined, and the best strategy to delay disease progression has yet to be identified. Advances in the field have shown that recipient cells may contribute to the replacement of cells in the arteries and myocardium of transplanted hearts. More specifically, the interaction between donor and recipient cells after organ transplantation has received great attention in an attempt to identify the pathogenesis of rejection and graft-vs-host disease *(21,22)*. More than 30 yr ago, it was recognized that transplanted organs become genetic chimeras. In an initial study in 1969, karyotyping was used to demonstrate that reticuloendothelial cells in the transplanted liver are replaced with recipient cells *(23)*. A landmark study followed in 1992 wherein it was reported that donor cells of dendritic cell origin could be identified in multiple recipient organs, including blood, lymph nodes, skin, intestine, and heart, suggesting that the chimeric state in long-term organ transplant recipients, i.e., liver and kidney, was not restricted to the organ, but was in fact systemic *(24,25)*. Microchimerism specifically refers to the composite immune system inclusive of cells from at least two sources, namely, recipient and donor *(21)*. Presently, the progenitor cell origin and fate of recipient cells in the transplanted human heart remains to be determined.

Recent studies have raised the possibility that undifferentiated cells may translocate from the recipient to the graft, contributing to ventricular remodeling *(9,10,26)*. However, the degree of cardiac chimerism is currently a matter of intensive discussion *(27)* since there are discrepancies in reported rates of chimerism in transplanted hearts *(15,16,28)*. Sex-mismatch cardiac transplantation, in which male patients receive hearts from female donors and vice versa, provide the opportunity to investigate whether stem cells or tissue-specific precursor cells migrate from the recipient to the graft. Female hearts allografted into male recipients are commonly analyzed for cardiac chimerism by determining Y chromosome-positive cells from the recipient present in the donor heart *(15,16)*. Fluorescence *in situ* hybridization using Y chromosome-specific hybridization probes can be used to detect cardiac chimerism and can be correlated with immunohistochemistry of cardiac-specific markers. Other detection systems have also been employed to study the rates of cardiac chimerism (*see* **Note 1**), including green fluorescent protein (GFP) expression *(29)*, MHC II detection *(30)*, and *LacZ* expression from bone marrow chimeric *LacZ* transgenic mice *(9,31–33)*. To date, the physiological consequences of cardiac chimerism remain obscure and the precise role of recipient-derived cardiomyocytes and vascular cells remains unknown. Thus, it is of vital importance to establish models and systems with which to examine this phenomenon in a controlled environment.

1.3. Ischemic Heart Disease

Myocardial infarction is the leading cause of death in both men and women in developed countries. Occlusion of a major artery results in the lack of adequate perfusion, or ischemia, causing an alteration in myocardial metabolism and decreased contractile function *(34)* generally proportionate to the extent of infarction and myocardial necrosis. Corresponding adaptive changes to the long-term effects of myocardial infarction include cardiomyocyte hypertrophy and atrophy, cardiac remodeling, myocardial fibrosis, and the loss of appropriate ventricular function. Heart failure primarily occurs following myocardial infarction owing to progressive ventricular remodeling, characterized by myocyte apoptosis, altered myocyte turnover, fibrous tissue deposition in the ventricular wall, and gradual expansion of the infarcted area, with dilation of the ventricular lumen *(35,36)*.

Approximately 50% of patients with congestive heart failure die within 5 yr of their initial diagnosis *(37)*. Currently, most available treatments are limited as they only delay progression of end-stage heart failure. Although cardiac transplantation is the ultimate destination treatment, its utilization is severely limited by donor organ availability. Susceptibility of allografts to rejection remains, as do other complications. Recently, interest has focused on the use of stem cells as potential therapy for myocardial regeneration following myocardial infarction. Experimental studies have shown that stem cells can be transformed into new cardiomyocytes and vascular endothelial cells in vitro when they are grown under optimized conditions *(3,38)*. Furthermore, reports document that the transplantation of undifferentiated cells into a damaged heart is a promising novel treatment, as stem cells have demonstrated the capability of adapting to the cardiac environment, regenerating the damaged cardiac tissue, restoring cardiac function, and improving blood flow to the damaged myocardium *(29,39)*. To date, numerous studies have shown evidence that bone marrow-derived stem cells possess the ability to differentiate into cardiac muscle cells *(9,40,41)*. Various animal models of the failing heart have been described in which myocardial infarction is caused by selective ligation of the coronary artery and for which stem cells are administered as a therapeutic maneuver. Rodent models have frequently been used in order to test the therapeutic impact of stem cells in regenerating infarcted myocardium; they have been introduced either by direct injection into heart muscle, or by injection into the coronary arteries, or through bone marrow transplantation *(10,39,42)*. Numerous bone marrow-derived cell types have been used to repair damaged areas of the heart owing to myocardial infarction with promising results. Embryonic and fetal stem cells, adult MSCs, and adult HSCs have all been recognized to possess the potential for cardiovascular repair post myocardial infarction. In recent years, MSC engraftment has also been targeted as a novel therapeutic approach for myocardial infarction owing to the capability of MSCs to differentiate into a myogenic lineage *(43–45)*. Current reports also suggest that HSCs are able to give rise to new myocardium and regenerate zones of infarction in damaged myocardium *(9,46)*.

Our laboratory has established two murine models to examine the role of endogenous bone marrow-derived progenitor cells in both a heterotopic heart transplant model and a myocardial infarction model of ischemia/reperfusion. These models incorporate the use of novel transgenic mice expressing GFP-positive bone marrow as recipient mice for both the heterotopic heart transplants and in the ischemia/reperfusion model in order to study the migration, localization, and fate of endogenous GFP-positive bone marrow-derived progenitor cells in the damaged transplanted and myocardial infarction heart, respectively (**Fig. 1**). The GFP cells can be detected using conventional 2D fluorescence; however, sophisticated 3D confocal and multiphoton microscopic analysis are powerful fluorescence imaging modalities that can provide both qualitative and quantitative assessments of the contribution of fluorescently labeled endogenous bone marrow-derived progenitor cells to the myocardium and vasculature of transplanted and infarcted hearts.

2. Materials

2.1. Murine Heterotopic Heart Transplant

1. Two pairs of jeweler's forceps, sizes 5 and 7, one straight, one curved.

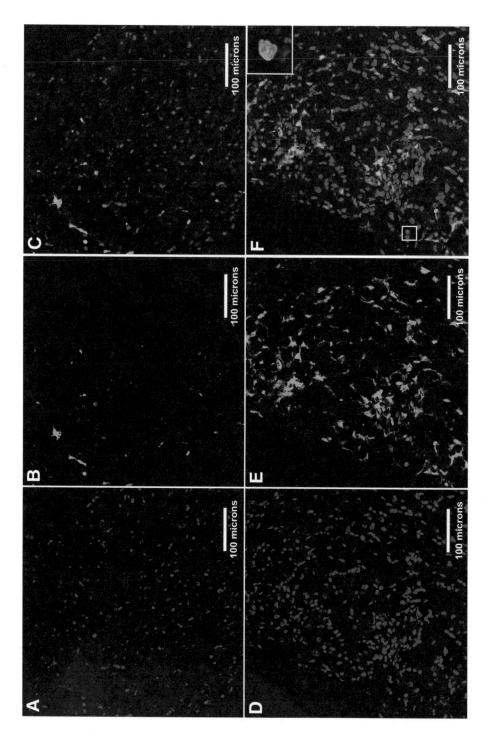

2. Two pairs of microsurgical scissors, one straight, one curved.
3. One microsurgical needleholder, spring-loaded.
4. One pair of minibulldog clamps including applicator.
5. One 3-mL syringe with a bend 30-gage needle.
6. Operating microscope (4–25× magnification).
7. Xylazine.
8. Ketamine.
9. Heparinized Ringer's solution.
10. Lacri-Lube ophthalmic ointment.
11. 8-0 Silk ties.
12. Isoflurane gas.
13. 11-0 Nylon suture.
14. Microfibrillar collagen (Avitene®).
15. 5/0 Vicryl.
16. Betadine antiseptic solution.
17. Buprenorphrine.

2.2. Ischemia/Reperfusion in Mouse Model

1. Ketaset (ketamine).
2. Xylamax (xylazine).
3. Aerrane (isoflurane).
4. Oxygen.
5. Polyethylene tubing PE 50.
6. Lacri-Lube ophthalmic ointment.
7. Saline.
8. Nair hair removal lotion.
9. Forceps.
10. Spatula.
11. Cannula.
12. Scalpel.
13. Spring scissors.
14. Spring scissors with round tip.

Fig. 1. *(opposite page)* Fluorescence images of nuclei and green fluorescent protein (GFP)-labeled bone marrow-derived recipient cells, respectively, in the native (**A–C**) and transplanted (**D–F**) mouse hearts 14 d post transplantation. Nuclei of cells (blue) were identified with Hoechst 33342 (**A** and **D**) and endogenous recipient GFP-labeled bone marrow-derived (green) recipient cells (**B** and **E**) were excited with a 488-nm laser line of a confocal microscope. Corresponding images of nuclei and GFP for both the native (**C**) and transplanted (**F**) hearts were merged to examine the preferential localization of the endogenous GFP-labeled recipient bone marrow-derived cells to the transplanted heart a compared with the native heart. At a higher magnification, the GFP-positive cells reveal GFP expression in the cytoplasm of the cells (**inset to F**).

15. Retractor.
16. Ventilator.
17. Cotton swabs.
18. Distilled water.
19. Masking tape.

3. Methods

3.1. Heterotopic Heart Transplant Surgery

In the heterotopic heart transplant model, the donor ascending aorta is sutured end to side to the recipient abdominal aorta, and the donor pulmonary artery is anastomosed to the recipient inferior vena cava (IVC). Hearts transplanted heterotopically behave functionally as aortocaval fistulae. Blood enters the donor, ascending aorta from the recipient abdominal aorta and is diverted into the coronary arteries by the closed aortic valve. After the myocardium is perfused, venous blood drains into the right atrium through the coronary sinus and is pumped back into the recipient IVC by way of the right ventricle. In this model, transgenic mice expressing GFP-positive bone marrow cells are used as recipient mice receiving hearts from normal, non-GFP-positive donor mice. Through this model, the migration, localization, and fate of recipient bone marrow-derived GFP-positive cells can be examined in the transplanted vs control native heart.

3.1.1. Donor Operation

1. The mouse is anesthetized with 10 mg/kg xylazine/120 mg/kg ketamine, ip.
2. The mouse is shaved, and the shaved area is cleaned with alcohol and Betadine antiseptic solution before being moved to the surgery table. Sterile drapes are placed on the surgery area, and aseptic technique is used throughout the surgery.
3. The abdominal cavity of the donor mouse is opened with a large longitudinal incision. Abdominal contents are moved to the left side of the animal, exposing the IVC.
4. Using a 3-mL syringe and a 30-gage needle, the IVC is cannulated and slowly perfused with up to 1 mL cold, heparinized Ringer's solution (30 μm/mL).
5. After ensuring that the liver has changed to a pale color, the aorta is cut and the thoracic cavity is opened by cutting through the ribs along both sides of the thoracic spine and through to the thoracic inlet. The anterior chest wall is moved superiorly and held in place with a hemostat. Heparinized Ringer's solution is administered via the IVC above the liver, which is clamped from below the heart.
6. The IVC and superior vena cava (SVC) are ligated with 8-0 silk ties. The ascending aorta is cut below the brachiocephalic artery. The main pulmonary artery is cut proximal to its bifurcation. The connective tissue between the ascending aorta and pulmonary artery is gently teased away at this stage. The pulmonary veins are ligated as a group with a single 8-0 silk tie. The donor heart is gently detached

from the remaining connective tissue with blunt dissection and placed in cold Ringer's solution on ice.

3.1.2. Recipient Operation

1. The recipient transgenic mouse expressing GFP-positive bone marrow is weighed, anesthetized with isoflurane inhalation anesthesia in an induction chamber set at 4% anesthesia, and prepped in the same manner as the donor. Ophthalmic ointment (Lacri-Lube) is put in the eyes to prevent drying, and the animal's ear is marked for identification. A well-insulated heating pad is positioned under the mouse so that the body temperature is maintained at 38°C.
2. The lumbar branches are ligated, and then the infrarenal aorta and IVC are carefully isolated and cross-clamped with two 4-mm microvascular clamps.
3. After retraction with an 11-0 nylon suture through the full thickness of the aorta, an elliptical aortotomy is made with a single cut using iris scissors.
4. A longitudinal venotomy is then made in the IVC by first puncturing the vessel with a 30-gage needles and then snipping with iris scissors parallel to the aortotomy. Both the aorta and IVC are flushed thoroughly with heparinized Ringer's solution. Two stay sutures are placed at both apices of the venotomy.
5. The donor heart is then removed from ice and placed in the right flank of the recipient mouse. After ensuring that the orientation of the donor pulmonary artery is correct, an end-to-side anastomosis between the donor pulmonary artery and recipient IVC is performed using continuous 11-0 nylon sutures. The posterior wall is sutured within the vessel lumen without repositioning the graft. The anterior wall is then closed externally using the same suture. Once the venous anastomosis is completed, the vein is gently stretched before the sutures are tied to avoid narrowing at the anastomotic site.
6. The arterial anastomosis between the donor aortic cuff and recipient aorta is performed in the same fashion as the venous anastomosis. A small quantity of microfibrillar collagen (Avitene) is placed around the arterial anastomosis before the clamp is released. Gentle pressure is applied to the site of anastomosis with a dry cotton swab for 1–2 min after the clamp is removed.
7. Once the anastomoses have been assessed for leaks, the bowel is returned to the abdominal cavity. The abdomen and skin are closed in a two-layer closure with 5/0 vicryl.
8. Animals are given fluids intraperitoneally, intravenously, and subcutaneously and are allowed to recover in an infant incubator with supplemental oxygen for a few hours. During surgery the mice are monitored visually for anesthetic depth and physical status, and corrective measures are taken when necessary.
9. Buprenorphine at 0.05 mg/kg sc is administered upon completion of the surgery and after 8–12 h if needed, following signs of postoperative pain as evidenced by:
   a. Decreased activity (lethargy).
   b. Decreased food and water intake.
   c. Rough hair coat, hunched posture.
   d. Vocalization when the incision is touched.

e. Isolation of the individual from the group.

10. Transplanted mice are monitored daily (heart palpitation) for the duration of the treatment period (approx 30 d post transplantation).

3.2. Myocardial Ischemia/Reperfusion Mouse Model

In the ischemia/reperfusion model, transgenic mice expressing GFP-positive bone marrow are subjected to a 30-min ligation of the left anterior descending (LAD) coronary artery, followed by reperfusion. Following a period of recovery (approx 30–90 d), the heart is examined to determine the role of endogenous bone marrow-derived GFP-positive cells in the repair of the areas of damage in the myocardium.

1. The mouse is weighed (transgenic mouse expressing GFP-positive bone marrow).
2. The appropriate amount of anesthetic (100 µL/10 g of weight) is administered to the mouse with a subcutaneous injection of a mixture of xylazine/ketamine in 0.9% saline. Use 100 µL/10 g of weight.
3. Ophthalmologic ointment is applied into the eyes to prevent the cornea from drying.
4. When the animal is fully anesthetized, the hair is removed from the chest to the abdominal area using Nair hair removal lotion. (Apply Nair on chest and abdomen, work it into the fur with backstrokes, wait 4 min, and then remove the hair with a wet piece of gauze.)
5. The fully anesthetized animal is placed on a plexiglass table (the table is on 30° slant) on its abdomen facing an operator, with legs widely spread, and the upper teeth are hooked onto a horizontal wire in order to keep the animal's mouth open during intubations.
6. The animal's mouth is opened using curved forceps and narrow spatula in order to pull the tongue out and sideway. A spatula is then inserted into the animal's mouth and gently pressed down onto the tongue, exposing the throat. An external light source is placed underneath the table in the area corresponding to the animal's throat in order to illuminate the mouth cavity and throat during surgery.
7. The mouse is then intubated by inserting an intravenous cannula into the trachea. (Use a 22-gage cannula for animals up to 30 g of weight and a 20-gage cannula for animals heavier than 30 g.)
8. The animal is placed on its back on a heated pad so that the operator faces the animal's left side of the chest. The cannula is connected to the ventilator outlet delivering a mixture of oxygen and isoflurane to keep the animal under deep anesthesia. (Volume is 0.5 ml of the mixture/stroke at the rate of 120 strokes/min.)
9. The mouse is secured by taping its legs down in order to prevent movement during the procedure and possible loss of ventilation.
10. A skin incision is made parallel with the midline and halfway between the midline and left elbow. The length of incision corresponds to the distance between the apex of the sternum and elbow.
11. The skin and subcutaneous muscles are separated from the layers of muscle underneath using serrated forceps. The edge of the transverse pectoral muscle

should be visible. The edge of the muscle is lifted with forceps, pulled up, and separated from the deep pectoral muscle underneath. Using the same technique, the deep pectoral muscle is pulled and separated, leaving the rib cage exposed. (Using suture pulled through the edge of the transverse pectoral muscle and applying constant pull keeps the rib cage exposed and helps with chest opening.)

12. Sharp pointed scissors are used to separate rib muscles longitudinally between the second and third ribs just above the left lung contour. Blunt pointed bone scissors are then inserted into the opening and underneath the chest wall. Avoid cutting any major blood vessels, and avoid an incision either too high or too close to the midline or close to the mammary arteries.

13. Open the chest and visualize the heart using a retractor. Be careful to monitor intubations and ventilation since the cannula can be easily extubated and ventilation lost owing to rough manipulation.

14. The LAD is ligated using a small piece of tubing (PE 50), approx 1 mm in length, and 8-0 polypropylene monofilament by driving the monofilament through the tubing and then going with the needle underneath the LAD. The tubing is tied down so it sits firmly on top of the LAD, applying pressure and blocking blood flow, resulting in ischemic myocardial injury. The duration of LAD ligation depends on the desired time of ischemia (e.g., 30 min).

15. The monsfilament is cut with forceps and fine scissors, the monofilament is cut and the tubing is removed to restore partial blood flow. Reperfuse the animal for a given period.

16. The animal is closed using a two-layer closure with 5/0 vicryl.

17. Mice are monitored daily for the predetermined experimental treatment period (approx 30–90 d) prior to sacrifice.

3.3. Assessment of Infarct Size Using Evans Blue Dye Staining

1. Upon sacrifice, hearts of infarcted mice are extracted.
2. The aortic arch is cannulated using an intravenous cannula.
3. Evans Blue Dye (EBD) is dissolved in phosphate-buffered saline (PBS; 0.15 M NaCl, 10 mM phosphate buffer, pH 7.4) with a concentration of the injected dye of 0.5 mg EBD/0.05 mL PBS.
4. EBD (50 µL) is slowly injected (16-gage cannula) into the aorta to perfuse the heart through the coronary arteries.
5. Infarcted areas appear pale in color, whereas normal, perfused areas are stained and appear blue with EBD.

3.4. Tissue Processing

1. Mice are terminally anesthetized with a subcutaneous injection of a mixture of xylazine/ketamine in 0.9% saline.
2. Both native and transplanted hearts as well as infarcted hearts are perfused with 6 mL of 0.9% saline followed by 6 mL of 2% paraformaldehyde (*see* **Note 2**) in PBS.
3. Hearts are excised and postfixed in 2% paraformaldehyde for 4 h, followed by cryoprotection through immersion in 20% sucrose in PBS overnight.

4. The following day, hearts are embedded in OCT, snap-frozen in liquid nitrogen and stored at –80°C.

5. OCT blocks are then cryosectioned and stored at –20°C until they are prepared for imaging (*see* **Notes 3** and **4**).

3.4. In Vivo Detection of GFP-Positive Bone Marrow Progenitor Cells

Fluorescent stains of fixed monolayer cultures or tissue sections can readily be visualized using confocal or multiphoton imaging. Conventional confocal microscopy is useful for routine imaging of relatively thin (<50 μm) sections of fixed cells or tissues. Multiphoton microscopy is most useful when one is imaging samples that are thick (>50 μm) and is advantageous over conventional confocal microscopy since it causes less photodamage and photobleaching. In our laboratory, the Leica TCS SP2 AOBS™ (Acousto-Optical Beam Splitter) confocal and multiphoton microscope is used to identify endogenous GFP-positive bone marrow-derived progenitor cells in heart tissue sections.

1. Set the appropriate objective in place (e.g., 20×, 40×, 63×). When using oil immersion objectives, place one drop of oil on the surface of the cover-slipped slide directly over the specimen (*see* **Notes 5–7**).

2. Using the coarse and fine focus knobs on the microscope, focus the specimen on the GFP-positive cells in the heart tissue.

3. Adjust the settings on the microscope to obtain the appropriate gain and light intensity to detect GFP-emission wavelengths (approx 509 nm) using the Leica FITC filter set (excitation wavelength 450–490 nm).

4. Confocal microscopy allows the user to perform optical Z-sections on biospecimens. By varying the distance between the pinhole and the specimen, users can generate an optical Z-series that dissects through the entire thickness of the specimen. The step size (how many Z-sections) and the thickness of each Z-section can be determined and set using the confocal software during image capture.

4. Notes

1. Recent studies have also incorporated in vivo techniques in animal models in which the peripheral stem cell population has been enriched and mobilized through treatment with various cytokines, such as granulocyte colony-stimulating factor (G-CSF) *(39)*. This cytokine can be used in conjunction with other synergistic cytokines, such as stem cell factor (SCF), for in vivo use in mice to increase stem cell mobilization in an effort to enhance stem cell recruitment to areas of damage (e.g., for injection of a 200-μL solution, G-CSF and SCF are combined at a concentration of 40 pg/mL G-CSF and 10 pg/mL SCF in PBS containing 0.1% bovine serum albumin and injected once a day for 3 or 5 d).

2. Although a wide variety of fixation methods can be utilized successfully, fixation in fresh 2% paraformaldehyde works very well for a wide variety of mono-

layer cultures and tissues. This method tends to produce the lowest amount of background intrinsic fluorescence.

3. After fluorescent staining of fixed tissues on slides, it is best to place the specimen beneath a cover slip using an antifade mounting medium, for example, Molecular Probes' SlowFade® antifade kits. Gently blot off the liquid remaining after the staining protocol, place a small drop of mounting medium over the sample, and place the cover slip over the area. The cover slip can be secured in place with nail polish.

4. Considerations when preparing tissue sections for confocal microscopy include the following:
   a. Avoid the use of tissues containing melanin, as this absorbs infrared light and prevents proper imaging of the specimen.
   b. Tissue sections should be placed as flat as possible against a cover slip, in order to minimize the required working distance during image capture.
   c. Choose probes with the highest fluorescence yield, in order to maximize the sensitivity of detection within autofluorescent tissues.

5. Handle lenses very carefully. Jarring a lens in any way can permanently destroy the alignment of the elements within it. Before examining a sample, ensure that there is no foreign material on the sample that could contaminate the lens surface. Prior to using the appropriate objective lens, make sure to check whether the lens is either water or oil immersion.

6. After using an oil immersion lens, clean the lens with appropriate lens paper and solution. Use several pieces of lens paper until there is no longer evidence of oil on the paper. Avoid pressing the lens paper with your finger onto the transparent part of the lens.

7. Do not mix immersion oils. If there is any other contaminant on your slide, clean it or do not use that slide. Contaminating the lens surface can lead to serious problems during imaging.

Acknowledgments

The authors wish to thank Dr. S. Corbel for creating and generously providing the GFP transgenic mice used in these studies. This work was funded by operating grants from the Canadian Institutes of Health Research (CIHR) and St. Paul's Hospital Foundation (to T.J.P.) and from CIHR and the Heart and Stroke Foundation of BC and Yukon (to B.M.M.). N.R. is a recipient of a David Hardwick Studentship and the University of British Columbia Faculty of Medicine Harry and Florence Dennison Fellowship in Medical Research.

References

1. Caplan, A. I. and Bruder, S. P. (2001) Mesenchymal stem cells: building blocks for molecular medicine in the 21st century. *Trends. Mol. Med.* **7,** 259–264.
2. Makino, S., Fukuda, K., Miyoshi, S., et al. (1999) Cardiomyocytes can be generated from marrow stromal cells in vitro. *J. Clin. Invest.* **103,** 697–705.

3. Pittenger, M. F., Mackay, A. M., Beck, S. C., et al. (1999) Multilineage potential of adult human mesenchymal stem cells. *Science* **284,** 143–147.

4. Grigoriadis, A. E., Heersche, J. N., and Aubin, J. E. (1988) Differentiation of muscle, fat, cartilage, and bone from progenitor cells present in a bone-derived clonal cell population: effect of dexamethasone. *J. Cell. Biol.* **106,** 2139–2151.

5. Prockop, D. J. (1997) Marrow stromal cells as stem cells for nonhematopoietic tissues. *Science* **276,** 71–74.

6. Goodell, M. A., Brose, K., Paradis, G., et al. (1996) Isolation and functional properties of murine hematopoietic stem cells that are replicating in vivo. *J. Exp. Med.* **183,** 1797–1806.

7. Corbel, S. Y., Lee, A., Yi, L., et al. (2003) Contribution of hematopoietic stem cells to skeletal muscle. *Nat. Med.* **9,** 1528–1532.

8. Jackson, K. A., Majka, S. M., Wang, H., et al. (2001) Regeneration of ischemic cardiac muscle and vascular endothelium by adult stem cells. *J. Clin. Invest.* **107,** 1395–1402.

9. Jackson, K. A., Majka, S. A., Wang, H., et al. (2001) Regeneration of ischemic cardiac muscle and vascular endothelium by adult stem cells. *J. Clin. Invest.* **107,** 1395–1402.

10. Orlic, D., Kajstura, J., Chimenti, S., et al. (2001) Bone marrow cells regenerate infarcted myocardium. *Nature* **410,** 701–705.

11. Orlic, D., Kajstura, J., Chimenti, S., et al. (2003) Bone marrow stem cells regenerate infarcted myocardium. *Pediatr. Transplant.* **7,** 86–88.

12. Goodell, M. A., Jackson, K. A., Majka, S. M., et al. (2001) Stem cell plasticity in muscle and bone marrow. *Ann. NY Acad. Sci.* **938,** 208–218; discussion 218–220.

13. Haynesworth, S. E., Goshima, J., Goldberg, V. M., et al. (1992) Characterization of cells with osteogenic potential from human marrow. *Bone* **13,** 81–88.

14. Soonpaa, M. H. and Field, L. J. (1998) Survey of studies examining mammalian cardiomyocyte DNA synthesis. *Circ. Res.* **83,** 15–26.

15. Soonpaa, M. H., Koh, G. Y., Pajak, L., et al. (1997) Cyclin D1 overexpression promotes cardiomyocyte DNA synthesis and multinucleation in transgenic mice. *J. Clin. Invest.* **99,** 2644–2654.

16. Laflamme, M. A., Myerson, D., Saffitz, J. E., et al. (2002) Evidence for cardiomyocyte repopulation by extracardiac progenitors in transplanted human hearts. *Circ. Res.* **90,** 634–640.

17. Quaini, F., Urbanek, K., Beltrami, A. P., et al. (2002) Chimerism of the transplanted heart. *N. Engl. J. Med.* **346,** 5–15.

18. Gao, S. Z., Schroeder, J. S., Alderman, E. L., et al. (1987) Clinical and laboratory correlates of accelerated coronary artery disease in the cardiac transplant patient. *Circulation* **76,** V56–61.

19. Gao, S. Z., Alderman, E. L., Schroeder, J. S., et al. (1988) Accelerated coronary vascular disease in the heart transplant patient: coronary arteriographic findings. *J. Am. Coll. Cardiol.* **12,** 334–340.

20. Lai, J. C., Tranfield, E. M., Walker, D. C., et al. (2003) Ultrastructural evidence of early endothelial damage in coronary arteries of rat cardiac allografts. *J. Heart Lung Transplant.* **22,** 993–1004.

21. Dong, C., Redenbach, D., Wood, S., et al. (1996) The pathogenesis of cardiac allograft vasculopathy. *Curr. Opin. Cardiol.* **11**, 183–190.
22. Triulzi, D. J. and Nalesnik, M. A. (2001) Microchimerism, GVHD, and tolerance in solid organ transplantation. *Transfusion* **41**, 419–426.
23. Ichikawa, N., Demetris, A. J., Starzl, T. E., et al. (2000) Donor and recipient leukocytes in organ allografts of recipients with variable donor-specific tolerance: with particular reference to chronic rejection. *Liver Transpl.* **6**, 686–702.
24. Kashiwagi, N., Porter, K. A., Penn, I., et al. (1969) Studies of homograft sex and of gamma globulin phenotypes after orthotopic homotransplantation of the human liver. *Surg. Forum* **20**, 374–376.
25. Starzl, T. E., Demetris, A. J., Trucco, M., et al. (1992) Systemic chimerism in human female recipients of male livers. *Lancet* **340**, 876,877.
26. Demetris, A. J., Murase, N., and Starzl, T. E. (1992) Donor dendritic cells after liver and heart allotransplantation under short-term immunosuppression. *Lancet* **339**, 1610.
27. Kocher, A. A., Schuster, M. D., Szabolcs, M. J., et al. (2001) Neovascularization of ischemic myocardium by human bone-marrow-derived angioblasts prevents cardiomyocyte apoptosis, reduces remodeling and improves cardiac function. *Nat. Med.* **7**, 430–436.
28. Taylor, D. A., Hruban, R., Rodriguez, E. R., et al. (2002) Cardiac chimerism as a mechanism for self-repair: does it happen and if so to what degree? *Circulation* **106**, 2–4.
29. Orlic, D., Kajstura, J., Chimenti, S., et al. (2001) Transplanted adult bone marrow cells repair myocardial infarcts in mice. *Ann. NY Acad. Sci.* **938**, 221–229; discussion 229,230.
30. Hasegawa, S., Becker, G., Nagano, H., et al. (1998) Pattern of graft- and host-specific MHC class II expression in long-term murine cardiac allografts: origin of inflammatory and vascular wall cells. *Am. J. Pathol.* **153**, 69–79.
31. Sata, M., Saiura, A., Kunisato, A., et al. (2002) Hematopoietic stem cells differentiate into vascular cells that participate in the pathogenesis of atherosclerosis. *Nat. Med.* **8**, 403–409.
32. Shimizu, K., Sugiyama, S., Aikawa, M., et al. (2001) Host bone-marrow cells are a source of donor intimal smooth- muscle-like cells in murine aortic transplant arteriopathy. *Nat. Med.* **7**, 738–741.
33. Saiura, A., Sata, M., Hirata, Y., et al. (2001) Circulating smooth muscle progenitor cells contribute to atherosclerosis. *Nat. Med.* **7**, 382,383.
34. Arai, A. E., Pantely, G. A., Thoma, W. J., et al. (1992) Energy metabolism and contractile function after 15 beats of moderate myocardial ischemia. *Circ. Res.* **70**, 1137–1145.
35. Pfeffer, J. M., Pfeffer, M. A., Fletcher, P. J., et al. (1991) Progressive ventricular remodeling in rat with myocardial infarction. *Am. J. Physiol.* **260**, H1406–1414.
36. White, H. D., Norris, R. M., Brown, M. A., et al. (1987) Left ventricular end-systolic volume as the major determinant of survival after recovery from myocardial infarction. *Circulation* **76**, 44–51.
37. Grogan, M., Redfield, M. M., Bailey, K. R., et al. (1995) Long-term outcome of patients with biopsy-proved myocarditis: comparison with idiopathic dilated cardiomyopathy. *J. Am. Coll. Cardiol.* **26**, 80–84.

38. Kehat, I., Kenyagin-Karsenti, D., Snir, M., et al. (2001) Human embryonic stem cells can differentiate into myocytes with structural and functional properties of cardiomyocytes. *J. Clin. Invest.* **108,** 407–414.

39. Orlic, D., Kajstura, J., Chimenti, S., et al. (2001) Mobilized bone marrow cells repair the infarcted heart, improving function and survival. *Proc. Natl. Acad. Sci. USA* **98,** 10,344–10,349.

40. Beltrami, A. P., Urbanek, K., Kajstura, J., et al. (2001) Evidence that human cardiac myocytes divide after myocardial infarction. *N. Engl. J. Med.* **344,** 1750–1757.

41. Bittner, R. E., Schofer, C., Weipoltshammer, K., et al. (1999) Recruitment of bone-marrow-derived cells by skeletal and cardiac muscle in adult dystrophic mdx mice. *Anat. Embryol. (Berl.)* **199,** 391–396.

42. Min, J. Y., Yang, Y., Converso, K. L., et al. (2002) Transplantation of embryonic stem cells improves cardiac function in postinfarcted rats. *J. Appl. Physiol.* **92,** 288–296.

43. Shake, J. G., Gruber, P. J., Baumgartner, W. A., et al. (2002) Mesenchymal stem cell implantation in a swine myocardial infarct model: engraftment and functional effects. *Ann. Thorac. Surg.* **73,** 1919–1925; discussion 1926.

44. Barbash, I. M., Chouraqui, P., Baron, J., et al. (2003) Systemic delivery of bone marrow-derived mesenchymal stem cells to the infarcted myocardium: feasibility, cell migration, and body distribution. *Circulation* **108,** 863–868.

45. Toma, C., Pittenger, M. F., Cahill, K. S., et al. (2002) Human mesenchymal stem cells differentiate to a cardiomyocyte phenotype in the adult murine heart. *Circulation* **105,** 93–98.

46. Orlic, D., Hill, J. M., and Arai, A. E. (2002) Stem cells for myocardial regeneration. *Circ. Res.* **91,** 1092–1102.

15

Endothelial Progenitor Cell Culture and Gene Transfer

Hideki Iwaguro and Takayuki Asahara

Summary

Bone marrow-derived endothelial progenitor cells (EPCs) are present in the systemic circulation, are augmented in response to certain cytokines and/or tissue ischemia, and home to as well as incorporate into sites of neovascularization. The EPC cell culture is extremely important for biological research of EPCs. The established culture system allows the selection of progenitor cells. This chapter addresses basic technique for the use of essential major items of EPC culture equipment and materials, such as ex vivo expansion and gene transfer. We discuss methodologies available for analysis of EPC cell therapy and gene-modified EPC therapy.

Key Words: Endothelial progenitor cells; angiogenesis; vasculogenesis; ischemia; gene transfer; vascular endothelial growth factor; neovasularization.

1. Introduction

Tissue regeneration by somatic stem/progenitor cells has been recognized as a maintenance or recovery system of many organs in the adult. The isolation and investigation of these somatic stem/progenitor cells have helped to explain how these cells contribute to postnatal organogenesis. On the basis of regenerative potency, these stem/progenitor cells are expected to develop as a key strategy in therapeutic applications for the damaged organs.

Recently, endothelial progenitor cells (EPCs) have been isolated from adult peripheral blood (1). EPCs are considered to share common stem/progenitor cells with hematopoietic stem cells and have been shown to derive from bone marrow (BM) and to incorporate into foci of physiological or pathological neovascularization (2–13). The finding that EPCs home to sites of

From: *Methods in Molecular Medicine, vol. 112: Molecular Cardiology: Methods and Protocols*
Edited by: Z. Sun © Humana Press Inc., Totowa, NJ

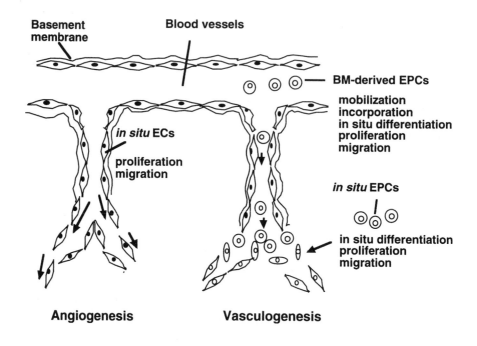

Fig. 1. Postnatal neovascularization in physiological or pathological events is consistent with the contribution to neovessel formation by angiogenesis and vasculogenesis at various rates according to the two mechanisms. Angiogenesis and vasculogenesis are caused by activation of *in situ* endotheial cells (ECs) and bone marrow (BM)-derived or *in situ* endothelial progenitor cells (EPCs), respectively.

neovascularization and differentiate into endothelial cells *in situ* is consistent with *vasculogenesis*, a critical paradigm well described for embryonic neovascularization. Recent findings in adults suggest that a reservoir of stem/progenitor cells contributes to postnatal vascular organogenesis. The discovery of EPCs has therefore drastically changed our understanding of adult blood vessel formation (**Fig. 1**).

EPC transplantation constitutes a novel therapeutic strategy that provides a robust source of viable endothelial cells (ECs) to supplement the contribution of ECs resident in the adult vasculature that migrate, proliferate, and remodel in response to angiogenic cues, according to the classic paradigm of angiogenesis developed by Folkman *(14)*. Just as classical angiogenesis may be impaired by certain pathologic phenotypes, EPC function (i.e., mobilization from the bone marrow and incorporation into neovascular foci) may be impaired by aging, diabetes, hypercholesterolemia, and hyperhomocysteinemia. Gene transfer to EPCs during ex vivo expansion represents a potential approach to enhance EPC function. We present research protocols for transferring vascular endothelial growth factor (VEGF) gene to EPCs to achieve angiogenic phenotypical modulation of EPC function.

2. Materials

1. 50- and 15-mL conical tubes.
2. DPBS, Ca^-, Mg^- with 0.5 mM EDTA (DPBSE). Store at 4°C.
3. Histopaque-1077. Store at 4°C (Sigma).
4. Ammonium chloride solution. Store at 4°C (Stem Cell Technologies).
5. DPBS, Ca^+, Mg^+. Store at 4°C (Clonetics).
6. 10-mL syringes with 18-gage needles.
7. Trypsin/EDTA solution store at 4°C (Clonetics).
8. Human fibronectin store at 4°C (Sigma).
9. Endothelial basal medium-2 (EBM-2) and EGM-2 MV store at 4°C (Clonetics).
10. 6-Well cell culture cluster (Corning).
11. Murine VEGF 164 gene.
12. *lacZ* (β-galactosidase) gene.
13. MTS Assay kit stable at 4°C for up to 3 mo (Promega, Madison, WI).
14. ELISA plate reader stable at 4°C for up to 1 mo (Bionetics Laboratory, Charleston, SC).
15. 96-Well cell culture cluster (Corning).
16. Fluorescent carbocyanine 1,1'-dioctadecyl-3,3,3',3'-tetramethylindo-carbocyanine perchlorate (DiI) at –20°C (Biomedical Technologies, Stoughton, MA).
17. Tumor necrosis factor (TNF)-α at 4°C (1 ng/mL).
18. Human umbilical vein endothelial cell (HUVEC).
19. X-gal solution: 5 mM Ferri/Ferro cyanide, 1 M $MgCl_2$, 5% deoxycholate, 5% Nonidet p-40, and 40 mg/mL X-gal solution.

3. Methods

The methods comprise include two steps: (1) mononuclear cell (MNC) selection, and (2) EPC culture.

3.1. MNCs Selection

1. Put 15 mL of DPBSE (*see* **Note 1**) into a 50-mL conical tube and collect 30–35 mL of peripheral blood from healthy human volunteers by dropping it slowly into the Histopaque tube at room temperature.
2. Centrifuge at 400g for 30 min at room temperature without a break, collect a monolayer of cells, and centrifuge at 450g for 10 min at 4°C with a low break.
3. To deplete platelets, centrifuge at 250g for 10 min at 4°C with a low break. Resuspend the cell pellet in ammonium chloride solution for 10 min on ice.
4. After washing with DPBSE, re-suspend endothelial cells (ECs) in basal medium-2 (EBM-2) complete medium.

3.2. EPC Culture

1. Following counting the number of MNC, incubate MNCs in EBM-2 (Clonetics, San Diego, CA) supplemented with 5% fetal bovine serum (FBS), human VEGF-A, human fibroblast growth factor-2, human epidermal growth factor, insulin-like growth factor-1, and ascorbic acid. Culture on human fibronectin (Sigma) coated culture dishes.
2. For human fibronectin coating, reconstitute 5 mg of human fibronectin with 5 mL of sterile water, and allow it to dissolve for at least 30 min at 37°C.
3. Put the fibronectin solution into a dish for 30 s and dry in the clean bench for more than 15 min. For coating a 4-well slide, or a 35-mm dish (or a dish made of glass), add 1.5% gelatin and 335 µL to 5 mL of fibrotectin solution. (Final concentration of gelatin is 0.5%.)
4. Generally, plate these MNCs $1–1.3 \times 10^7$ in a 35-mm^2 dish (*see* **Note 2**).
5. On d 4, after washing cells with DPBS twice, collect cells by pipeting into a 50-mL conical tube. Centrifuge at 250g for 5 min at 4°C, resuspend cell pellets in EBM-2 complete media, and seed 1×10^6 cells into a 35-mm^2 dish. By d 7, the culture should be maintained in EBM-2 in a 5% CO_2 incubator *(4,6)*.

3.2.1. EPC Gene Transfer and In Vitro Study

The methods described below outline (1) EPC gene transfer, (2) proliferative activity assay, and (3) in vitro incorporation of Tf-EPCs into the HUVEC monolayer.

3.2.2. EPC Gene Transfer

After 7 d in culture, cells were transduced with an adenovirus encoding the murine VEGF 164 gene (Ad/VEGF) or *lacZ* gene (Ad/β-gal) *(15)*. To establish optimal conditions for EPCs, adenovirus gene transfer serum concentration, virus incubation time, and virus concentration were evaluated using X-gal staining to detect ß-galactosidase expression (**Fig. 2**).

Human EPCs were transfected with 1000 MOI of Ad/VEGF or Ad/β-gal for 3 h of incubation in 1% serum media. After an adenovirus transduction, the cells were washed with phosphate-buffered saline (PBS) and incubated in EBM-2 media for 24 h prior to transplantation experiments.

3.2.3. Proliferative Activity Assay

1. At 24 h after gene transfer, reseed EPCs transduced with Ad/VEGF (Tf/V-EPCs), Ad/β-gal (Tf/β-EPCs), or nontransduced EPCs (non-Tf/EPCs) on 96-well plates coated with human fibronectin to determine the proliferative activity using the 3-(4,5-dimethylthiazol-2-yl)-5-(3-carboxymethoxyphenyl)-2-(4-sulfophenyl)-2H-tetrazolium assay (*see* **Note 3**).
2. After 48 h in culture, add methotrexate/phenazine methosulfate (MTS/PMS) solution to each well, and incubate for 3 h. Light absorbance at 490 nm was detected by an ELISA plate reader.

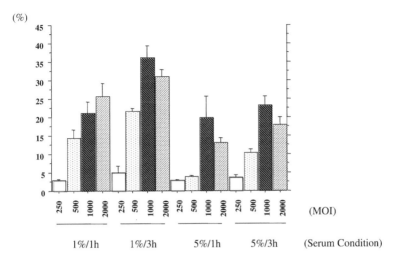

Fig. 2. Profile of transfection efficiencies for Ad/β-gal in ex vivo expanded human EPCs. Four different multiplicities of infection (MOIs: 250, 500, 1000, and 2000) were tested in two different media conditions (1% or 5% serum EBM-2), for 1 or 3 h of incubation. Error bars represent SEM of triplicate experiments. Following these preliminary experiments, human EPCs were transduced with 1000 MOI Ad/VEGF or Ad/β-gal for 3 h in 1% serum media (*see* **Note 2**). *$p < 0.01$, non-Tf vs Tf/β-gal.

In our previous experiments *(15)*, the MTS assay was employed to determine proliferative activity of transduced EPCs. By using 5% serum conditioned media, we found that the proliferative activity of Ad/VEGF-transduced EPCs exceeded the proliferative activity of Ad/β-gal (0.48 ± 0.03 vs 0.37 ± 0.01 corrected absorbance at 490 nm, $p < 0.01$) and nontransduced EPCs (non-Tf = 0.32 ± 0.02, $p < 0.05$) in vitro (**Fig. 3**).

3.2.4. In Vitro Incorporation of Td-EPCs Into the HUVEC Monolayer

At 24 h after gene transfer, Tf/V-EPCs and Tf/β-EPCs were stained with fluorescent carbocyanine DiI. DiI-labeled EPCs (*see* **Note 4**) were incubated in a monolayer of HUVECs in 4-well culture slides for 12 h with or without pretreatment with TNF-α (1 ng/mL) *(16)*.

1. Three hours after incubation, remove nonadherent cells by washing with PBS, apply new media, and maintain the culture for an additional 24 h.
2. Count the total number of adhesive EPCs in each well in a blinded manner under a ×200 magnification field of a fluorescent microscope.
3. At 24 h after transduction, label EPCs with the fluorescent marker DiI for cell tracking. Incubate DiI-labeled, VEGF-transduced EPCs in a HUVEC monolayer for 12 h with or without pretreatment with TNF-α (1 ng/mL) (**Fig. 4A**).

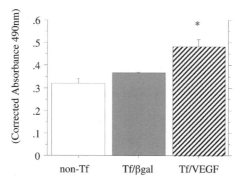

Fig. 3. Proliferative activity assay. The proliferative activity of EPCs transduced in 5% serum was measured by MTS assay after 48 h in culture. The increase in mitogenic response of EPCs transduced with Ad/VEGF (Tf/V-EPCs) was statistically significant in comparison with EPCs transduced with Ad/β-gal (Tf/β-EPCs) and nontransduced EPCs (non-Tf). *$p < 0.01$, Tf/β-gal vs non-Tf.

4. After 3 h of incubation, remove nonadherent cells by washing with PBS, and count DiI-marked cells adherent to the HUVEC monolayer manually.

In our previous experiments *(15)*, in the quiescent HUVEC monolayer, adhesion of DiI-labeled EPCs was not significantly different between Tf/V-EPCs and Tf/β-EPC transplanted animals (2.7 ± 0.2 vs 2.2 ± 0.3, p = ns; **Fig. 4B**). In activated HUVECs, however, adhesion of DiI-labeled Tf/V-EPCs exceeded that of Tf/β-EPCs (4.3 ± 0.4 vs 2.9 ± 0.3, $p < 0.01$). Alternatively, the same cells were incubated in new media and maintained for 24 h in the HUVEC monolayer to confirm incorporation in vitro and in vivo (*see* **Note 5**). In the quiescent HUVEC monolayer, incorporation of DiI-labeled Tf/V-EPCs exceeded that of Tf/β-EPCs (7.0 ± 0.5 vs 3.5 ± 0.5, $p < 0.01$; **Fig. 4B**). In activated HUVECs, incorporation of DiI-labeled Tf/V-EPCs also exceeded that of Tf/β-EPCs (13.8 ± 0.8 vs 5.3 ± 0.6, $p < 0.001$).

4. Notes

1. Basic DPBS solution: add 45 g of sodium chloride, 13.11 g of sodium phosphase (monobasic), and 57.41 g of sodium phosphase (dibasic) to 5 L of sterile water. For making the DPBSE solution, add 186.1 g of EDTA to 800 mL of sterile water, and mix EDTA solution with the DPBS solution for 0.5 M DPBSE solution. (Stirring and adjust pH 8.0.)
2. Cell culture number of the initial plates (approximate):
   A 10-cm dish: 3.0–5.0×10^7 cells.

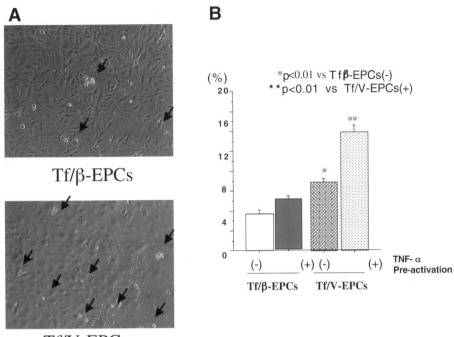

Fig. 4. In vitro incorporation of Td-EPCs in HUVEC monolayer. (**A**) Representative macroscopic photographs of Tf/V-EPCs and Tf/β-EPCs in a HUVEC monolayer at 24 h after transduction with Ad/VEGF or Ad/β-gal, respectively. Upper panel, Tf/β-EPCs. Lower panel, Tf/V-EPCs in HUVEC monolayer, both pretreated with tumor necrosis factor-α (TNF-a) stimulation. White bars indicate 50-μm length. (**B**) Quantitative analysis of EPC adhesion observed at 3 h and incorporation observed at 24 h after transduction with (+) and without (-) pretreatment with TNF-α. *$p < 0.01$, Tf/β-EPCs vs Tf/V-EPCs.

       A 35-mm dish: $0.8–1.0 \times 10^7$ cells.

       A 4-well dish: $2.0–8.0 \times 10^6$ cells.

3. MTS (3-(4,5-dimethylthiazol-2-yl)-5-(3-carboxymethoxyphenyl)-2-(4-sulfophenyl)-2H-tetrazolium) assay: nonradioactive cell proliferation is a method for determining the number of viable cells in proliferation or chemosensitivity assays. The following procedure is recommended for the preparation of reagents sufficient for one 96-well plate containing cells cultured in a 100 μL volume. Then add 20 μL of combined MTS/PMS solution (basic 100 μL of PMS solution/2.0 mL of MTS solution) into each well of the 96-well assay plate containing the sample, and incubate the plate for 1–4 h at 37°C in a humidified 5% CO_2 atmosphere.

4. DiI-acetylated-LDL incorporation: purified low-density lipoprotein was acetylated (Ac) and then labeled with the fluorescent probe DiI for labeling endothelial cells and macrophages. Aseptically dilute the DiI-Ac-LDL to 10 µg/mL in standard media, add it to live cells, and incubate for 2–4 h at 37°C. Remove media containing DiI-Ac-LDL, wash twice with DPBS, and count cells for each experiment.

5. In vivo cell transplantation: we found, for the first time, that VEGF gene-transferred EPCs improved the impaired neovascularization in an animal model of limb ischemia *(15)*. Transplantation of heterologous EPCs transduced with adenovirus encoding human VEGF 165 (Tf/V-EPC) not only improved neovascularization and blood flow recovery but also had meaningful biological consequences, i.e., limb necrosis and autoamputation were reduced by 63.7% in comparison with Tf/β-EPC animals. Notably, the dose of EPCs needed to achieve limb salvage in these in vivo experiments was 30 times less than that required in the previous experiments using unmodified EPCs.

Acknowledgments

The authors thank Ms. Kanako Ota for her tremendous contribution to the manuscript preparation.

References

1. Asahara, T., Murohara, T., Sullivan, A., et al. (1997) Isolation of putative progenitor endothelial cells for angiogenesis. *Science* **275,** 964–967.
2. Asahara, T., Masuda, H., Takahashi, T., et al. (1999) Bone marrow origin of endothelial progenitor cells responsible for postnatal vasculogenesis in physiological and pathological neovascularization. *Circ. Res.* **85,** 221–228.
3. Takahashi, T., Kalka, C., Masuda, H., et al. (1999) Ischemia- and cytokine-induced mobilization of bone marrow-derived endothelial progenitor cells for neovascularization. *Nature Med.* **5,** 434–438.
4. Asahara, T., Takahashi, T., Masuda, H., et al. (1999) VEGF contributes to postnatal neovascularization by mobilizing bone marrow-derived endothelial progenitor cells. *EMBO J.* **18,** 3964–3972.
5. Kalka, C., Masuda, H., Takahashi, T., et al. (2000) Vascular endothelial growth factor165 gene transfer augments circulating endothelial progenitor cells in human subjects. *Circ. Res.* **86,** 1198–1202.
6. Kalka, C., Tehrani, H., Laudenberg, B., et al. (2000) Mobilization of endothelial progenitor cells following gene therapy with VEGF$_{165}$ in patients with inoperable coronary disease. *Ann. Thorac. Surg.* **70,** 829–834.
7. Shi, Q., Rafii, S., Wu, MH-D., et al. (1998) Hammond WP. Evidence for circulating bone marrow-derived endothelial cells. *Blood* **92,** 362–367.
8. Hatzopoulos, A. K., Folkman, J., Vasile, E., Eiselen, G. K., and Rosenberg, R. D. (1998) Isolation and characterization of endothelial progenitor cells from mouse embyros. *Development* **125,** 1457–1468.

9. Gunsilius, E., Duba, H. C., Petzer, A. L., et al. (2000) Evidence from a leukaemia model for maintenance of vascular endothelium by bone-marrow-derived endothelial cells. *Lancet* **355,** 1688–1691.

10. Gehling, U. M., Ergun, S., Schumacher, U., et al. (2000) In vivo differntiation of endothelial cells from AC133-positive progenitor cells. *Blood* **95,** 3106–3112.

11. Crosby, J. R., Kaminski, W. E., Schatteman, G., et al. (2000) Endothelial cells of hematopoietic origin make a significant contribution to adult blood vessel formation. *Circ. Res.* **87,** 728–730.

12. Moldovan, N. I., Goldschmidt-Clermont, P. J., Parker-Thornburg, J., Shapiro, S. D., and Kolattukudy, P. E. (2000) Contribution of monocytes/macrophages to compensatory neovascularization. The drilling of metalloelastase-positive tunnels in ischemic myocardium. *Circ. Res.* **87,** 378–384.

13. Murohara, T., Ikeda, H., Duan, J., et al. (2000) Transplanted cord blood-derived endothelial precursor cells augment postnatal neovascularization. *J. Clin. Invest.* **105,** 1527–1536.

14. Folkman, J. (1993) Tumor angiogenesis, in *Cancer Medicine*, 3rd ed. (Holland, J. F., Frei, E., III, Bast, R. C., Jr., et al., eds.), Lea & Febiger, Philadephia, PA, pp. 153–170.

15. Iwaguro, H., Yamaguchi, J., Kalka, C., et al. (2002) Endothelial progenitor cell vascular endothelial growth factor gene transfer for vascular regeneration. *Circulation* **105,** 732–738.

16. Simmons, P. J., Masinovdky, B., Longenecker, B. M., Berenson, R., Torok-Storb, B., and Gallatin, W. M. (1992) Vascular cell adhesion molecule-1 expressed by bone marrow stromal cells mediates the binding of hematopoietic progenitor cells. *Blood* **80,** 388–395.

IV

GENE ANALYSIS IN THE INJURED AND HYPERTROPHIED HEART

16

Delineation of Sequences Essential for Specific Promoter Activation During Pressure Overloaded Hypertrophy or Factor-Induced Hypertrophy

Chellam Rajamanickam and Radhakrishnan Jeejabai

Summary

Earlier studies from our laboratory have demonstrated the appearance of a high M_r (182-kDa) phosphoprotein during early stages of development of cardiac hypertrophy in the sera of animals subjected to aortic constriction. Furthermore, it has been reported that the injection of purified 182-kDa protein into normal animals led to the development of hypertrophy, and the injection of polyclonal antibodies into the aorta constricted animals completely, abolished the development of hypertrophy, and downregulated the expression of the β-Myosin heavy chain (MHC) gene. To identify the *cis*-acting regulatory element(s), which controls induction of the β-MHC gene in acute pressure-overloaded cardiac hypertrophy induced by the 182-kDa protein, the β-MHC promoter fragments of various lengths linked to the chloramphenicol acetyl transferase (CAT) reporter were injected into the left ventricular apex of adult rats, which underwent aortic constriction/182-kDa protein injection or were sham-operated. Activation of the β-MHC gene by the 182-kDa protein was studied by a chimeric gene constructed by fusion of the 5' regulatory regions of the β-MHC gene to bacterial CAT, demonstrating that at least 431 bp of the β-MHC promoter (+103 to −328) with one E-box motif, along with upstream regulatory sequences such as the TATA box, N-Fe, C-rich, and M-CAT elements are required for β-MHC gene expression in vivo during cardiac hypertrophy induced by the 182-kDa protein.

Key Words: β-Myosin heavy chain gene; cardiac hypertrophy; aortic constriction; CAT assay; 182-kDa protein; promoter deletion.

From: *Methods in Molecular Medicine, vol. 112: Molecular Cardiology: Methods and Protocols*
Edited by: Z. Sun © Humana Press Inc., Totowa, NJ

1. Introduction

Cardiac hypertrophy is the primary chronic compensatory mechanism responding to increased hemodynamic load, yet the underlying mechanisms leading to its development are poorly understood. The gene for β-myosin heavy chain (MHC) gene has been studied extensively, and its induction is characteristic of pressure overloaded cardiac hypertrophy. Earlier studies from our laboratory have demonstrated the appearance of a high M_r (182-kDa) phosphoprotein in the sera of animals subjected to aortic constriction *(1)*. The injection of purified 182-kDa protein into normal animals led to the development of hypertrophy *(2)*, and the injection of polyclonal antibodies into the aorta constricted animals completely, abolished the development of hypertrophy, and downregulated the expression of the β-MHC gene *(3)*. To identify the *cis*-acting regulatory element(s), which controls induction of the β-MHC gene in acute pressure overload induced by 182-kDa protein, β-MHC promoter fragments of various lengths linked to the chloramphenicol acetyl transferase (CAT) reporter were injected into the left ventricular apex of adult rats, which underwent aortic constriction/182-kDa protein injection or were sham-operated. Activation of the β-MHC gene by the 182-kDa protein was studied by a chimeric gene constructed by fusion of the 5' regulatory regions of the β-MHC gene to bacterial CAT.

2. Materials

1. Albino rats of Wistar derived strain (weight range of 120 ± 5 g).
2. Cesium chloride.
3. Dithiothreitol (DTT): thermo labile—prepare 200 mM stock in sterile MQ water, and store at –20°C.
4. Ethidium bromide: prepare a stock of 10 mg/mL in sterile water, and store in dark bottles at 4°C.
5. Acetyl coenzyme A (CoA): prepare a 20 mM stock in sterile MQ water, and store aliquots at –20°C.
6. EGTA: prepare a stock of 0.5 M EGTA in sterile MQ water, and adjust the pH to 8.0 with 5 N NaOH. The salt will not go into solution until the pH of the solution is adjusted to approx 8.0 by the addition of NaOH.
7. Chloramphenicol: prepare a stock of 30 mg/mL in 100% ethanol, and store aliquots at –20°C. Use 30 μg/mL as the working concentration.
8. RNase A: prepare a stock of 10 mg/mL in 10 mM Tris-HCl, pH 7.5, and 15 mM NaCl; store aliquots at –20°C.
9. S1 nuclease and exonuclease III (MBI Fermentas).
10. S1 nuclease buffer (7.4X): 300 mM potassium acetate (pH 4.6 at 25°C), 2.5 M NaCl, 10 mM $ZnSO_4$, and 50% glycerol.
11. Exonuclease III reaction buffer (10X): 660 mM Tris-HCl, pH 8.0 and 6.6 mM $MgCl_2$.

12. Homogenization buffer for CAT assay: 25 m*M* Tris-HCl, pH 7.8, 15 m*M* MgSO$_4$, 4 m*M* EGTA, pH 8.0, and 1 m*M* DTT (prepare freshly, and add DTT after autoclaving).
13. 10X Phosphate-buffered saline (PBS): 0.8% NaCl, 0.02% KCl, 0.11% Na$_2$HPO$_4$·7H$_2$O, and 0.02% KH$_2$PO$_4$.
14. 1 *M* Tris-HCl, pH 7.5.
15. 1 *M* Tris-HCl, pH 7.2.
16. 0.5 *M* EGTA: prepare a stock of 0.5 *M* EGTA in MQ water, adjust the pH with 5 *N* NaOH, and autoclave. The salt will not go into solution until the pH of the solution is adjusted to approx 8.0 by the addition of NaOH.
17. ^{14}C-labeled chloramphenicol (Radiochemical Centre, Amersham, UK).
18. Ethyl acetate.
19. Chloroform.
20. Methanol.
21. Thin-layer chromatography (TLC) plate and chamber.
22. X-ray film.
23. Tissue homogenizer.
24. Murine β-MHC gene promoter bearing plasmid β5pJR CAT (kind gift of Prof. Jeffrey Robbins).
25. *Escherichia coli* harboring the Cam$^+$ plasmid (to be used as positive control for CAT assay).

3. Methods

The following methods are described in detail:
1. Induction of cardiac hypertrophy in experimental animals by aortic constriction as well as intravenous injection of the 182-kDa protein.
2. Preparation of plasmid constructs for in vivo gene injection.
3. Determination of the minimum length of the β-MHC promoter that is still inducible in vivo during hypertrophy induced by the 182-kDa protein.

3.1. Induction of Cardiac Hypertrophy in Experimental Animals

3.1.1. Aortic Constriction

Cardiac hypertrophy in rats was induced following the method of Rakusan and Poupa *(4)* with slight modifications. Under light diethyl ether anesthesia, a left thoractomy in the third inter costal space was performed to expose the aortic arch. After the ascending aorta had been carefully dissected free, a tantalum hemoclip (Edward Weck, cat. no. 523135) was applied onto the proximal ascending aorta just distal to the coronary ostia, by using a specially designed applicator to occlude the aorta partially. In all the animals the aorta was constricted to the same degree of occlusion that produced hypertrophy without heart failure. The incision was closed with surgical thread. The sham operation was performed similarly on control animals except that no clip was applied on the ascending aorta. The animals were sacrificed at various time intervals after aortic constriction, and the increase in the ratio of heart weight to body weight was calculated.

3.1.2. Intravenous Injection of 182-kDa Protein

Cardiac hypertrophy was induced by intravenous injection of 75 mg of purified 182-kDa protein in 20 mM Tris-HCl, pH 7.2, and 1 mM EDTA buffer (three injections on alternate days).

3.2. Preparation of Plasmid Constructs for Injection Studies

The plasmid β5pJR CAT (β5.11) contains approx 5 kb of the gene, upstream region and the complete nontranslated sequences with the intron–exon organization conserved, fused to the CAT gene of the vector JRCATX (**Fig. 1**). Promoterless reporter vectors such as pSV$_0$CAT and pSV$_2$CAT were from the laboratory collection. The plasmids β0.7 (+103 to –600) of the β-MHC promoter sequence and β0.5 (+103 to –328) as well as plasmids with deletions (clones 1, 2, and 3) were also used (**Fig. 2**).

3.2.1. Generation of Unidirectional Deletions in Plasmid DNA

1. Digest 10 µg of plasmid DNA with a pair of restriction enzymes one of which generates a blunt (for example, *Hae*III) or 5'-overhanging end (for example, *Nde*I), on the side planned for deletions are to proceed (*see* **Note 1**).
2. Cut with a second enzyme that produces a four-base 3'-overhang (for example, *Pst*I) close to the priming site, after ensuring that the first digestion is complete.
3. Perform the digestions for at least 3 h to ensure complete digestion.
4. Extract the reaction mixture with 1 vol of phenol/CHCl$_3$ (25:24:1) and then with 1 vol of CHCl$_3$/isoamyl alcohol (24:1).
5. Precipitate DNA by adding 0.1 vol of 3 M sodium acetate, pH 5.2, and 3 vol 100% ice-cold ethanol. Mix and centrifuge at 12,000 rpm for 10 min. Wash the pellet with 1 mL of 70% ethanol cooled to –20°C.
6. Dissolve the dry pellet (10 µg) in 1.2 µL of 10X exonuclease III reaction buffer. Add sterile MQ water to 12 µL.
7. Put 7.5 µL of S1 nuclease mix (6.75 µL of 7.4X S1 nuclease buffer and sterile MQ water to 50 µL) in tubes numbered for different time points (three different time points, viz., 40 s, 80 s, and 120 s) and place the tubes on ice.
8. Warm the DNA solution at 30°C in a water bath, add 100 U exonuclease III (0.5 µL), and mix rapidly (*see* **Note 2**).
9. Remove 4-µL aliquots from the bath at specific time intervals (*see* **Note 2**), and stop the digestion by adding them to the 7.5 µL S1 nuclease mix kept on ice.
10. After all samples are taken, remove the tubes from ice, heat at 68°C for 10 min, and place on ice.

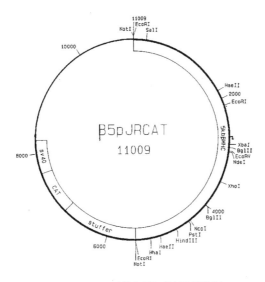

Fig. 1. Plasmid map of β5pJR CAT (β5.11 construct).

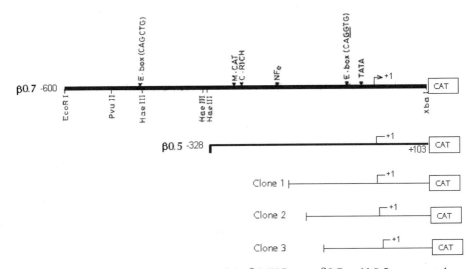

Fig. 2. Upstream regulatory elements of the β-MHC gene. β0.7 and b0.5 constructs harbor 710 bp and 431 bp, respectively, of the upstream regulatory elements of the β-MHC gene. Clones 1, 2, and 3 have approx 250–300 bp of the β-MHC promoter sequence.

11. To make the DNA blunt-ended, add 7.5 μL S1 nuclease mix (6.75 μL of 7.4X S1 nuclease buffer, 0.5 μL [50 U] of S1 nuclease, and sterile MQ water to 50 μL), and incubate for 30 min at 30°C.

15. Then add 1.1 µL of 0.5 *M* EDTA (50 m*M* EDTA final concentration), and heat at 70°C for 10 min to inactivate the S1 nuclease.

16. Precipitate the DNA with ethanol, resuspend in sterile MQ water, and load on a 0.8% agarose gel *(5)*.

3.3. Determination of Minimum Length of the β-MHC Promoter That Is Still Inducible In Vivo During Hypertrophy Induced by 182-kDa Protein

3.3.1. Expression of Full-Length β-MHC Gene Promoter

The β-MHC gene is expressed in a muscle-specific fashion, and its transcripts are found in the ventricles and in the slow skeletal muscle fibers, which can respond to developmental and hormonal cues. Three *cis*-acting elements in the proximal promoter region, termed M-CAT, C-rich, and βe3, have been implicated by *in vitro* transient transfection studies as playing critical roles in the muscle-specific regulation of the gene *(6)*. Earlier reports from our lab have shown that direct injection of purified 182-kDa serum protein into normal animals led to the development of cardiac hypertrophy and the induction of β-MHC characteristic of pressure overloaded hypertrophy *(2)*. To determine whether the sequence included in the β5.11 harboring the full-length β-MHC promoter construct responds to the hypertrophy induced by the 182-kDa protein, reporter gene expression was determined by a CAT assay. Hypertrophy was induced in rats by aortic constriction and protein injection as described in **Subheading 3.1.** Then 75 µg of pure β5.11 construct harboring the full-length β-MHC promoter fused with the CAT reporter gene in 0.9% NaCl was injected (*see* **Note 3**) into the ventricular apex of the heart 2 d after aortic constriction/ 6 d after protein injection. The animals were sacrificed on the fifth day after injection, and CAT activity was studied *(7)* in the ventricular tissues of the heart.

The CAT assay was performed as follows:

1. Mince the heart tissue, and homogenize in 1 mL of homogenization buffer.

2. Centrifuge the suspension at 6000*g* for 10 min at 4°C, and use the supernatant for the CAT assay.

3. Take 10% of the supernatant, and incubate at 65°C for 10 min to inactivate endogenous acetyl transferases, and then centrifuge at 10,000*g* for 5 min. After centrifugation, mix 91.5 µL of clear supernatant with 30 µL of 1 *M* Tris-HCl, pH 7.5, 8 µL ^{14}C-labeled chloramphenicol (0.2 µCi; Radiochemical Centre), and 20 µL of 4 m*M* acetyl-CoA.

4. Incubate the reaction mixture at 37°C for 4 h.

5. Extract the acetylated chloramphenicol with 1 mL of ethyl acetate.

6. Dry under vacuum, suspend in 20 µL ethyl acetate, spot on a TLC plate *(7)*, and run in a chamber equilibrated with chloroform and methanol (95:5) for 30 min.

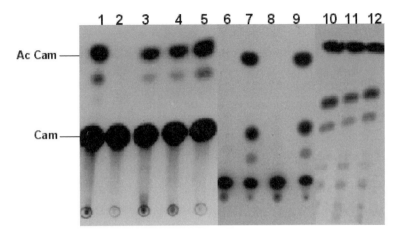

Fig. 3. CAT activity of the β-MHC promoter. Lane 1, pSV2 CAT vector injected (positive control); lane 2, Sham-operated β5.11 construct injected; lane 3, aorta-constricted β5.11 construct injected; lane 4, 182-kDa protein-injected β5.11 construct injected; lane 5, *E. coli* extract harboring CAT gene in pUC 18 plasmid (positive control); lane 6, sham-operated β0.7 construct injected; lane 7, aorta-constricted β0.7 construct injected; lane 8, sham-operated β0.5 construct injected; lane 9, aorta-constricted β0.7 construct injected; lane 10, 182-kDa protein-injected β0.7 construct injected; lane 11, 182-kDa protein-injected β0.5 construct injected; lane 12, *E. coli* extract harboring CAT gene in pUC 18 plasmid (positive control).

7. After the run, air-dry the TLC plate, and expose it to X-ray film in a dark room for 7 d. Develop the film.

The positive control used was *E. coli* extract derived from *E. coli* harboring the Cam[+] plasmid.

The results shown in **Fig. 3** indicate that promoter activity was high in the 182-kDa protein-injected and aorta-constricted animals but absent in sham-operated animals, indicating that the β5.11 construct was able to promote expression of promoter-dependent CAT activity during 182-kDa protein-induced cardiac hypertrophy.

3.3.2. Expression of β0.7/β0.5 Constructs

The *cis–trans* interactions that underlie 182-kDa protein-induced β-MHC expression are not known. Three *cis*-acting elements in the β-MHC gene promoter, which are highly conserved between species, show a complex protein binding pattern in vitro (*8*) and play an important role in the gene's regulation, as determined by transient assay systems. At least one of these elements, the βe3 region, is important for the induction of β-MHC in response to physiological stimuli (the α1-adrenergics) in vitro *(9)*. To determine the *cis* elements required for the β-MHC gene's response to 182-kDa protein, the β5.11 construct having the 5-kb promoter sequence of the β-MHC gene was restricted to about 700-bp (+103 to –600) sequence (β0.7) and a 431-bp (+103 to –328) sequence (β0.5), both of which contain all the upstream regulatory elements except that two E-box sequences are present in the 700-bp upstream sequence, whereas a single E-box sequence is present in the 431-bp sequence.

These constructs (β0.7 and β0.5) with the reporter gene were injected into aorta-constricted, 182-kDa protein-injected, and sham-operated animals, and CAT activity was studied as described in **Subheading 3.3.1.** The results showed that both the β0.7 and β0.5 constructs were able to produce promoter-dependent CAT activity in aorta-constricted and protein-injected animals but not in sham-operated animals (**Fig. 3**).

3.3.3. Cardiac Muscle-Specific Expression of β-MHC Gene in Response to Hypertrophy Induced by the 182-kDa Protein Can Be Mediated by the Proximal Promoter

The β0.5 construct, which carries only 431 bp of the sequence 5' to the transcriptional start site, was able to promote expression during 182-kDa protein-induced cardiac hypertrophy. To determine whether this short basal promoter can be narrowed down further and still be induced by the 182-kDa protein, nested deletions were carried out with this plasmid using exonuclease III. After deletion, plasmid subclones with approx 250–300 bp of β-MHC promoter region were obtained (**Fig. 2**).

3.3.4. Expression of the 250–300-bp β-MHC Promoter Constructs

Plasmid constructs with 250–300 bp of the β-MHC promoter region were injected into the hearts of protein injected and aorta-constricted rats. All three plasmid constructs carrying varying lengths of the β-MHC promoter were unable to express the CAT gene in this study.

Radioactivity associated with acetylated and nonacetylated forms of chloramphenicol was determined on the developed film. The autoradiogram (**Fig. 4**) indicated the absence of promoter activity of β-MHC in all the animals and confirmed that these clones were not able to induce expression of β-MHC during hypertrophy induced by injection of the 182-kDa protein. The same was the case with aorta-constricted animals, showing that at least 431 bp of the β-MHC promoter (+103 to –328) with only one E-box motif, along with upstream regulatory sequences (such as TATA box, N-Fe, C-rich, and M-CAT elements) are required for β-MHC gene expression in vivo during cardiac hypertrophy induced by the 182-kDa protein.

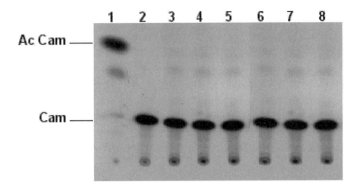

Fig. 4. CAT activity of approx 250–300 bp of the β-MHC promoter. Lane 1, *E. coli* extract (positive control); lane 2, sham-operated β5.11 CAT-injected; lanes 3–5, aorta-constricted/clones (clones 1, 2, and 3) with approx 250–300 bp β-MHC promoter injected; lanes 6–8, 182-kDa protein-injected/clones (clones 1, 2, and 3) with approx 250–300 bp β-MHC promoter injected.

4. Notes

1. The 5'-overhanging end will be susceptible to exonuclease III digestion. If there are no restriction sites available on the side on which the deletions are to proceed, it should be incorporated by a subcloning method. The enzyme that produces a four-base 3'-overhang close to the priming site will be resistant to cleavage by exonuclease III. It is important to ensure that digestion is complete. If the 3'-cutter doesn't cut properly, then the deletions will proceed from both directions.

2. Exonuclease III digests duplex DNA at nicks, producing single-stranded gaps, but it is not active on 3'-protruding ends of DNA that are at least four bases long or on single-stranded DNA. Exonuclease III activity depends on temperature, salt concentration, purity of DNA, and the molar ratio of DNA to enzyme in the reaction mixture. Hence optimal enzyme concentration and the specific time intervals that produce unidirectional deletions without digesting the whole sample should be standardized prior to each specific experiment.

3. The quality of the vector DNA plays a critical role in achieving successful expression. Usually, the DNA is purified by two rounds of CsCl density gradient centrifugation, by anion-exchange chromatography, Qiagen column, or (more recently) by triple-helix affinity chromatography *(10)* to make the DNA free of protein, RNA, and chemical contamination. Evans blue (0.25%) is mixed with the plasmid DNA to localize the site of injection. For in vivo gene injection, 26-gage needles (insulin syringes) can be used.

Acknowledgments

The authors thank Prof. Dr. Jeffrey Robbins for the β-MHC gene clone, β5pJRCAT.

References

1. Mariappan, M., Selvamurugan, N., and Rajamanickam C. (1990) Purification and characterization of a high-molecular-weight protein induced in rat serum during the development of cardiac hypertrophy. *Arch. Biochem. Biophys.* **281,** 287–297.
2. Rajamanickam, C., Sakthivel, S., Babu, G. J., Lottspeich, F., and Kadenbach, B. (2001) Cardiac isoform of alpha-2 macroglobulin, a novel serum protein, may induce cardiac hypertrophy in rats. *Basic. Res. Cardiol.* **96,** 23–33.
3. Prabhakar, R. and Rajamanickam, C. (1993) Serum protein of 135 kDa molecular weight-a molecular signal for cardiac hypertrophy. *Arch. Biochem. Biophys.* **302,** 425–430.
4. Rakusan, K. and Poupa, O. (1966) Differences in capillary supply of hypertrophic and hyperplastic hearts. *Cardiology* **49,** 293–298.
5. Henikoff, S. (1984) Unidirectional digestion with exonuclease III creates targeted breakpoints for DNA sequencing. *Gene* **28,** 351–359.
6. Rindt, H., Knotts, S., and Robbins, J. (1995) Segregation of cardiac and skeletal muscle-specific regulatory elements of the beta-myosin heavy chain gene. *Proc. Natl. Acad. Sci. USA* **92,** 1540–1544.
7. Seed, B. and Sheen, J. Y. (1988) A simple phase-extraction assay for chloramphenicol acyltransferase activity. *Gene* **67,** 271–277.
8. Thompson, W. R., Nadal-Ginard, B., and Mahdavi, V. (1991) A MyoD1-independent muscle-specific enhancer controls the expression of the beta-myosin heavy chain gene in skeletal and cardiac muscle cells. *J. Biol. Chem.* **266,** 22,678–22,688.
9. Kariya, K., Karns, L. R., and Simpson, P. C. (1994) An enhancer core element mediates stimulation of the rat β-myosin heavy chain promoter by an α1-adrenergic agonist and activated β-protein kinase C in hypertrophy of cardiac myocytes. *J. Biol. Chem.* **269,** 3775–3782.
10. Wils, P. V., Escriou, A., Warnery, F., et al. (1977) Efficient purification of plasmid DNA for gene transfer using triple-helix affinity chromatography. *Gene Ther.* **4,** 323–330.

17

Evaluation of the Cardiac Isoform of α_2-Macroglobulin as a Factor Inducing Cardiac Hypertrophy

Chellam Rajamanickam and Radhakrishnan Jeejabai

Summary

Earlier studies from our laboratory showed that a 182-kDa high-molecular-weight protein appeared during early stages of development of cardiac hypertrophy in animals subjected to aortic constriction. Later it was confirmed that this protein is a cardiac isoform of α_2-macroglobulin belonging to the macroglobulin family. Furthermore, it has been demonstrated that direct injection of the purified 182-kDa protein intravenously (through the tail vein) into the normal animals led to the development of cardiac hypertrophy. It was accompanied by enlargement of cardiac myocytes and induction of β-myosin heavy chain (MHC) and MLC-2 gene expression. Multiple injections of 182-kDa protein-specific polyclonal antibody into the circulation of aorta-constricted animals completely abolished the development of hypertrophy and downregulated the expression of β-MHC and myosin light chain (MLC)-2. The full-length cDNA of the 182-kDa protein cloned in eukaryotic expression vector, namely, pcDNA 3.1(–) could induce cardiac hypertrophy upon direct injection into rat heart. Hypertrophy was monitored by determining the heart weight/body weight ratio and also by Northern blot analysis of muscle-specific marker genes such as β-MHC, MLC-2, and antrial natriuretic factor. Also, induction of promoter activity of β-MHC and *c-fos* genes analyzed by chloramphenicol acetyl transferase assay confirmed the induction of cardiac hypertrophy upon direct injection of the full-length cDNA of the 182-kDa protein.

Key Words: α_2-Macroglobulin; cardiac hypertrophy; aortic constriction; CAT assay; Northern blot analysis; 182-kDa protein; RT-PCR.

From: *Methods in Molecular Medicine, vol. 112: Molecular Cardiology: Methods and Protocols*
Edited by: Z. Sun © Humana Press Inc., Totowa, NJ

1. Introduction

Earlier studies from our laboratory on a 182-kDa high-molecular-weight protein that appeared during early stages of development of cardiac hypertrophy in animals subjected to aortic constriction, suggested that this protein is a cardiac isoform of α_2-macroglobulin belonging to the macroglobulin family *(1)*. Furthermore, it has been demonstrated that direct injection of the purified 182-kDa protein intravenously (through the tail vein) into normal animals led to the development of cardiac hypertrophy accompanied by enlargement of cardiac myocytes *(2)* and induction of the β-myosin heavy chain (MHC) and myosin light chain (MLC)-2 gene expression characteristic of pressure-overloaded cardiac hypertrophy *(1)*. Multiple injections of 182-kDa protein-specific polyclonal antibody into the circulation of aorta-constricted animals completely abolished the development of hypertrophy and downregulated the expression of β-MHC and MLC-2 *(3)*. In humans, during cardiac ailments, 182-kDa protein levels have been shown to have some correlation with the left ventricular mass. These studies further suggest that the 182-kDa protein could be used as a molecular marker to identify the early stage of cardiac hypertrophy *(4)*.

Several groups have attempted to evaluate the potential of direct gene transfer into cardiac tissue by expressing various reporter constructs *(5–8)*, and the technique was widely used to map the regulatory elements of genes in cardiac tissue *(9–11)*. Here we demonstrate that the full-length cDNA of the 182-kDa protein obtained from hypertrophied rat heart mRNA, cloned in an appropriate eukaryotic expression vector, pcDNA3.1(–), and injected directly into the rat heart, led to the development of cardiac hypertrophy.

2. Materials

1. Platinum *pfx* DNA polymerase.
2. PGEM T-Easy vector (Promega).
3. Plasmids such as pcDNA3.1(–) (Invitrogen).
4. Murine β-MHC gene promoter bearing plasmid β5pJR chloramphenicol acetyl transferase (CAT; kind gift of Prof. Jeffrey Robbins).
5. *c-fos* promoter-bearing plasmid.
6. GeneAmp polymerase chain reaction (PCR) system 2400 (Perkin Elmer).
7. Tissue homogenizer.
8. Albino rats of a Wistar-derived strain (weight range of 100 ± 5 g).
9. Diethyl ether; 70% ethanol; 20% sodium dodecyl sulfate (SDS).
10. Solution D (prepare immediately before use): 4 *M* GTC, 25 m*M* sodium citrate, pH 7.0, 0.5% sarcosyl, and 100 m*M* β-mercapto ethanol.
11. Agarose and formaldehyde.
12. 10X MOPS buffer: 0.2 *M* MOPS, 50 m*M* sodium acetate, and 10 m*M* EDTA.
13. 20X SSC: 3 *M* NaCl and 0.3 *M* sodium citrate.

14. 100X Denhardt's solution: 2% w/v bovine serum albumin (BSA), 2% w/v Ficoll, and 2% w/v PVP.
15. Prehybridization buffer: 6X SSC, 50% formamide, 5X Denhardt's solution, 10% dextran sulfate, and 100 µg/mL denatured salmon sperm DNA.
16. Hybridization washing solutions:
    a. Washing solution I: 2X SSC/0.2% SDS.
    b. Washing solution II: 1X SSC/0.2% SDS.
    c. Washing solution III:0.5X SSC/0.2% SDS.
17. Homogenization buffer for CAT assay: 25 mM Tris-HCl, pH 7.8, 15 mM MgSO$_4$, 4 mM EGTA, pH 8.0, and 1 mM dithiothreitol (DTT).
18. 10X Phosphate-buffered saline (PBS): 0.8% NaCl, 0.02% KCl, 0.11% Na$_2$HPO$_4$·7H$_2$O, and 0.02% KH$_2$PO$_4$.
19. 1 M Tris-HCl, pH 7.5.
20. ^{14}C-labeled chloramphenicol (Radiochemical Centre, Amersham, UK).
21. Acetyl coenzyme A (CoA): prepare a stock of 20 mM acetyl CoA in sterile MQ water, filter-sterilize, and store aliquots at –20°C.
22. Cesium chloride.
23. DTT: prepare a 200-mM stock in sterile MQ water, filter-sterilize, and store aliquots at –20°C.
24. Ethidium bromide: prepare a stock of 10 mg/mL in sterile water, and store in dark bottles at 4°C.
25. EGTA: prepare a stock of 0.5 M EGTA in MQ water, adjust pH to 8.0 with 5 N NaOH, and autoclave. The salt will not go into solution until the pH of the solution is adjusted to approx 8.0 by the addition of NaOH.
26. Chloramphenicol: prepare a stock of 30 mg/mL in 100% ethanol, and store aliquots at –20°C. Use 30 µg/mL as the working concentration.
27. RNase A: prepare a stock of 10 mg/mL in 10 mM Tris-HCl, pH 7.5, and 15 mM NaCl; store aliquots at –20°C.
28. Ethyl acetate.
29. Chloroform.
30. Methanol.
31. Thin-layer chromatography (TLC) plate and chamber.
32. X-ray film.
33. Solutions for SDS-PAGE, Coomassie Brilliant Blue R-250.
34. Sephadex G50.
35. Gibco-BRL Superscript™ first-strand synthesis system for RT-PCR.
36. PCR primers:
    Forward:
        F1: 1 5'-AGGACCAGATCTCTGGCGGGGAGTAGGG-3' 28.
        OF5: 1431 5'-ACCAAGCAGAAGCTTCCTGCAC-3' 1452.
        F4: 2066 5'-AAGAGGACATGTACGGCTTCC-3' 2087.
    Reverse:
        OR3: 1451 5'-TGCAGGAAGCTTCTGCTTGGTG-3' 1430.
        OR2: 2634 5'-TGCCCTGGACGCGGTGTG-3' 2619.
        R1: 4524 5'-GAGGTCAGGGCTCTGGCGAAACAC-3' 4501.

3. Methods

The methods followed describe the construction of full-length cDNA of 182-kDa protein, a cardiac isoform of α_2-macroglobulin, its expression in vivo in the rat heart and evaluation of the development of hypertrophy in the animals injected with full-length cDNA of the 182-kDa protein cloned in an eukaryotic expression vector, pcDNA 3.1(–) (*see* **Note 1**).

3.1. Construction of Full-Length cDNA of the 182-kDa Protein

3.1.1. Cloning Strategy

The total cellular RNA obtained from the hypertrophied rat heart (on the third day after aortic constriction) by the guanidium thiocyanate method of Chomczynski and Sacchi *(12)* was used to construct the full-length cDNA through RT-PCR (*see* **Note 2**). Based on the results obtained from the partial amino acid sequencing of the 182-kDa protein, which was generously done by Prof. Dr. Friedrich Lottspiech (Max-Planck-Institut for Biochemistry, Germany) and also on the sequence of α_2-macroglobulin developed by Gehring et al. *(13)*, gene-specific primers were designed in such a way that the RT-PCR products obtained spanned the entire region of the full-length cDNA of the 182-kDa protein including the 5' untranslated region (UTR) region. The Gibco-BRL Superscript™ first-strand synthesis system was used to synthesize first-strand cDNA following the manufacturer's protocol. The first-strand cDNA was then amplified on the GeneAmp PCR system 2400 (Perkin Elmer) using platinum *Pfx* DNA polymerase to obtain several products. The conditions are as follows:

1. R1 and F4: 35 cycles with 30 s denaturation at 94°C, 30 s annealing at 60°C, and 3 min extension at 72°C.
2. OR2 and OF5: 35 cycles with 30 s denaturation at 94°C, 30 s annealing at 60°C, and 3 min extension at 72°C.
3. OR3 and F1: 35 cycles with 30 s denaturation at 94°C, 30 s annealing at 64°C, and 2 min extension at 72°C.

All the RT-PCR products were then cloned into pGEM-T Easy vector after the A-tailing procedure in the manufacturer's protocol.

3.1.2. Primers

See **Subheading 2., item 36.**

3.1.3. Full-Length Assembly of the cDNA

Three successful RT-PCR reactions yielded products that could span the full-length cDNA of the 182-kDa protein. All the products were initially cloned in pGEM-T Easy vector (*see* **Note 3**); and later, using the unique restriction sites available in the existing sequence, they were assembled to yield a full-length cDNA. Initially the two products of the N-terminal region were joined using the *Hin*dIII restriction site to obtain a larger product of 2.59 kb of the N-terminal region. This was then fused to the C-terminal product of 2.5 kb using the site *Esp*I to get a full-length cDNA. For cloning purposes, the unique sites in the pGEM-T Easy vector were used to maintain the orientation of the clones (**Fig. 1**).

3.2. Expression of Full-Length cDNA of the 182-kDa Protein In Vivo

3.2.1. Plasmids for Injection

The full-length cDNA along with its 5′UTR that was originally cloned in the pGEM-T Easy vector was subcloned in eukaryotic expression vector, pcDNA 3.1(–) (Invitrogen). Restriction digestion of the p182-pGEM-T Easy vector with *Not*I released the full-length insert, which was then subcloned in the *Not*I site of the pcDNA 3.1(–) vector by standard protocols *(14)*. This clone construct with appropriate orientation was then selected (**Fig. 2**) and isolated in a large scale *(14)* for direct gene injection into the heart to induce hypertrophy. The empty pcDNA3.1(–) vector was used as a negative control in all the injection experiments.

3.2.2. Injection Techniques

1. Anesthetize the rats with diethyl ether, place in a supine position, and tape the upper limbs to a table.
2. Clean the chest skin with 70% ethanol, and make a 1–1.5-cm incision along the left side of the sternum.
3. Cut open the throat at the point of the most pronounced cardiac pulsation.
4. Use forceps to widen the chest, and press the abdomen and the right side of the chest to push the heart out of the thoracic cavity.
5. Inject about 100 µg of supercoiled plasmid DNA suspended in physiological saline through a 26-gage needle (*see* **Note 4**) into the apex of the heart.
6. Following the injection, place the heart back into the thoracic cavity, close the chest with sutures using surgical thread, apply sulfanin, and allow the rat to recover.

3.2.3. Tissue Homogenization

After in vivo gene injection of p182-pcDNA 3.1(–), the animals were sacrificed at different time points, as indicated in the figure legends for different experiments such as Northern blot, reporter gene, and electron micrographic analyses. At the time of sacrifice, the heart tissue was perfused with ice-cold phosphate-buffered saline and resected. The ventricles alone were taken,

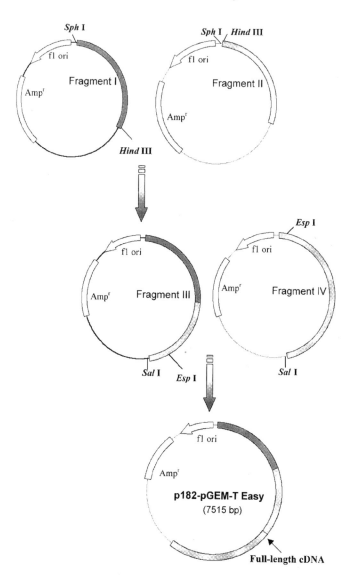

Fig. 1. Cloning-assembly of full-length cDNA of the 182-kDa protein. (Reprinted from **ref. *13a***, with permission from Springer-Verlag.)

drained of buffer solution, weighed immediately, and minced, and the total RNA was isolated *(12)*.

3.3. Western Blot Analysis

To determine whether the protein expressed was secretory (*see* **Note 5**), levels of 182-kDa protein in the sera of p182 pcDNA 3.1(–)-injected animals were

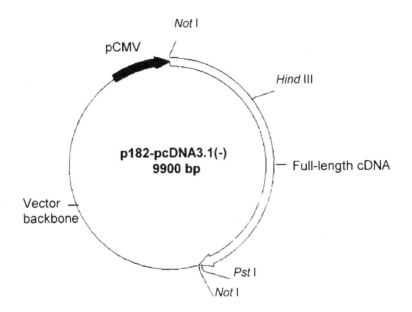

Fig. 2. Expression construct (p182 pcDNA 3.1[–]) used for in vivo injection studies.

analyzed by Western blot *(15)* using antibody specific for the 182-kDa protein. The 182-kDa protein was detected on the first day and monitored until the fourth day on a Coomassie stained 10% SDS-polyacrylamide gel electrophoresis (PAGE) (**Fig. 3A**) that was later confirmed by Western blot analysis using anti-182 kDa (**Fig. 3B**). The protein could not be detected in the serum at later stages, i.e., after the sixth day, which supports the data obtained using the heart weight to body weight ratio showing regression of hypertrophy.

3.4. Evaluation of Development of Cardiac Hypertrophy

3.4.1. Heart Weight/Body Weight Ratio

To evaluate the hypertrophy-inducing potential of a full-length cDNA for the 182-kDa protein, we monitored the development of hypertrophy in the animals that were injected directly with the plasmid DNA into the heart.

Comparison of heart weight/body weight ratios of the control and test plasmid injected animals, presented in **Table 1** showed up to a 20% increase in the heart weight to body weight ratio in animals sacrificed 3 d after plasmid injection; decrease was seen after. Cardiac tissues from these animals were used for further analysis.

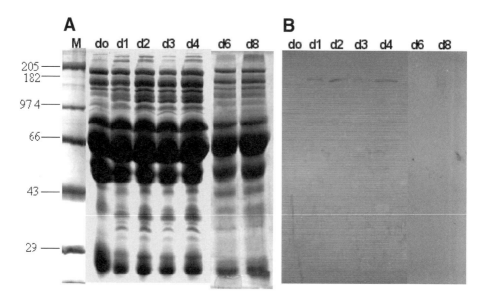

Fig. 3. Western blot analysis of rat serum at different time points (days) after direct gene injection with the expression construct p182-pcDNA 3.1(–). Coomassie stained pattern (**A**) and Western blot (**B**) carried out with the antibody raised against the 182-kDa protein. (Reprinted from **ref.** *13a* with permission from Springer-Verlag.)

3.4.2. Northern Blot Analysis

To substantiate the hypertrophy-inducing potential of the full-length cDNA for the 182-kDa protein, the effect of this in vivo expressed protein on the expression of muscle-specific genes such as that of β-MHC, MLC-2, and ANF, which are induced in pressure-overloaded hypertrophy, was investigated by Northern blot analysis. Expression of the injected plasmid was also analyzed. For Northern analysis, 25 µg of total RNA was size-fractionated in a 1.2% formaldehyde agarose gel and transferred onto a nylon membrane *(16)*. Hybridization was carried out as described in the Amersham instructions *Membrane Transfer and Detection Methods* at 42°C overnight. Then the RNA was washed in hybridization washing solutions I, II, and III for 30 min each at room temperature. Autoradiography was performed with AX X-ray film (Konica).

Considerable increases in β-MHC and MLC-2 mRNA levels and to some extent ANF levels (**Fig. 4**) were observed. Glyceraldehyde 3-phosphate dehydrogenase, a housekeeping gene, showed a constant level of expression in all the samples, indicating that the 182-kDa protein induced only the muscle-specific genes and not any other constitutively expressed genes.

Table 1
Heart Weight/Body Weight (HW/BW) Ratio of Animals Injected With p182-pcDNA 3.1(–) (Test) and pcDNA 3.1 (–) (Control)

	Day					
	1	2	3	6	9	12
Ratio of HW/BW × 100						
Control	0.361 ± 0.004	0.347 ± 0.003	0.350 ± 0.004	0.366 ± 0.002	0.336 ± 0.003	0.352 ± 0.003
Test	0.384 ± 0.002	0.376 ± 0.004	0.420 ± 0.004	0.395 ± 0.001	0.356 ± 0.001	0.364 ± 0.002
% of Hypertrophy	106	108	120	108	106	103

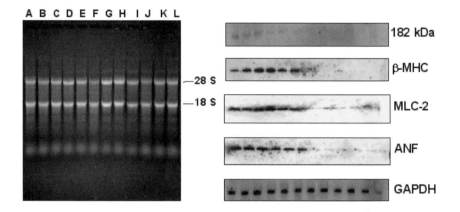

Fig. 4. Northern blot analysis of total RNA from cardiac tissue after direct gene injection; Lanes A–F, test injected; lanes G–L, control injected (days 1, 2, 3, 6, 9, and 12). (Reprinted from **ref. *13a*** with permission from Springer-Verlag.)

3.4.3. Reporter Gene Expression by Using Hypertrophy-Specific Marker Genes as Promoters

To substantiate the results on development of cardiac hypertrophy as observed by heart weight/body weight ratio and by Northern blot analysis, induction of hypertrophy-specific marker genes such as the β-MHC and *c-fos* genes upon direct injection of the full-length cDNA of the 182-kDa protein into the heart in vivo, was analyzed by reporter gene activity. Activity of CAT as the reporter gene upon injection of the specific promoter, fused with the reporter gene construct along with a 182-kDa protein cDNA expression vector construct was monitored.

3.4.3.1. CAT ASSAY FOR β-MHC PROMOTER ACTIVITY

Cardiac hypertrophy was induced in the rat by injection of p182-pcDNA 3.1(–), and CAT activity was measured (*17*) in the ventricular tissues of the same animals after injection of the β-MHC promoter fused reporter gene construct, 3 d after p182-pcDNA 3.1(–) injection. The CAT assay was performed as follows:

1. Mince the heart tissue, and homogenize in 1 mL of homogenization buffer.
2. Centrifuge the suspension at 6000*g* for 10 min at 4°C, and use the supernatant for the CAT assay.
3. Take 10% of the supernatant, incubate at 65°C for 10 min to inactivate endogenous acetyl transferases and then centrifuge at 10,000*g* for 5 min.

4. After centrifugation, mix 91.5 µL of clear supernatant with 30 µL of 1 *M* Tris-HCl, pH 7.5, 8 µL ^{14}C-labeled chloramphenicol (0.2 µCi), and 20 µL of 4 m*M* acetyl-CoA.
5. Incubate the reaction mixture at 37°C for 4 h.
6. Extract the acetylated chloramphenicol with 1 mL of ethyl acetate.
7. Dry under vacuum, suspend in 20 µL ethyl acetate, spot on a TLC plate *(17)*, and run in a chamber equilibrated with chloroform and methanol (95:5) for 30 min.
8. After the run, air-dry the TLC plate, and expose it to an X-ray film in a dark room for 7 d. Develop the film.

In another experiment, a construct harboring a 1.5-kb N-terminal region of the cDNA of the 182-kDa protein cloned in pcDNA 3.1(–) was also injected to check hypertrophy induction and subsequently β-MHC promoter activity as described in **Subheading 3.4.3.** The pcDNA 3.1(–) vector without the 182-kDa protein cDNA was injected as the control. The β5pJR CAT plasmid was then injected on the third day in both groups, and the CAT assay was performed.

CAT activity could be measured only in the animals injected with full-length cDNA (**Fig. 5A**) and not in the other two subjects. These results clearly demonstrate and confirm induction of β-MHC gene, upon p182-pcDNA 3.1(–) injection, characteristic of pressure-overloaded cardiac hypertrophy, substantiating the Northern analysis of induction of β-MHC gene. The results further indicate that the partial 1.5-kb N-terminal region of the cDNA is not sufficient to induce cardiac hypertrophy, and hence the promoter activity, and only a full-length cDNA that could synthesize a mature protein in its native conformation is needed for the induction of cardiac hypertrophy.

3.4.3.2. CAT Assay for *c-fos* Promoter Activity

Induction of *c-fos* has been observed as an early event in the pressure-overloaded rat heart *(18)*. Earlier studies in the lab have also revealed that *c-fos* is induced within 30 min with high-level expression up to 6 h after aortic constriction *(19)*. Cardiac hypertrophy was induced in the rat by the injection of p182-pcDNA 3.1(–) as described, and CAT activity was checked in the ventricular tissues of the same animals injected with the *c-fos* promoter fused reporter gene construct, after p182-pcDNA 3.1(–) injection. The ventricular tissue was assayed for CAT activity at two different time points, namely, 3 and 6 h.

In another experiment, a construct harboring a 1.5-kb N-terminal region of the cDNA of the 182-kDa protein cloned in pcDNA 3.1(–) was also injected to check hypertrophy induction and subsequently *c-fos* promoter activity as such. The pcDNA 3.1(–) vector without 182-kDa protein cDNA was injected as the control.

CAT activity could be measured only in the animals injected with the full-length cDNA at 6 h (**Fig. 5B**) and not in all other subjects. These results clearly

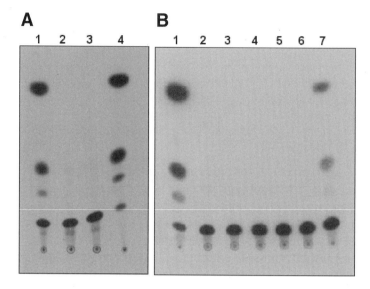

Fig. 5. (A) CAT assay for β-MHC promoter activity. About 100 mg of purified β5pJR CAT was injected into the myocardium of the following animals, and a CAT assay was performed. Lane 1, full-length cDNA of 182-kDa protein-injected animals; lane 2, partial N-terminal region (1.5 kb) of the cDNA of 182-kDa protein-injected animals; lane 3, empty pcDNA 3.1(–) injected animals; lane 4, pUC18 CAT *E. coli* extract. **(B)** CAT assay for *c-fos* promoter activity. Lane 1, pUC18 CAT *E. coli* extract; lane 2, empty pcDNA 3.1(–) + p600CAT3 (3 h); lane 3, partial N-terminal region (1.5 kb) of the cDNA of 182-kDa + p600CAT3 (3 h); lane 4, full-length cDNA of 182-kDa protein + p600CAT3 (3 h); lane 5, empty pcDNA 3.1(–) + p600CAT3 (6 h); lane 6, partial N-terminal region (1.5 kb) of the cDNA of 182-kDa + p600CAT3 (6 h); lane 7, full-length cDNA of 182-kDa protein + p600CAT3 (6 h). (Reprinted from **ref.** *13a* with permission from Springer-Verlag.)

demonstrate that induction of the *c-fos* gene, characteristic of pressure-over-loaded cardiac hypertrophy, is prominent only at 6 h and not at 3 h. Furthermore, the results also indicate that the partial 1.5-kb N-terminal region of the cDNA is not sufficient to induce cardiac hypertrophy and subsequently c-*fos* promoter activation, similar to that observed in β-MHC promoter induction.

3.4.4. Electron Microscopic Studies

To give firm evidence for the development of hypertrophy in response to cardiac injection of the eukaryotic expression vector containing the cDNA of the 182-kDa protein, histological evidence using the scanning electron microscope was sought (**Fig. 6**).

A B

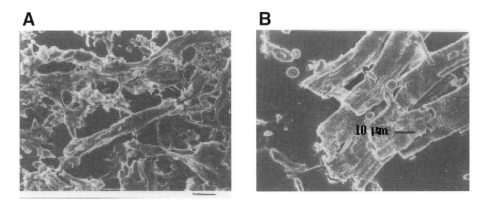

Fig. 6. Scanning electron micrographs of heart sections from (**A**) a normal animal and (B) a p182-pcDNA 3.1(–)-injected animal.

Scanning electron micrographs of the cardiac myofibrils obtained from the hearts of normal as well as cDNA of 182 kDa protein injected animals (3 d after injection of cDNA) show a clear visible evidence of expansion of the myofibrils in cDNA-injected animals.

4. Notes

1. The feasibility of direct gene transfer into the adult mammalian heart to characterize the activity of a cellular gene and to modulate overall cardiac function in vivo was also analyzed by several groups. Molkentin et al. *(20)* have demonstrated that transfection of the full-length cDNA of an activated NF-AT3, a transcription factor, into cardiomyocytes is sufficient to evoke a hypertrophic response in vivo. Zhang et al. *(21)* reported that a variant of transforming growth factor-β-activated kinase (TAK1) expressed in the myocardium of transgenic mice was sufficient to produce myocardial hypertrophy. Higaki et al. *(22)* have demonstrated that local overexpression of cardiac angiotensin-converting enzyme by in vivo gene transfer into the heart could promote autocrine/paracrine angiotensin II-mediated cardiac hypertrophy in vivo.

5. The problem of focal expression can be overcome by cloning the full-length cDNA along with the signal peptide, thus rendering the protein that is synthesized secretory so that the protein that is released into the circulation may exert its function.

2. Cloning of the full-length cDNA by screening a cDNA library depends on the size of the mRNA and its abundance. For rare messages the RT-PCR approach can be exploited. Screening of expression libraries with antibody probes will be troublesome since many polyclonal antibodies crossreact with the *E. coli* proteins. Initially, the primary antibody should be treated for 1–2 h at 4°C with *E.*

coli proteins so as to avoid a nonspecific reaction, but this will also not be as efficient as the DNA probe.

3. There are alternate vectors for cloning PCR products other than pGEM T. Different expression vectors for cloning in mammalian cells are also available. The function of the expression vector is to direct transcription of the administered gene into RNA, translation of the therapeutic product from RNA, and proper posttranslational modification or compartmentalization of the product.

4. For in vivo gene injection, 26-gage needles (insulin syringes) can be used. A critical parameter for achieving successful expression is the quality of the expression vector DNA. The plasmids used for injection studies should be free of protein, RNA, and chemical contamination. Usually, the DNA can be purified by two rounds of CsCl density gradient centrifugation, by anion-exchange chromatography, or, as shown more recently, by triple-helix affinity chromatography *(23)*. 0.25% Evans blue is mixed with the plasmid DNA to localize the site of injection. Other protocols such as purification using a Qiagen column can also be employed.

Acknowledgments

The authors thank Prof. Dr. F. Lottspeich and Prof. Dr. B. Kadenbach for their contribution in sequencing the 182-kDa protein.

References

1. Rajamanickam, C., Sakthivel, S., Babu, G. J., Lottspeich, F., and Kadenbach, B. (2001) Cardiac isoform of α-2 macroglobulin, a novel serum protein, may induce cardiac hypertrophy in rats. *Basic Res. Cardiol.* **96,** 23–33.

2. Jegadeesh Babu, G. (1993) Regulation of gene expression during cardiac hypertrophy. Ph.D., thesis, Madurai Kamaraj University, Madurai 625 021, India.

3. Prabhakar, R. and Rajamanickam, C. (1993) Serum protein of 135 kDa molecular weight—a molecular signal for cardiac hypertrophy. *Arch. Biochem. Biophys.* **302,** 425–430.

4. Rajamanickam, C., Sakthivel, S., Joseph, P. K., and Janarthanan, R. A. (1998) A novel serum protein of molecular weight 182 kDa: a molecular marker for an early detection of increased left ventricular mass in patients with cardiac hypertrophy. *J. Cardiovasc. Risk.* **5,** 335–338.

5. Aokki, M., Morishita, R., Muraishi, A., et al. (1997) Efficient *in vivo* gene transfer into the heart in the rat myocardial infarction model using the HVJ (heam agglutinating virus of Japan)—Liposome method. *J. Mol. Cell. Cardiol.* **29,** 949–959.

6. Buttrick, P. M., Kass, A., Kitsis, R. N., Kaplan, M. L., and Leinwand, L. A. (1992) Behavior of genes directly injected into the rat heart *in vivo*. *Circ. Res.* **70,** 193–198.

7. Li, K., Welikson, R. E., Vikstrom, K. L., and Leinwand, L. A. (1997) Direct gene transfer into the mouse heart. *J. Mol. Cell. Cardiol.* **29,** 1499–1504.

8. Prentice, H., Kloner, R. A., Yuwei, Li., Newman, L., and Kedes, L. (1995) Ischemic/reperfused myocardium can express recombinant protein following direct DNA or retroviral injection. *J. Mol. Cell. Cardiol.* **28,** 133–140.

9. Aoyagi, T. and Izumo, S. (1993) Mapping of the pressure response element of the *c-fos* gene by direct DNA injection into beating hearts. *J. Biol. Chem.* **268,** 27,176–27,179.

10. Bassel-Duby, R., Grohe, C. M., Jessen, M. E., et al. (1993) Sequence elements required for transcriptional activity of the human myoglobin promoter in intact myocardium. *Circ. Res.* **73**, 360–366.

11. Hasegawa, K., Lee, S. S. J., Jobe, S. M., Markham, B. E., Kitsis, R. N. (1997) *cis*-Acting sequences that mediate induction of β-myosin heavy chain gene expression during left ventricular hypertrophy due to aortic constriction. *Circulation* **96**, 3943–3953.

12. Chomczynski, P. and Sacchi, N. (1987) Single-step method of RNA isolation by acid guanidinium thiocyanate-phenol-choloform extraction. *Anal. Biochem.* **162**, 156–159.

13. Gehring, M. R., Shiels, B. R., Northemann, W., et al. (1987) Sequence of rat liver α-2 macroglobulin and acute phase control of its messenger RNA. *J. Biol. Chem.* **262**, 446–454.

13a. Rajan, S. Radhakrishnan, J., and Rajamanickam, C. (2003) Direct injection and expression in vivo of full-length cDNA of the cardiac isoform of α-2 macroglobulin includes cardiac hypertrophy in the rat. *Basic Res. Cardiol.* **98**, 39–49.

14. Sambrook, J., Fritsch, E. F., and Maniatis, T. (1989) *Molecular Cloning: A Laboratory Manual*, 2nd ed. Cold Spring Harbor Laboratory Press, Cold Spring Harbor, NY.

15. Towbin, H., Staehelin, T., and Gordon, J. (1979) Electrophoretic transfer of proteins from polyacrylamide gels to nitrocellulsose sheets: procedure and some applications. *Proc. Natl. Acad. Sci. US.* **76**, 4350–4354.

16. Ausubel, F. M., Brent, R., Kingston, R. E., et al. (1989) *Current Protocols in Molecular Biology.* John Wiley, New York.

17. Seed, B. and Sheen, J. Y. (1988) A simple phase-extraction assay for chloramphenicol acyltransferase activity. *Gene* **67**, 271–277.

18. Komuro, I., Kurabayashi, M., Takaku, F., and Yazaki, Y. (1988) Expression of cellular oncogenes in the myocardium during the developmental stage and pressure-overloaded hypertrophy of the rat heart. *Circ. Res.* **62**, 1075–1079.

19. Jegadeesh Babu, G., Prabhakar, R., Kartha, C. C., and Rajamanickam, C. (1994) Expression of proto-oncogenes, genes for muscle specific isoforms and heat shock protein (HSP) -70 gene in hypertrophied cardiac muscles from patients with atrial septal defect or Tetralogy of Fallot. *Biochem. Mol. Biol. Int.* **34**, 627–637.

20. Molkentin, J. D., Lu, J. R., Antos, C. L., et al. (1998) A calcineurin-dependent transcriptional pathway for cardiac hypertrophy. *Cell* **93**, 215–228.

21. Zhang, D., Gaussin, V., Taffer, G. E., et al. (2000) TAK1 is activated in the myocardium after pressure overload and is sufficient to provoke heart failure in transgenic mice. *Nature Med.* **6**, 556–563.

22. Higaki, J., Aoki, M., Morishita, R., et al. (2000) *In vivo* evidence of the importance of cardiac angiotensin-converting enzyme in the pathogenesis of cardiac hypertrophy. *Arterioscler. Thromb. Vasc. Biol.* **20**, 428–434.

23. Wils, P. V., Escriou, A., Warnery, F., et al. (1977) Efficient purification of plasmid DNA for gene transfer using triple-helix affinity chromatography. *Gene Ther.* **4**, 323–330.

18

Detection of Apoptosis in Cardiovascular Diseases

Arwen L. Hunter, Jonathan C. Choy, and David J. Granville

Summary

The past decade has seen a surge in research devoted to understanding the role of cell death in the pathogenesis of various forms of cardiovascular disease. In particular, apoptosis has received much attention owing to the tightly regulated biochemical nature of this form of cell death and the realization of potential therapeutic opportunities. The current chapter describes a few of the more widely used protocols for detecting and quantifying apoptosis in cardiovascular tissues. Specifically, this chapter describes terminal deoxynucleotidyl transferase dUTP nick-end labeling (TUNEL) staining for DNA fragmentation, Hoechst staining for chromatin condensation, annexin V labeling of phosphatidylserine externalization, and Western blot and immunofluorescence detection of caspase cleavage and activation, respectively.

Key Words: Annexin V; apoptosis; atherosclerosis; blood vessel; cardiomyopathy; caspase; cell death; DNA fragmentation; endothelial cell; heart; Hoechst; mitochondria; myocardial infarction; myocarditis; myocyte; protease; smooth muscle cell; restenosis; TUNEL; vascular injury.

1. Introduction

Apoptosis is a tightly controlled form of cell death characterized by cell shrinkage, DNA fragmentation, and membrane blebbing, resulting in the packaging of the cell into membrane-enclosed vesicles. These vesicles are then engulfed by surrounding "professional" (macrophages) or "nonprofessional" phagocytes. Although numerous apoptotic pathways exist, most forms of apoptosis are regulated in large part by Bcl-2 pro- and antiapoptotic proteins and are mediated by caspases, a family of cysteinyl-aspartate proteases that cleave multiple substrates, resulting in the systematic dismantling of the cell

From: *Methods in Molecular Medicine, vol. 112: Molecular Cardiology: Methods and Protocols*
Edited by: Z. Sun © Humana Press Inc., Totowa, NJ

(1,2). Apoptosis is believed to play a key role in the pathogenesis of many cardiovascular disorders such as myocardial infarction, hypertrophy, myocarditis, atherosclerosis, restenosis, transplant rejection, and many other ailments *(1,3–8)*. Thus intense research has been devoted to deciphering the role of cell death in the pathogenesis of various types of cardiovascular disease. In the heart, the loss of cardiac myocyte viability, even if at low frequencies, can have drastic pathophysiological consequences owing to the terminally differentiated and irreplaceable nature of these cells. Alternatively, the role of apoptosis in atherogenesis is less clear. Although intimal smooth muscle apoptosis may be beneficial in limiting intimal hyperplasia, at later stages cell death may contribute to plaque instability. Similarly, the role of endothelial cell death in cardiovascular pathogenesis requires further elucidation.

The current chapter describes, in detail, the standard methods used to detect apoptosis in cardiovascular diseases. It is important to realize that many of the intrinsic cell suicide pathways are redundant, and it is likely that not all these pathways will be activated when a cell is undergoing apoptosis. Furthermore, the mechanisms by which cell death occurs are dependent on the cell type and stimulus. The present chapter outlines methods used to detect common features of the apoptotic phenotype that are typically used for the study of apoptosis in cardiovascular diseases.

Terminal deoxynucleotidyl transferase dUTP nick-end labeling (TUNEL) staining is one of the most widely used procedures to detect DNA fragmentation. This technique utilizes enzymatic addition of labeled dUTP to the 3' ends of DNA strand breaks by the DNA repair enzyme terminal deoxynucleotidyl transferase (TdT) *(9,10)*. The labeled nucleotides are then detected by enzymatically conjugated antibodies that recognize these labels, allowing quantitative analysis by flow cytometry or visualization by either light or fluorescence microscopy. **Figure 1** shows a schematic representation of the TUNEL staining method. Visualization by microscopy is particularly useful as it permits the localization of DNA fragmentation to specific cell populations *in situ* (**Fig. 2**).

Chromatin condensation is a hallmark of apoptosis. Staining DNA with nuclear dyes permits the visualization of chromatin condensation. Hoechst is a fluorescent dye that binds to the minor groove of DNA. In addition, this dye is cell-permeable, thereby making this protocol rapid and simple. The condensed chromatin appears as small, bright, fragmented nuclei (**Fig. 2**).

Annexin V labeling detects the externalization of phosphatidylserine (PS) on the outer membrane of apoptotic cells. PS is normally localized on the inner leaflet of viable cells. During apoptosis, this localization of PS is lost, leading to its accumulation on both the outer and inner leaflets *(11)*. The exposure of PS is a prophagocytotic signal that triggers the engulfment of apoptotic cells by both professional phagocytes and neighboring cells. Annexin V is an anti-

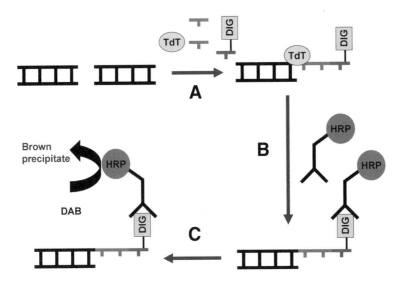

Fig. 1. Schematic of TUNEL staining. **(A)** DNA strand breaks that are abundant during apoptosis are labeled by terminal deoxynucleotide transferase (TdT)-mediated addition of digoxigenin (DIG)-conjugated dUTP. **(B)** DIG-conjugated dUTP is recognized by anti-DIG antibodies conjugated to HRP. **(C)** Visualization of DNA strand breaks is accomplished by the conversion of 3,3'-diaminobenzidene (DAB), a substrate for HRP, to a brown precipitate.

body that specifically recognizes PS. By staining nonpermeabilized cells with a fluorescently conjugated annexin V, the procedure detects PS on the outer leaflet of cells. The addition of propidium iodide (PI) allows the distinction between apoptotic and necrotic cells since disruption of membrane integrity during necrosis results in the staining of nuclei with PI. Thus annexin V-positive cells are interpreted as apoptotic, and cells positive for both annexin V and PI are interpreted as necrotic.

There are numerous pathway-specific apoptotic assays, many of which take advantage of the modification and/or redistribution of apoptotic proteins and their substrates within the cell upon apoptosis induction. Commonly, these events are assessed by sodium dodecyl sulfate-polyacrylamide gel electrophoresis (SDS-PAGE) and Western blot analysis or by immunofluorescence. Caspase processing is often targeted in these assays, as it is implicated in several apoptotic pathways. Caspase activation, which involves the proteolytic processing of procaspases into active enzymatic subunits, is easily visualized using immunoblotting by either the appearance of cleavage fragments or by diminution of the pro-form *(12)*. Caspase activity can also be assessed using caspase protease activity assays. Whole cell lysates are sufficient for examin-

TUNEL   Hoechst

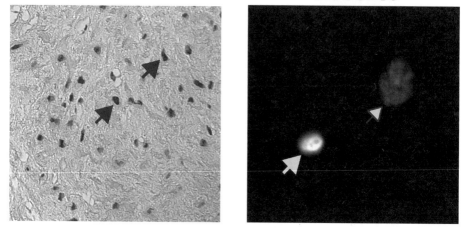

Fig. 2. Assessment of TUNEL and Hoechst staining. Positive TUNEL staining is interpreted as brown staining localized to the nucleus (black arrows). Chromatin condensation is visualized in apoptotic smooth muscle cells as condensed, bright nuclei (white arrow). This is in contrast to healthy cells, which display a large, uniform nuclear morphology with lighter staining (white arrowhead).

ing caspase activation by both of these methods. Preparation of whole cell lysates is described in detail below. It is often desirable to examine several caspases (caspase-2, -3, -6, -7, -8, -9, and -10) known to be involved in different caspase-dependent apoptotic cascades *(13)*.

2. Materials

2.1. In Situ *TUNEL Labeling of Paraffin-Embedded Slides*

1. Phosphate-buffered saline (PBS): 2.69 mM KCl, 137 mM NaCl, 1.47 mM KH_2PO_4, 8.1 mM Na_2HPO_4, pH 7.6.
2. Xylene.
3. Ethanol.
4. 3% H_2O_2 (diluted from 30% H_2O_2 in distilled H_2O).
5. Proteinase K (diluted in PBS).
6. Equilibration buffer: 200 mM potassium cacodylate, pH 6.6, 25 mM Tris-HCl, pH 6.6, 0.2 mM dithreitol (DTT), 0.25 mg/mL bovine serum albumin (BSA), 2.5 mM cobalt chloride.
7. TdT (Boehringer).
8. Reaction mixture: 50 U/mL TdT and 1:50 dilution of digoxigenin (DIG) DNA labeling mixture (Boehringer) in equilibration buffer.

 9. Horseradish peroxidase (HRP)-conjugated anti-DIG antibody.
10. 3,3'-Diaminobenzidine (DAB).
11. Hematoxylin.

2.2. TUNEL on Cell Cultures

 1. 10% Neutral buffered formalin or 4% paraformaldehyde.
 2. PBS: 2.69 mM KCl, 137 mM NaCl, 1.47 mM KH$_2$PO$_4$, 8.1 mM Na$_2$HPO$_4$, pH 7.6.
 3. 0.01% Triton X-100 (diluted in PBS).
 4. Proteinase K (diluted in PBS).
 5. Equilibration buffer: 200 mM potassium cacodylate, pH 6.6, 25 mM Tris-HCl, pH 6.6, 0.2 mM DTT, 0.25 mg/mL BSA, 2.5 mM cobalt chloride.
 6. TdT (Boehringer).
 7. Reaction mixture: 50 U/mL TdT and 1:50 dilution of DIG DNA labeling mixture (Boehringer) in equilibration buffer.
 8. HRP-conjugated anti-DIG antibody.
 9. DAB.
10. Hematoxylin.

2.3. Hoechst Nuclear Staining

 1. PBS: 2.69 mM KCl, 137 mM NaCl, 1.47 mM KH$_2$PO$_4$, 8.1 mM Na$_2$HPO$_4$, pH 7.6.
 2. Fixative: 10% neutral buffered formalin or 4% paraformaldehyde.
 3. Hoechst 33342 (Molecular Probes, Eugene, OR).

2.4. Annexin V Labeling

 1. Annexin V staining buffer: 10 mM HEPES, 140 mM NaCl, 2.5 mM CaCl$_2$, pH 7.6.
 2. PBS: 2.69 mM KCl, 137 mM NaCl, 1.47 mM KH$_2$PO$_4$, 8.1 mM Na$_2$HPO$_4$, pH 7.6.
 3. Alexa-488–conjugated annexin V (Molecular Probes).
 4. PI (Molecular Probes).

2.5. Preparation of Whole Cell Lysates From Nonadherent Cells, Adherent Cells, and Tissue Sections

 1. PBS: 2.69 mM KCl, 137 mM NaCl, 1.47 mM KH$_2$PO$_4$, 8.1 mM Na$_2$HPO$_4$, pH 7.6.
 2. Whole cell lysate buffer: 1% Nonidet P-40 (NP-40), 20 mM Tris-base, pH 8.0, 137 mM NaCl, 10% glycerol, supplemented with 1 mM phenylmethylsulfonyl fluoride (PMSF), 0.15 U/mL aprotinin, and 1 mM sodium orthovanadate immediately prior to use.
 3. Cell scrapers.
 4. Tissue homogenizer.

2.6. Western Blot Detection of Caspase Processing

1. Lysates (prepared as described in **Subheadings 3.4.1.–3.4.3.**).
2. 2X SDS/sample buffer: 100 mM Tris-base, 25% glycerol, 2% SDS, 0.01% bromophenol blue, 10% β-mercaptoethanol, pH 6.8.
3. 10% Separating polyacrylamide agarose gel with 4% stacking polyacrylamide agarose gel.
4. Running buffer: 25 mM Tris-base, 192 mM glycine, 1% SDS.
5. Nitrocellulose membrane (Amersham).
6. Transfer buffer: 20 mM Tris-base, pH 8.0, 150 mM glycine, 20% methanol.
7. Blocking buffer: 125 mM NaCl, 25 mM Tris-base, pH 8.0, 5% skim milk, 0.01% Tween-20.
8. Primary antibody against caspase of interest and complementary secondary antibody conjugated to HRP.
9. Enhanced chemiluminescence (ECL) developing solution (Amersham).
10. X-ray film.

2.7. Caspase Protease Assay

1. Lysates (prepared as described in **Subheadings 3.4.1.–3.4.3.**).
2. 96-Well flat-bottomed plate.
3. Reaction buffer: 1% NP-40, 20 mM Tris-base, pH 7.5, 137 mM NaCl, 10% glycerol.
4. Whole cell lysate buffer: 1% NP-40, 20 mM Tris-base, pH 8.0, 137 mM NaCl, 10% glycerol, supplemented with 1 mM PMSF, 0.15 U/mL aprotinin, and 1 mM sodium orthovanadate immediately prior to use.
5. Caspase substrate (Calbiochem) (*see* **Note 1**).
6. Fluorescent plate reader (PerSeptive Biosystems).

3. Methods

3.1. TUNEL Staining

This section describes methods for *in situ* TUNEL staining of paraffin-embedded tissues (**Subheading 3.1.1.**) and TUNEL staining of cells in culture (**Subheading 3.1.2.**).

3.1.1. In Situ *TUNEL Labeling of Paraffin-Embedded Slides*

1. Fix tissues in 10% neutral buffered formalin overnight, and embed in paraffin (*see* **Note 2**).
2. Cut 3 μm tissue sections onto glass slides.
3. Incubate slides in 60°C oven overnight.
4. Deparaffinize and rehydrate slides in a series of xylene and ethanol washes as follows:
   a. Xylene 3X 5 min using fresh xylene for each wash.
   b. 100% Ethanol 2X 5 min using fresh ethanol for each wash.
   c. 90% Ethanol 1X 5 min.

    d. 70% Ethanol 1X 5 min.

    e. Distilled H_2O (dH_2O) 1X 5 min.

5. Block endogenous peroxide by incubation of tissue in 100 µL of 3% H_2O_2 for 20 min at room temperature (RT) (*see* **Note 3**).

6. Wash 3X with PBS for 2 min each wash.

7. Digest DNA-associated proteins by incubating tissues in 100 µL of 20 µg/mL proteinase K for 15 min (*see* **Note 4**).

8. Wash 3X with PBS for 5 min each wash.

9. Add 75 µL of equilibration buffer to tissue for at least 1 min at RT.

10. Label DNA breaks by incubating tissue in 75 µL of TdT diluted in reaction buffer for 1 h at 37°C (*see* **Note 4**).

11. Stop TdT reaction by washing slides in PBS 3X for 5 min each wash.

12. Detect DIG-conjugated dUTP by incubating tissue in 100 µL of HRP-conjugated anti-DIG for 30 min at RT. The concentration of this antibody will vary, depending on the vendor. Thus concentration optimization needs to be determined by the operator.

13. Wash tissue 2X with PBS for 5 min each wash.

14. Wash tissue 2X with dH_2O for 5 min each wash.

15. Visualize staining by incubating tissue in 100 µL of the HRP substrate DAB for 5–10 min (*see* **Note 3**).

16. Wash off DAB with dH_2O 2X 5 min.

17. Counterstain nuclei in hematoxylin (5–10 s).

18. Wash off hematoxylin with dH_2O.

19. Dehydrate tissue in series of ethanol and xylene washes:

    a. 70% Ethanol for 1 min.

    b. 90% Ethanol for 1 min.

    c. 100% Ethanol 2X 1 min using fresh ethanol for each wash.

    d. Xylene 2X 1 min, using fresh xylene for each wash.

20. Cover slip.

21. Slides are ready to be visualized.

3.1.2. TUNEL on Cell Cultures

The procedure for TUNEL staining of cell cultures is similar to that utilized in paraffin-embedded sections. Therefore, the distinctions between the two procedures will be outlined and the majority of the experimental protocol will refer to **Subheading 3.1.1.**

1. Culture cells and perform experiments in 8-well tissue culture chamber slides.

2. Wash cells 1X in PBS.

3. Fix cells in 10% neutral buffered formalin or 4% paraformaldehyde for 15 min.

4. Wash cells 2X in PBS for 5 min each wash.

5. Permeabilize cells by incubating in 0.01% Triton X-100 for 15 min at RT.

6. Wash cells 2X in PBS for 5 min each wash.

7. Follow **steps 9–21** as outlined in **Subheading 3.1.1.**

3.2. Hoechst Nuclear Staining

1. Wash cells 1X with PBS.
2. Fix cells with 10% neutral buffered formalin or 4% paraformaldehyde for 15 min at RT (*see* **Note 5**).
3. Wash cells 1X with PBS.
4. Incubate cells in 1 µg/mL Hoechst 33342 for 10 min at RT.
5. Wash cells 1X in PBS.
6. Mount in aqueous mounting medium.
7. Visualize using fluorescence microscopy (excitation 350 nm, emission 460 nm).

3.3. Annexin V Labeling

This is a live cell staining procedure; therefore it should be performed rapidly without fixation (*see* **Note 6**).

1. Wash cells 1X in PBS.
2. Incubate cells in Alexa-488–conjugated annexin V (1:50 dilution) and 1 µg/mL PI diluted in annexin V staining buffer for 15 min at 37°C (*see* **Note 7**).
3. Wash cells 2X in annexin V staining buffer.
4. Visualize in phenol-free medium or PBS (emission 495 nm and excitation 519 nm).

3.4. Immunodetection of Caspase Processing

This section describes the preparation of whole cell lysates from nonadherent cells (**Subheading 3.4.1.**), adherent cells (**Subheading 3.4.2.**), and tissue segments (**Subheading 3.4.3.**), as well as their subsequent analysis for caspase processing by immunodetection (**Subheading 3.4.4.**) and by caspase protease activity (**Subheading 3.4.5.**).

3.4.1. Preparation of Whole Cell Lysates From Nonadherent Cultured Cells

1. Pellet cells by centrifugation.
2. Gently wash cell pellets 2X with ice-cold PBS, and resuspend the pellet in 1 mL of whole cell lysis buffer (*see* **Note 8**) for 20 min on ice.
3. Centrifuge samples for 10 min at 15,800g at 4°C.
4. Aliquot supernatant and store at –80°C.

3.4.2. Preparation of Whole Cell Lysates From Adherent Cultured Cells

1. Transfer conditioned media from plates of cultured adherent cells to centrifuge tubes, and pellet detached cells by centrifugation (*see* **Note 9**).
2. Wash adherent cells and pelleted detached cells twice with ice-cold PBS. Be gentle, so as not to dislodge cells.

3. Treat adherent cell plates, with 0.5–1.0 mL of whole cell lysis buffer for 20 min on ice (*see* **Note 8**).
4. Scrape cells from plate and transfer cell lysates to 1.5 mL microfuge tubes.
5. Centrifuge samples for 10 min at 15,800g at 4°C.
6. Resuspend detached cell pellets from conditioned media (from **step 2**) in the cell lysate obtained from the plate for the particular treatment (*see* **Note 9**).
7. Lyse cells on ice for 20 min, and centrifuge for 10 min at 15,800g at 4°C.
8. Aliquot supernatant and store at –80°C.

3.4.3. Preparation of Whole Cell Lysates From Tissue Sections

1. Homogenize 100–500 mg frozen tissue samples in 1.0 mL lysis buffer, and leave on ice for 20 min.
2. Remove insoluble materials by centrifugation for 10 min at 15,800g at 4°C, and then transfer the supernatant to new tubes.
3. Aliquot and store lysates at –80°C.

3.4.4. Western Blot Detection of Caspase Processing

1. Mix lysates prepared as described above in **Subheading 3.4.3.** 1:1 in 2X SDS sample buffer.
2. Boil samples for 5 min, and cool samples on ice.
3. Load 20–50 mg of whole cell lysate per lane of an SDS-PAGE minigel.
4. Electrophorese samples at 20 mA/gel until dye front reaches the bottom of the gel in running buffer.
5. Transfer proteins to nitrocellulose blotting membrane at 250 mA in transfer buffer for 2–4 h.
6. Incubate blot in blocking buffer for 1 h at RT.
7. Incubate blot for 1 h with primary antibody diluted in blocking buffer at RT. Check the supplier's recommendation for antibody concentration.
8. Wash blot 4X 5 min in washing buffer with shaking at RT.
9. Incubate blot with appropriate secondary antibody conjugated to HRP diluted in blocking buffer for 1 h at RT. Check with supplier for appropriate concentration.
10. Wash blot 4X 5 min in washing buffer with shaking at RT.
11. Treat blot with ECL solution for 1 min.
12. Expose to X-ray film for 15 s to 30 min. A longer exposure time may be required to detect cleavage fragments.
13. Examine blots for the appearance of caspase cleavage products (*see* **Note 10**).

3.4.5. Caspase Protease Assay

1. Dilute caspase substrates to 1 mg/mL working solution in reaction buffer.
2. In a 96-well plate, add 100 µL of whole cell lysis buffer per assay well.
3. Add 50 µL of cell lysates (~1 mg/mL) prepared as described in **Subheadings 3.4.1.–3.4.3.** Add 50 µL of whole cell lysis buffer to act as a blank. It is recommended that samples be added in triplicate wells.

4. Incubate at 37°C for 15 min.
5. Add 4 μL of the 1 mg/mL caspase substrate prepared in **step 1**.
6. Read fluorescence at time zero (*see* **Note 1**).
7. Incubate at 37°C.
8. Read fluorescence at various time points (i.e., 0.25, 0.5, 1.0, 2.0, and 4.0 h).
9. Calculate caspase activity using the Michaelis–Menten equation. The Michaelis constant (K_m) is specific for each caspase–substrate combination and should be indicated by the supplier.

4. Notes

1. Because caspases differ in their abilities to cleave specific sequences, caspase substrates should be selected for the caspase of interest. The excitation and emission wavelengths, as well as the Michaelis constants will differ for each caspase substrate. This information should be obtained from the supplier prior to commencing the assay. It should also be noted that, for convenience, several caspase assay kits are commercially available.

2. Positive control slides or tissues must be included in every run. Normal spleen contains numerous apoptotic leukocytes and can be used for positive control. Negative control slides must also be included in every run. These can include spleen incubated with reaction mixture without the addition of TdT for 1 h at 37°C.

   To ensure the specificity of staining, nuclear localization of staining and assessment of nuclear morphology are routinely employed. TUNEL positivity should be localized to nuclei. Cytoplasmic staining indicates either nonspecific staining or detection of necrotic cells owing to DNA fragmentation in the presence of nuclear disruption. TUNEL positivity in the cytoplasm of macrophages may also indicate the phagocytosis of apoptotic cells by these phagocytes.

3. Excessive background staining is typically related to the DAB development time. Although incubation with DAB for 5–10 min is recommended, this step should be optimized by the user. Certain tissues have high endogenous peroxidase activity. Therefore, increasing the incubation with 3% H_2O_2 may reduce background staining caused by this process.

4. A lack of staining may result from inefficient digestion of DNA-associated proteins or low concentration/activity of TdT. The concentration of these components can be optimized by the operator.

5. If the density of total cells is reduced after the procedure, many of the apoptotic cells that become detached may have washed off. In this case, cells can either be washed more gently, or the supernatant of the treated cells can be cytospun with harvested (trypsinized) adherent cells and stained in the same manner as described.

6. If a known apoptotic inducer is utilized, and a high frequency of annexin V-positive and PI-positive cells remains, the procedure may need to be performed more rapidly. Since this is a live staining method, maintenance of these cells outside a proper incubator may lead to cell damage. In addition, the concentra-

Table 1
Approximate Sizes of Caspase
Cleavage Products[a]

	Molecular weight (kDa)	
Caspase	Pro-form	Cleavage subunits
2	49	12, 13, 18
3	32	12, 17
6	33	11, 18
7	34	11, 20
8	55	10, 18
9	46	10, 35
10	59	12, 17,25

[a]Caspases are cleaved from the pro-forms into cleavage subunits upon activation. These cleavage events can be visualized by Western blot analysis.

tion of annexin V may need to be adjusted by the operator to ensure optimum staining of different cell types.

7. If limited staining is observed, the concentration of annexin V can be increased in **Subheading 3.3., step 2**. In addition, the intensity of fluorescent dyes decreases with increased exposure time to excitation wavelengths (photobleaching). Therefore, the length of time the stained cells are exposed to light should be limited. Finally, antifade reagents that reduce the sensitivity of fluorescent dyes can be purchased. The cells can be maintained in solutions containing these reagents in **Subheading 3.3., step 4** if need be.

8. The volume of whole cell lysis buffer can be adjusted depending on the cell number. It is recommended that 100–200 μL be used per 10^6 pelleted cells. For adherent cells the volume must be adjusted based on the surface area of the plate. Typically use 0.5–1 mL of buffer for 100-mm Petri dishes or 0.2–0.4 mL of buffer for 35-mm Petri dishes.

9. Many cells will detach upon apoptosis; therefore it is important to collect these cells from the conditioned media. We recommend that pelleted cells from the media be lysed in the lysis buffer from their respective treatments. This ensures that all cells are lysed in an equal volume of buffer and are thus equally represented in the lysate.

10. It is important to remember that some caspases also show intermediate cleavage products and that the sizes of these cleavage products can vary depending on which protease was responsible for their cleavage. Furthermore, antibodies typically only recognize the pro-form plus one cleavage product. It is important to check with the antibody supplier as to which cleavage fragments are recognized by each primary antibody (**Table 1**).

Acknowledgments

This work was supported in part by grants from the Canadian Institutes for Health Research (CIHR), The Canada Foundation for Innovation (CFI), the Michael Smith Foundation for Health Research (MSFHR), the St. Paul's Hospital Foundation, and the British Columbia Transplant Society. D.J.G. is a Canada Research Chair in Cardiovascular Biochemistry and an MSFHR Scholar. A.L.H. is a recipient of a CIHR/MSFHR Transplantation Training Program Research Award. J.C.C. is a recipient of a CIHR Doctoral Research Award, a Michael Smith Foundation for Health Research Traineeship, and an Honorary Killam Pre-Doctoral Fellowship. A.L.H. and J.C.C contributed equally to this chapter.

References

1. Granville, D. J., Carthy, C. M., Hunt, D. W., and McManus, B. M. (1998) Apoptosis: molecular aspects of cell death and disease. *Lab. Invest.* **78,** 893–913.
2. Granville, D. J. and Gottlieb, R. A. (2002) Mitochondria: regulators of cell death and survival. *Sci. World J.* **2,** 1569–1578.
3. Tedgui, A. and Mallat, Z. (2003) Apoptosis, a major determinant of atherothrombosis. *Arch. Mal. Coeur. Vaiss.* **96,** 671–675.
4. Gonzalez, A., Fortuno, M. A., Querejeta, R., et al. (2003) Cardiomyocyte apoptosis in hypertensive cardiomyopathy. *Cardiovasc. Res.* **59,** 549–562.
5. Gottlieb, R. A. (2003) Mitochondrial signaling in apoptosis: mitochondrial daggers to the breaking heart. *Basic Res. Cardiol.* **98,** 242–249.
6. Miller, L. W., Granville, D. J., Narula, J., and McManus, B. M. (2001) Apoptosis in cardiac transplant rejection. *Cardiol. Clin.* **19,** 141–154.
7. Yanagawa, B., Esfandiarei, M., Carthy, C., et al. (2003) Life and death signaling pathways in CVB3-induced myocarditis in *Myocarditis: From Bench to Bedside.* (Cooper, L. T., ed.), Humana, Totowa, NJ, pp. 161–197.
8. Choy, J. C., Granville, D. J., Hunt, D. W., and McManus, B. M. (2001) Endothelial cell apoptosis: biochemical characteristics and potential implications for atherosclerosis. *J. Mol. Cell. Cardiol.* **33,** 1673–1690.
9. Gold, R., Schmied, M., Giegerich, G., et al. (1994) Differentiation between cellular apoptosis and necrosis by the combined use of in situ tailing and nick translation techniques. *Lab. Invest.* **71,** 219–225.
10. Gold, R., Schmied, M., Rothe, G., et al. (1993) Detection of DNA fragmentation in apoptosis: application of in situ nick translation to cell culture systems and tissue sections. *J. Histochem. Cytochem.* **41,** 1023–1030.
11. Martin, S. J., Reutelingsperger, C. P., McGahon, A. J., et al. (1995) Early redistribution of plasma membrane phosphatidylserine is a general feature of apoptosis regardless of the initiating stimulus: inhibition by overexpression of Bcl-2 and Abl. *J. Exp. Med.* **182,** 1545–1556.

12. Kohler, C., Orrenium, S., and Zhivotovsky, B. (2002) Evaluation of caspase activity in apoptotic cells. *J. Immuno. Methods.* **265,** 97–110.

13. Nicholson, D. W. (1996) Caspase structure, proeolytic substrates, and function during apoptotic cell death. *Cell. Death Differ.* **6,** 1028–1042.

19

Detection of Cardiac Signaling in the Injured and Hypertrophied Heart

Xiaoning Si, Maziar Rahmani, Ji Yuan, and Honglin Luo

Summary

Cardiac hypertrophy is a compensatory response to a variety of physiological or pathological stimuli. However, prolonged hypertrophic responses may eventually lead to heart failure, arrhythmia, and sudden death. A number of intracellular signaling pathways have been implicated to play a critical role in the regulation of cardiac hypertrophy. In this chapter, the mitogen-activated protein kinase signaling pathway is used to illustrate conventional assays to detect the expression, phosphorylation, and activation of signaling proteins during cardiac hypertrophy, including Western blot, immunohistochemical staining, and immune complex kinase assays. Newly emerging techniques for analyzing cell signaling are also discussed in this chapter. Identifying and characterizing the expression and activation of these signaling proteins will provide important insights into the mechanisms that regulate hypertrophic cell growth and assist in development of new therapeutic approaches to limit cardiac hypertrophy.

Key Words: Signaling pathway; cardiac hypertrophy; Western blot; immunohistochemical staining; immunoprecipitation; immune complex kinase assay.

1. Introduction

In response to hormonal or pathophysiological stimuli, the heart undergoes hypertrophic growth as an adaptive response. However, sustained cardiac hypertrophy may ultimately lead to heart failure and death. An increasing number of intracellular signaling pathways have been implicated in the induction of cardiac hypertrophy, including heterotrimeric G proteins (1), small GTP

From: *Methods in Molecular Medicine, vol. 112: Molecular Cardiology: Methods and Protocols*
Edited by: Z. Sun © Humana Press Inc., Totowa, NJ

binding proteins *(2,3)*, calcineurin *(4,5)*, mitogen-activated protein kinases (MAPKs) *(6–10)*, protein kinase C *(1,11)*, glycogen synthase kinase-3 *(9,12,13)*, signal transducer and activator of transcription *(14)*, and nuclear factor-κB *(15)*. Activation of these signaling pathways directly modifies transcriptional regulatory factors, promoting the regulation of cardiac gene expression. In this chapter, we use the MAPK signaling pathway to illustrate general methods for detecting cardiac signal transduction in the regulation of cardiac hypertrophy.

1.1. The MAPK Signaling Pathway and Cardiac Hypertrophy

MAPKs consist of a superfamily of highly related serine/threonine kinases, which includes at least extracellular signal-regulated kinases 1 and 2 (ERK1/2) *(16)*, c-Jun NH2-terminal kinase/stress-activated protein kinase (JNK/SAPK) *(17)*, p38 MAP kinase *(17)*, and big MAP kinase 1 (BMK1, also known as ERK5) *(18)*. MAPK signaling cascades are activated through three kinase modules composed of a MAPKK kinase (MAPKKK, or MEKK), a MAPK kinase (MAPKK, or MEK, MKK), and a MAPK *(19)*. In response to extracellular stimuli, these kinase modules are differentially activated and transduce signals from the cell membrane to the nucleus. MAPKs are directly phosphorylated by upstream dual-specificity protein kinases (MEK) at both a threonine and adjacent tyrosine residue within a Thr-X-Tyr motif. For example, ERK1/2 and BMK1/ERK5 proteins are phosphorylated by MEK1/2 and MEK5, respectively, at a Thr-Glu-Tyr (TEY) motif. p38 kinases are activated by MKK6 and MKK3 within a Thr-Gly-Tyr (TGY) motif, whereas JNK/SAPK proteins are activated by the upstream MAPK kinases MKK4 and MKK7 on a Thr-Pro-Tyr (TPY) motif. Once activated, MAPKs directly phosphorylate a wide variety of substrates including transcription factors (e.g., c-Myc, c-Jun, activating transcription factor-2 [ATF-2], murine embryonic fibroblast 2C [MEF2C], activation protein-1 [AP-1], GATA4, cAMP-responsive element binding protein [CREB], and Elk-1), protein kinases, and cytoskeletal proteins. Consequently, they regulate a variety of cellular processes, including cell proliferation, cell differentiation, stress response, and cell death *(19)*. In cardiomyocytes, the MAPK signaling cascade is activated by G protein-coupled receptors (GPCR), receptor tyrosine kinase, protein kinase C, or stress stimuli *(17)*. The MAPK-signaling cascades are illustrated in **Fig. 1**.

Although there remains a lack of consensus regarding the function of the ERK1/2 pathway in cardiac hypertrophy, increasing evidence has suggested that the ERK signaling pathway plays an important role in the regulation of cardiac hypertrophic responses both in vitro and in vivo. In response to mechanical stretching, GPCR, and mitogens, ERK1/2 are activated in cultured cardiomyocytes *(7)*. In aortic-banded mice, ERK1/2 are activated by pressure-

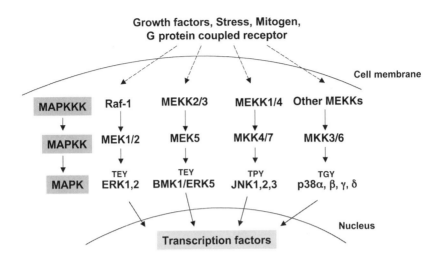

Fig. 1. Mitogen-activated protein kinase (MAPK) signaling pathways. BMK1, big MAPK (also known as ERK5); JNK, c-Jun NH_2-terminal kinase; MAPKK (MEK or MKK), MAPK kinase; MAPKKK, MAPK kinase kinase; MEKK, MEK kinase; TEY, Thr-Glu-Tyr; TGY, Thr-Gly-Tyr; TPY, Thr-Pro-Tyr.

overload hypertrophy *(10,20)*. Recent studies also demonstrate that BMK1/ERK5, a MAPK closely related to ERK1/2, is activated by chronic pressure overload and by acute mechanical stretch in vivo *(10)*. Constitutively active MEK1 or ERK stimulates hypertrophic gene expression, such as atrial natriuretic factor (ANF) and β-myosin heavy chain in cardiomyocytes, whereas dominant-negative or pharmacologic inhibition (e.g., the MEK1 inhibitors PD98059 or U0126) effectively blocks GPCR agonist-induced hypertrophy *(21–23)*. It was further demonstrated that ERK1/2 are required for sarcomeric organization induced by hypertrophy agonists *(24)*. Importantly, recent studies on MEK1 transgenic mice demonstrate a hypertrophic phenotype, indicating that the MEK-ERK1/2 signaling pathway is sufficient to induce a hypertrophic response in vivo (6).

Four p38 MAPK isoforms (α, β, γ, and δ) have been identified so far, P38α and p38β being the most important ones expressed in the human heart *(17)*. Accumulating evidence has strongly suggested that p38 activation is a necessary signaling event regulating the cardiac hypertrophic response, both in vitro and in vivo. In cardiomyocytes, cellular stress (such as reactive oxygen species, hyperosmotic shock, hypoxia/reoxygenation, and proinflammatory cytokines) and GPCR (such as phenylephrine, angiotensin II, and endothelin-1) are potent activators of p38 kinases *(17)*. In vivo, p38 MAPKs are activated by pressure overload in mouse aortic-binding models and in human heart failure *(9,25)*. In addition, overexpression of constitutively active MKK3 or MKK6, the direct upstream kinases of p38, in neonatal cardiomyocytes is sufficient to induce hypertrophy and ANF expression *(25,26)*. Inhibition of p38 kinase activity using the specific inhibitors SB202190 and SB203580 blocks agonist-induced hypertrophic responses in culture *(24,26)*. Adenovirus-mediated gene delivery of a dominant-negative p38 MAPK to neonatal cardiomyocytes significantly reduced agonist-induced hypertrophic response *(25)*.

Recent studies have implicated JNKs as critical regulators of cardiac hypertrophy both in cell culture and in the human heart. In cultured cardiomyocytes, JNK activation has been associated with cellular stress or GPCR activation *(17,27)*. JNKs have also been linked to pressure overload-induced cardiac hypertrophy in animal and human heart failure *(8,9)*. Overexpression of constitutively active MEKK1 or MKK4 induces cardiac hypertrophic promoter expression, whereas transfection of a dominant-negative MEKK1 diminishes ANF promoter activity *(28,29)*. Adenovirus-mediated gene delivery of a dominant-negative MKK4 significantly attenuates agonist or aortic banding-induced cardiac hypertrophy in vivo *(8)*.

In this chapter, we describe the methods for (1) preparing cardiac homogenates and cell lysates, (2) analyzing the phosphorylation status of signaling proteins by Western blot, (3) evaluating the phosphorylation state of signaling proteins through immunohistochemical staining, and (4) detecting kinase activities by immune complex kinase assays.

2. Materials

2.1. Sample Preparation

1. Radioimmunoprecipitation assay (RIPA) lysis buffer: 20 mM Tris-HCl, pH 7.5, 150 mM NaCl, 1% Nonidet P-40, 50 mM NaF, 0.1 mM Na$_3$VO$_4$, 0.5% sodium deoxycholate, 1 mM EDTA, 0.1% sodium dodecyl sulfate (SDS). Store at 4°C. (*see* **Note 1**).
2. Modified oncogen science lysis buffer (MOSLB): 50 mM sodium pyrophosphate, 50 mM NaF, 50 mM NaCl, 5 mM EDTA, 5 mM EGTA, 100 µM Na$_3$VO$_4$, 10 mM HEPES, pH 7.4, 0.1% Triton X-100. Store at 4°C.
3. Phosphate-buffered saline (PBS): 137 mM NaCl, 2.7 mM KCl, 4.3 mM Na$_2$HPO$_4$, 1.4 mM KH$_2$PO$_4$, pH 7.3. Store at room temperature.
4. Protease inhibitor cocktail (Sigma).
5. Bradford protein assay reagent (Bio-Rad).

2.2. Western Blot

1. Tris-buffered saline (TBS): 25 mM Tris-HCl, pH 7.5, 150 mM NaCl. Store at room temperature.

2. Wash buffer (TBS/T buffer): 0.1% Tween-20 in TBS. Store at room temperature.
3. Blocking buffer: 5% (w/v) nonfat dry milk in TBS/T buffer. Prepare freshly before use.
4. Primary antibodies: ERK1/2 antibody (1:1000, Cell Signaling, cat. no. 9102), phospho-ERK1/2 antibody (1:2000, Cell Signaling, cat. no. 9106), p38 antibody (1:1000, Cell Signaling, cat. no. 9212), phospho-p38 antibody (1:2000, Cell Signaling, cat. no. 9216), JNK antibody (1:1000, Cell Signaling, cat. no. 9252), phospho-JNK antibody (1:1000, Cell Signaling, cat. no. 9251), ERK5 antibody (1:1000, Cell Signaling, cat. no. 3372), and phospho-ERK5 antibody (1:1000, Cell Signaling, cat. no. 3371).
5. Horseradish peroxidase (HRP)-conjugated secondary antibodies (1:2000, Cell Signaling).
6. Enhanced chemiluminescent (ECL) reagent (Amersham).
7. Stripping buffer: 62.5 mM Tris-HCl, pH 6.7, 1% SDS. (Add 35 µL β-mercaptoethanol per 10 mL stripping buffer before use.) Store at room temperature.

2.3. Immunohistochemical Staining

1. 10 mM Sodium citrate buffer, pH 6.0. Store at room temperature.
2. 3% H_2O_2 in methanol. Store at room temperature.
3. Blocking solution: 5% normal goat or horse serum in TBS/T buffer.
4. Avidin–biotin–HRP complex (ABC) reagent (Vector).
5. Primary antibodies: ERK1/2 antibody (1:100, Cell Signaling, cat. no. 9102), phospho-ERK1/2 antibody (1:100, Cell Signaling, cat. no. 9106), p38 antibody (1:50, Cell Signaling, cat. no. 9212), phospho-p38 antibody (1:50, Cell Signaling, cat. no. 9216), phospho-JNK antibody (1:100, Cell Signaling, cat. no. 9251).
6. Diaminobenzidine (DAB) solution (Sigma). Store in the dark at –20°C.
7. 1% Acid alcohol: 1% HCl in 100% ethanol. Store at room temperature.
8. Others: 0.5% $CuSO_4$, lithium carbonate, xylene, ethanol, hematoxylin.

2.4. Immune Complex Kinase Assays

1. Protein G plus/protein A agarose beads (Calbiochem).
2. Kinase assay buffer: 20 mM HEPES, pH 7.5, 150 mM NaCl, 10 mM $MgCl_2$, 0.1% Triton X-100, 10% glycerol, 1 mM Na_3VO_4. Store at 4°C.
3. 2X SDS-polyacrylamide gel electrophoresis (PAGE) sample buffer: 125 mM Tris-HCl, pH 6.8, 20% glycerol, 4% SDS, 0.1% β-mercaptoethanol, 0.01% bromophenol blue. Store at –20°C.
4. [γ-^{32}P]ATP.
5. Antibodies: ERK1/2 antibody, p38 antibody, JNK antibody, ERK5 antibody (all from Santa Cruz).
6. Substrates: glutathione S-transferase (GST)-c-Jun for JNK activity assay (Upstate Biotechnology), myelin basic protein (MBP) for ERK1/2 or ERK5 assay (Santa Cruz), and GST-activating transcription factor-2 (ATF-2) for p38 assay (Santa Cruz).

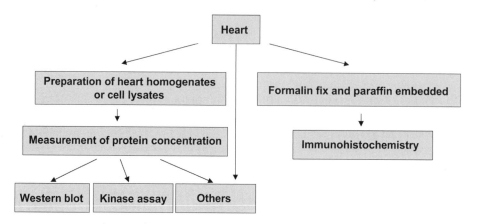

Fig. 2. Flowchart for detecting signaling proteins in the hypertrophied heart.

3. Methods

The overall experimental methods are outlined in **Fig. 2**.

3.1. Sample Preparation

3.1.1. Preparation of Cardiac Homogenates (see **Note 2**)

1. Homogenize frozen hearts in ice-cold RIPA lysis buffer containing freshly added protease inhibitor cocktail (one tablet per 10 mL lysis buffer).
2. Centrifuge the homogenates at 12,000g for 10 min at 4°C to pellet tissue debris.
3. Collect supernatant, and measure protein concentration by the Bio-Rad Bradford protein assay.
4. Aliquot, and store samples at –80°C.

3.1.2. Preparation of Cell Lysates (see **Note 2**)

1. Wash cultured cardiomyocytes twice with ice-cold PBS.
2. Add MOSLB lysis buffer containing a freshly added protease inhibitor cocktail to cells, and incubate on ice for 10 min.
3. Scrape the cells with a cell scraper, and transfer the cell debris and lysis buffer to a chilled microfuge tube.
4. Centrifuge the lysates at 12,000g for 10 min at 4°C.
5. Transfer supernatant into a clean tube, and measure protein concentration by the Bio-Rad Bradford protein assay.
6. Aliquot, and store lysates at –80°C. Avoid repeated freeze–thaw cycles.

3.2. Western Blot (see Note 3)

Western blot analyses with phosphospecific antibodies have been widely used to measure the phosphorylation status of MAPK signaling proteins in cell lysates or tissue homogenates.

1. Equal amounts of protein are subjected to SDS-PAGE and then transferred to nitrocellulose membranes.
2. Optional: wash nitrocellulose membrane with TBS for 5 min at room temperature.
3. Incubate membrane with blocking buffer for 1 h at room temperature.
4. Dilute the phosphospecific primary antibodies (*see* **Note 4**) to the recommended concentration in 2.5% nonfat dry milk in TBS/T buffer. Incubate membrane in primary antibody dilution for 1–2 h at room temperature or overnight at 4°C with agitation.
5. Wash the membrane three times for 10 min each with TBS/T wash buffer.
6. Incubate membrane with HRP-conjugated secondary antibody for 1 h at room temperature or overnight at 4°C with agitation. For a mouse monoclonal antibody, a goat/antimouse HRP-conjugated antibody is recommended; for a rabbit polyclonal antibody, a goat/antirabbit HRP-conjugated antibody is recommended.
7. Wash the membrane three times for 10 min each with TBS/T wash buffer.
8. Incubate membrane with ECL reagent for 1 min at room temperature with gentle agitation.
9. Drain membrane of excess developing solution, wrap in plastic wrap, and expose to X-ray film.
10. Strip membrane and probe for antibodies against total signaling proteins (e.g., ERK1/2, p38, JNK, and ERK5). Membrane stripping:
    a. After film exposure, wash membrane twice for 10 min each in TBS/T wash buffer.
    b. Incubate membrane for 10 min at 50°C in stripping buffer containing β-mercaptoethanol with gentle shaking.
    c. Wash membrane three times for 10 min each in wash buffer.
    d. The membrane is now ready to reuse for Western blot starting from **step 3**.
11. Quantify the phosphorylation status by densitometric analysis using NIH Image software, and normalize to the expression of total signaling proteins.

3.3. Immunohistochemical Staining (see Note 5)

Through the use of phosphospecific antibodies, immunohistochemical staining provides an excellent opportunity to examine directly the activation state of signaling proteins in tissue samples.

3.3.1. Deparaffinization and Rehydration

1. Deparaffinize sections in three changes of xylene for 5 min each.
2. Rehydrate sections in two washes of 100% ethanol for 10 min each, followed by two washes of 95% ethanol for 10 min each.
3. Wash sections twice in dH_2O for 5 min each, and place in PBS for 5 min.

3.3.2. Antigen Retrieval

1. Fully immerse slides in preboiled 10 mM sodium citrate buffer, and heat slides to boiling three times for 5 min each.
2. Cool slides for 30 min.
3. Wash sections in dH$_2$O twice for 5 min each.

3.3.3. Blocking and Binding

1. Block endogenous peroxidase activity by incubating sections in 3% H$_2$O$_2$ in methanol for 10 min.
2. Wash sections three times in TBS/T wash buffer for 5 min each.
3. Block sections with 100 µL blocking solution for 1 h at room temperature in a humidity chamber.
4. Remove blocking solution, and add 100 µL diluted primary antibody (diluted in blocking solution) to each section, and incubate overnight at 4°C in a humidity chamber.
5. Wash slides three times in TBS/T wash buffer for 5 min each.
6. Add 100 µL diluted secondary antibody (diluted in blocking solution) to each tissue section, and incubate for 30 min in a humidity chamber at room temperature.
7. Wash slides three times in TBS/T wash buffer for 5 min each.

3.3.4. Detection

1. Prepare ABC reagent according to the manufacturer's instructions and incubate for 30 min at room temperature prior to use.
2. Add 100 µL ABC reagent per tissue section, and incubate for 30 min at room temperature.
3. Wash sections three times in wash buffer for 5 min each.
4. Prepare the DAB solution as 50 mg DAB added to 100 mL 0.1 M Tris buffer (*see* **Note 6**).
5. Add 100 µL DAB solution per section, and incubate for 5 min or less. (As soon as the section turns brown, immerse slides in dH$_2$O.)
6. Wash sections twice in dH$_2$O for 5 min each.
7. Place slides in 0.5% CuSO$_4$ for 5 min at room temperature.
8. Rinse slides thoroughly in dH$_2$O.

3.3.5. Counterstaining and Dehydration

1. Place slides in hematoxylin for 1 min and rinse thoroughly in dH$_2$O.
2. Dip slides in 1% acid alcohol solution for 5 s and rinse thoroughly in dH$_2$O.
3. Dip slides in lithium carbonate for 15 s, and rinse thoroughly in dH$_2$O.
4. Dehydrate sections in two changes of 95% ethanol for 10 s each.
5. Dehydrate sections in two changes of 100% ethanol for 10 s each.
6. Clear in two changes of xylene for 10 s each and mount on a cover slip.

3.4. Immune Complex Kinase Assays

Immune complex kinase assays provide a direct measurement of kinase activities by detecting the ability to phosphorylate the substrates (*see* **Note 7**).

3.4.1. Immunoprecipitation

1. To prepare protein G plus/protein A agarose beads, wash the beads twice with PBS and restore to a 50% slurry with PBS (*see* **Note 8**).
2. Optional: preclear the lysates by adding 30 μL of protein G plus/protein A agarose beads (50% slurry) per 1 mg of cell lysate, and incubate at 4°C for 10 min on a rocker or orbital shaker. Remove the protein G plus/protein A beads by centrifugation at 4000*g* for 3 min at 4°C. Transfer the supernatant to a fresh centrifuge tube (*see* **Note 9**).
3. Dilute the lysates to approx 1 mg/mL total cell protein with PBS to reduce the concentration of the detergents in the buffer.
4. Add 2–5 μg of recommended antibodies to 500 μg of the lysate.
5. Gently mix the lysate/antibody mixture for 1–2 h at 4°C on a rocker/orbital shaker.
6. Capture the immunocomplex by adding 30 μL protein G plus/protein A beads, and gently rock on a rocker or orbital shaker for 1 h to overnight at 4°C.
7. Collect the agarose beads by centrifugation at 4000*g* for 5 min at 4°C. Carefully aspirate the supernatant and discard. Wash the beads three times with 1 mL ice-cold RIPA buffer. Repeat the centrifugation step.

3.4.2. Kinase Assay (see **Note 10**)

1. Wash the agarose beads with kinase assay buffer, repeat the centrifugation step, and remove the supernatant. Keep the beads on ice (*see* **Note 11**).
2. Incubate the pellets for 30 min at 30°C with 20 μL kinase buffer that contains 25 μ*M* ATP, 2.5 μCi [γ-^{32}P]-ATP, and the appropriate protein substrate (1.0 mg/mL) with vortexing every 5 min (*see* **Note 12**).
3. Stop the reaction by adding 20 mL of 2X SDS-PAGE sample buffer.
4. Boil the agarose beads for 5 min to dissociate the immunocomplexes from the beads. Collect the supernatant fraction by centrifugation at 12,000*g* for 5 min.
5. Separate the proteins by SDS-PAGE.
6. Briefly rinse the gel in dH$_2$O, and cut the gel below the 14-kDa marker to remove unincorporated [γ-^{32}P]-ATP (*see* **Note 13**).
7. Transfer the gel to a nitrocellulose membrane, and proceed to autoradiography (*see* **Note 14**).
8. Examine the expression of immunoprecipitated signaling proteins on the same membrane by Western blot.
9. Quantify kinase activities by densitometric analysis using the National Institutes of Health Image software, and normalize to immunoprecipitated protein levels.

3.5. Other Techniques

Recent advances in genomics and proteomics have increased the available options to study the cardiac signaling pathways in hypertrophied heart. *Transgenic mouse models* provide us with novel and reliable in vivo systems to look into the functions of certain genes in the cardiac signaling.

Crude lysates prepared from the hypertrophied heart can also be fractionated by either sucrose-gradient centrifugation or chromatography prior to coimmunoprecipitation. Both *2D electrophoresis* and *mass spectrometry* provide powerful tools to reveal the molecular identities of coimmunoprecipitated signaling proteins.

Expression profiling of hypertrophied cardiac genes can be obtained by traditional methods including *subtractive hybridization* and *differential display* techniques and also by recent approaches including *microarray, real-time polymerase chain reaction (PCR),* and *serial analysis of gene expression (SAGE)* techniques. Protein phosphorylation is an important posttranslational modification for many cellular signaling proteins. Protein phosphorylation profiling utilizing the *AntibodyArrays™* technique developed by Hypromatrix (www.hypromatrix.com) allows researchers to perform a quick screening of the phosphorylation status of hundreds of well-characterized signaling proteins. Also, a sensitive and quantitative assay, *phosphoELISA™*, has been introduced by Biosource (www.biosource.com) for efficient detection of the phosphorylation status of proteins without the hassle of immunoprecipitation, SDS-PAGE, or transfer.

Cardiomyocyte culture provides a useful in vitro approach to study cardiac signaling in hypertrophied heart. Constitutively active or dominant–negative mutants of signaling proteins can be introduced into cultured cardiomyocytes by *liposome-based transfection* methods or by *adenoviral infection*, which is much more efficient for gene delivery. Furthermore, the downregulation of specific genes can be achieved by either the *RNA interference (RNAi)* technique or the *antisense RNA technique*. Additionally, this cell-based system allows us to design controlled experiments to focus on particular signaling pathways, while also being very useful for pharmacological inhibitor studies.

4. Notes

1. Do not add sodium deoxycholate when preparing lysates for kinase assay.
2. All the procedures involving cardiac homogenate and cell lysate preparation should be done at 4°C using precooled reagents.
3. If there is a high background in the Western blot, we recommend (1) increasing the blocking time up to 3 h at room temperature or overnight at 4°C, (2) diluting antibodies in TBS/T buffer containing 5% nonfat dry milk, (3) decreasing the concentration of primary antibodies, (4) reducing the incubation time with pri-

mary antibodies, or (5) increasing the washing time. In contrast, if there is low protein signal in the Western blot, we recommend: (1) increasing the concentration of primary antibodies, (2) diluting primary antibodies in TBS/T buffer without milk, (3) increasing the incubation time with primary antibodies, or (4) decreasing the washing time.

4. ERK5 phosphorylation can also be detected by band-shift assay using the total ERK5 antibody. Phosphorylation of ERK5 results in a retardation in electrophoretic mobility of immunoreactive ERK5 on a Western blot. A correlation has been consistently seen between the shifted fraction of phosphorylated ERK5 and the activity of ERK5 as measured by protein kinase assay.

5. Negative, positive, or internal controls should be included to validate the immunohistochemical staining results.

6. **Caution:** DAB is a suspected carcinogen and must be handled with care.

7. In addition to phosphorylating their substrates, some kinases are capable of autophosphorylation.

8. It is recommended to cut off the micropipet tip when manipulating agarose beads to avoid disruption of the beads.

9. Preclearing the lysate will reduce nonspecific binding of proteins to the beads.

10. We recommend that each assay should include a positive control (purified active enzyme) and two negative controls (sample with no kinase and sample with no substrate).

11. Buffer composition may differ slightly depending on the kinase under study.

12. The occasional vortexing step is important to keep the beads suspended in the reaction mixtures.

13. Rinsing the gel with distilled water can remove the unincorporated $[\gamma\text{-}^{32}P]$ ATP from the running buffer, thereby reducing the background signals.

14. If the signal is low, instead of transferring the gel to a membrane, dry the gel and then expose it directly to X-ray film.

Acknowledgment

We thank Dr. Bruce McManus and Ms. Elizabeth K.-Y. Walker for invaluable assistance and critical reading of the manuscript.

References

1. Molkentin, J. D. and Dorn, I. G. 2nd. (2001) Cytoplasmic signaling pathways that regulate cardiac hypertrophy. *Annu. Rev. Physiol.* **63,** 391–426.

2. Aikawa, R., Komuro, I., Yamazaki, T., et al. (1999) Rho family small G proteins play critical roles in mechanical stress-induced hypertrophic responses in cardiac myocytes. *Circ. Res.* **84,** 458–466.

3. Clerk, A. and Sugden, P. H. (2000) Small guanine nucleotide-binding proteins and myocardial hypertrophy. *Circ. Res.* **86,** 1019–1023.

4. Sugden, P. H. (1999) Signaling in myocardial hypertrophy: life after calcineurin? *Circ. Res.* **84,** 633–646.

5. Williams, R. S. (2002) Calcineurin signaling in human cardiac hypertrophy. *Circulation* **105,** 2242–2243.

6. Bueno, O. F., De Windt, L. J., Tymitz, K. M., et al. (2000) The MEK1-ERK1/2 signaling pathway promotes compensated cardiac hypertrophy in transgenic mice. *EMBO J.* **19,** 6341–6350.

7. Bueno, O. F. and Molkentin, J. D. (2002) Involvement of extracellular signal-regulated kinases 1/2 in cardiac hypertrophy and cell death. *Circ. Res.* **91,** 776–781.

8. Choukroun, G., Hajjar, R., Fry, S., et al. (1999) Regulation of cardiac hypertrophy in vivo by the stress-activated protein kinases/c-Jun NH(2)-terminal kinases. *J. Clin. Invest.* **104,** 391–398.

9. Haq, S., Choukroun, G., Lim, H., et al. (2001) Differential activation of signal transduction pathways in human hearts with hypertrophy versus advanced heart failure. *Circulation* **103,** 670–677.

10. Takeishi, Y., Huang, Q., Abe, J., et al. (2001) Src and multiple MAP kinase activation in cardiac hypertrophy and congestive heart failure under chronic pressure-overload: comparison with acute mechanical stretch. *J. Mol. Cell. Cardiol.* **33,** 1637–1648.

11. Takeishi, Y., Ping, P., Bolli, R., Kirkpatrick, D. L., Hoit, B. D., and Walsh, R. A. (2000) Transgenic overexpression of constitutively active protein kinase C epsilon causes concentric cardiac hypertrophy. *Circ. Res.* **86,** 1218–1223.

12. Haq, S., Choukroun, G., Kang, Z. B., et al. (2000) Glycogen synthase kinase-3beta is a negative regulator of cardiomyocyte hypertrophy. *J. Cell. Biol.* **151,** 117–130.

13. Hardt, S. E. and Sadoshima, J. (2002) Glycogen synthase kinase-3beta: a novel regulator of cardiac hypertrophy and development. *Circ. Res.* **90,** 1055–1063.

14. Booz, G. W., Day, J. N., and Baker, K. M. (2002) Interplay between the cardiac renin angiotensin system and JAK-STAT signaling: role in cardiac hypertrophy, ischemia/reperfusion dysfunction, and heart failure. *J. Mol. Cell. Cardiol.* **34,** 1443–1453.

15. Hirotani, S., Otsu, K., Nishida, K., et al. (2002) Involvement of nuclear factor-kappaB and apoptosis signal-regulating kinase 1 in G-protein-coupled receptor agonist-induced cardiomyocyte hypertrophy. *Circulation* **105,** 509–515.

16. Lange-Carter, C. A., Pleiman, C. M., Gardner, A. M., Blumer, K. J., and Johnson, G. L. (1993) A divergence in the MAP kinase regulatory network defined by MEK kinase and Raf. *Science* **260,** 315–319.

17. Sugden, P. H. and Clerk, A. (1998) "Stress-responsive" mitogen-activated protein kinases (c-Jun N-terminal kinases and p38 mitogen-activated protein kinases) in the myocardium. *Circ. Res.* **83,** 345–352.

18. Lee, J. D., Ulevitch, R. J., and Han, J. (1995) Primary structure of BMK1: a new mammalian map kinase. *Biochem. Biophys. Res. Commun.* **213,** 715–724.

19. Widmann, C., Gibson, S., Jarpe, M. B., and Johnson, G. L. (1999) Mitogen-activated protein kinase: conservation of a three-kinase module from yeast to human. *Physiol. Rev.* **79,** 143–180.

20. Rapacciuolo, A., Esposito, G., Caron, K., Mao, L., Thomas, S. A., and Rockman, H. A. (2001) Important role of endogenous norepinephrine and epinephrine in the

development of in vivo pressure-overload cardiac hypertrophy. *J. Am. Coll. Cardiol.* **38,** 876–882.

21. Gillespie-Brown, J., Fuller, S. J., Bogoyevitch, M. A., Cowley, S., and Sugden, P. H. (1995) The mitogen-activated protein kinase kinase MEK1 stimulates a pattern of gene expression typical of the hypertrophic phenotype in rat ventricular cardiomyocytes. *J. Biol. Chem.* **270,** 28,092–28,096.

22. Kodama, H., Fukuda, K., Pan, J., et al. (2000) Significance of ERK cascade compared with JAK/STAT and PI3-K pathway in gp130-mediated cardiac hypertrophy. *Am. J. Physiol. Heart Circ. Physiol.* **279,** H1635–1644.

23. Yue, T. L., Gu, J. L., Wang, C., et al. (2000) Extracellular signal-regulated kinase plays an essential role in hypertrophic agonists, endothelin-1 and phenylephrine-induced cardiomyocyte hypertrophy. *J. Biol. Chem.* **275,** 37,895–37,901.

24. Clerk, A., Michael, A., and Sugden, P. H. (1998) Stimulation of the p38 mitogen-activated protein kinase pathway in neonatal rat ventricular myocytes by the G protein-coupled receptor agonists, endothelin-1 and phenylephrine: a role in cardiac myocyte hypertrophy? *J. Cell. Biol.* **142,** 523–535.

25. Wang, Y., Huang, S., Sah, V. P., et al. (1998) Cardiac muscle cell hypertrophy and apoptosis induced by distinct members of the p38 mitogen-activated protein kinase family. *J. Biol. Chem.* **273,** 2161–2168.

26. Nemoto, S., Sheng, Z., and Lin, A. (1998) Opposing effects of Jun kinase and p38 mitogen-activated protein kinases on cardiomyocyte hypertrophy. *Mol. Cell. Biol.* **18,** 3518–3526.

27. Komuro, I., Kudo, S., Yamazaki, T., Zou, Y., Shiojima, I., and Yazaki, Y. (1996) Mechanical stretch activates the stress-activated protein kinases in cardiac myocytes. *FASEB J.* **10,** 631–636.

28. Thorburn, J., Xu, S., and Thorburn, A. (1997) MAP kinase- and Rho-dependent signals interact to regulate gene expression but not actin morphology in cardiac muscle cells. *EMBO J.* **16,** 1888–1900.

29. Ramirez, M. T., Sah, V. P., Zhao, X. L., Hunter, J. J., Chien, K. R., and Brown, J. H. (1997) The MEKK-JNK pathway is stimulated by alpha1-adrenergic receptor and ras activation and is associated with in vitro and in vivo cardiac hypertrophy. *J. Biol. Chem.* **272,** 14,057–14,061.

20

Affymetrix Oligonucleotide Analysis of Gene Expression in the Injured Heart

Bobby Yanagawa, Lydia Taylor, Theresa A. Deisher, Raymond Ng, George F. Schreiner, Timothy J. Triche, Decheng Yang, and Bruce M. McManus

Summary

Microarrays have helped researchers gain much insight into gene expression profiles in the context of many diseases including those in the injured heart. Our genomic investigations have been focused on elucidation of host gene responses to enterovirus infection. We have gained valuable technical expertise in using Affymetrix oligonucleotide arrays, also known as GeneChip®s, and cDNA spotted arrays to probe differential gene expression in both cultured cells and in heart tissue. Here, we provide a technique-focused supplement to the *Affymetrix GeneChip® Expression Analysis Manual* for sample preparation, processing, and array hybridization. We provide expanded explanations to highlight important points within the existing protocol and offer variations to standard procedures when appropriate. For investigators using myocardial tissues for microarray experiments, we further address the necessity of and methods for *in situ* flushing of the vasculature, tissue homogenization, and considerations for limits of expression detection in rare cells. It is our intention to provide useful technical information, based on our experience, to assist those researchers using Affymetrix GeneChips in their own genomic research.

Key Words: Affymetrix; GeneChip®; microarray; genomics; heart.

1. Introduction

Affymetrix oligonucleotide arrays, also known as GeneChips, have helped to revolutionize microarray experimentation by creating an extremely small-

From: *Methods in Molecular Medicine, vol. 112: Molecular Cardiology: Methods and Protocols*
Edited by: Z. Sun © Humana Press Inc., Totowa, NJ

featured microarray on which to probe known sequences in an enclosed platform. These arrays facilitate the simultaneous detection of transcriptional changes in a 500-fold range *(1)*, thereby enabling quantification and direct comparison of relative transcription levels across nearly limitless numbers of samples. This technique, among others, has become important as one facet of a functional framework for the vast amount of information produced by genome sequencing in biological and biomedical realms *(2)*. For example, significant findings regarding transcriptional profiles in the human aging process *(3,4)* and their patterns in human cancers *(5)*, as well as identification of human housekeeping genes *(6)*, and T-cell transcripts *(7)*, have all been possible based on the Affymetrix platform.

The Affymetrix microarray consists of a silicon slide with short (25-mer) oligonucleotide sequences "built" directly onto the surface using the same technology that revolutionized the microprocessor industry—photolithographics *(8,9)*. In essence, the power of light is harnessed to catalyze intermolecular reactions in building the oligonucleotide chains, thereby producing the smallest feature size on the market *(10)*. Thus, the most recent human GeneChip, the Human Genome U133 Plus 2.0 Array, is able to provide quantitative information across a range of transcript abundance levels of over 47,000 genes and expressed sequence tags (ESTs) using more than 1,300,000 different oligonucleotide features. Each gene or EST is probed in multiple copies using known sequences, allowing for the distinction of closely related sequences including polymorphisms, as well as splice variants. Thus, this technology lends itself to evaluation of message expression detection, but, in addition, the system has utility in sequence variation detection. In the latter applications, the creation of probes from known sequences allows mutations and isoforms to be probed, including both single-base changes and insertions/deletions.

For Affymetrix expression detection microarrays, each gene or EST is probed with as many as 16 25-mer sequences, depending on the array type, randomly distributed over the microarray surface. Probes are selected from novel gene-specific sequences with optimal hybridization behavior, biased toward the 3' end (to enhance information collection from samples using poly-A extraction methods) and avoiding palindromes *(1)*. Additionally, each 25-mer oligonucleotide probe has a reference probe constructed adjacent to it, with the central nucleotide containing a single-base mismatch. This *perfect match/mismatch* design permits an accounting for possible cross-hybridization and controls for nonspecific binding and location-dependent hybridization differences. Target RNAs are determined to be present if the hybridization intensities of the perfect match probes are significantly above the background level after subtraction of the mismatch hybridization level.

Affymetrix microarrays have several advantages, and cDNA microarrays also have their desirable features (**Table 1**). Affymetrix arrays have a com-

Table 1
Strengths of Oligonucleotide and Spotted cDNA Microarrays

Strength	Explanation
Oligonucleotide microarray	
Cartridge system	Protects, consistent reaction volumes, ease of use
Small feature size	Large number of transcripts assayed per experiment
Designer probes	Uniform hybridization behavior and the ability to distinguish closely realted sequences increases quantitative ability
Both pyrimidines used for labeling	Prevent detection error owing to sequence-dependent labeling differences from use of only one of the four nucleotides
cDNA mircoarray	
EST exploration	Ability to measure transcription of larger number of unassigned ESTs
Cost	Inexpensive as compared with Affymatrix oligonucleotide micoarray platform
Flexibility	Ability to create custom arrays easily
Direct labeling technique	Creates linear signal detection, ensuring linear abundance measurement

Abbreviation: EST, expressed sequence tag.

paratively smaller feature size, permitting the assaying of larger numbers of transcripts in a single experiment. The advantages of designer probe sequences, outlined above, allow uniform hybridization behavior and the ability to distinguish closely related sequences, thereby enriching transcript quantitation. Additionally, the enclosure of the Affymetrix microarray has allowed not only a fixed reagent volume and sample retrieval while preventing user-imposed damage, but also the automated and controlled washing and staining critical for assay reproducibility. **Table 1** outlines a comparison of some of the advantages of oligonucleotide and spotted cDNA microarrays.

Our laboratories have been using the Affymetrix platform to study gene expression patterns for coxsackievirus B3 (CVB3)-induced myocarditis. The coxsackievirus B group is the serogroup ranked number one in the causation of clinically important myocardial diseases *(11)*; thus, CVB3 infection of the myocardium is of significance in relation to the societal burden of cardiovascular disease *(12)* and in relation to understanding viral pathogenesis *(13–16)*. As a comparative assay to earlier microarray studies of murine CVB3 myocarditis carried out by our laboratory *(17)*, we have used Affymetrix GeneChips to study gene expression profiles during the viremic, inflammatory, and reparative stages of enteroviral infection. To focus on host–virus interactions outside of the complexity of the in vivo model, we also used GeneChips to examine the very early (30 min to 9 h post infection) transcriptional events that may influence overall pathogenesis in CVB3 infection in an in vitro model. Dissection of those events that are virus-induced and those that are host-protective is currently underway.

Important considerations need to be taken into account when one is profiling gene expression in rare cells within the intact heart. On a cellular basis, the mouse ventricles are comprised of approx 30% cardiac myocytes, 40% cardiac fibroblasts, 15% endothelial cells, 10% smooth muscle cells, and less than 5% combined hematopoietic cells, pericytes, progenitors, and other cell types (*18–21*). The ability to detect changes in gene expression among the rare cell types is limiting and may require digestion of the heart to single-cell suspension, followed by fluorescent or magnetic cell sorting and pooling of the purified cell phenotype. This approach may be necessary for adequate profiling for cells comprising less than 5% of the total cardiac cell number, except when one is looking for the highest expressed genes specific for that cell type. For instance, macrophages and dendritic cells account for less than 1% of the cell number of nonmanipulated hearts based on immunohistochemistry for macrophages and cell morphology. However, of the 13 cluster designations included on the Affymetrix mouse chip that recognize either cell type, only very weak CD86 signals can be detected in 7-wk-old male C57Bl6/J mice (Deisher et al., in review).

In initiating the Affymetrix protocol, total RNA is isolated from either cell or tissue preparations and used as a template for double-stranded cDNA creation by a linear reverse transcriptase-polymerase chain reaction (RT-PCR) reaction using poly-T primers containing a T7 RNA polymerase promoter sequence. The cDNA is then transcribed and labeled with biotin by in vitro transcription (IVT) using T7 RNA polymerase. The biotin-labeled cRNA transcripts are employed subsequently to hybridize DNA oligonucleotide sequences on the microarray surface. This method is advantageous for several reasons. First, total RNA can be used, as this procedure selectively amplifies the poly-A RNA, thereby enriching the poly-A portion of the sample. Second, both cDNA and IVT amplifications are linear, thus retaining relative transcript abundance ratios. Third, the transcription reaction uses biotinylated CTP and UTP, both RNA pyrimidine nucleotides, creating uniformly labeled resultant transcripts and thus eliminating potential experimental noise caused by the labeling variability of sequence differences that are inherent when one is using a single-labeled nucleotide. Last, the use of RNA rather than DNA target sequences for hybridization to the microarray-bound DNA probe sequences makes use of the RNA–DNA duplex, a more stable complex than the DNA–DNA duplex (*22*), consequently allowing increased hybridization stringency conditions. Following creation of biotin-labeled cRNA, it is fragmented into approximately 35–200 base-long fragments to permit physical/steric access of all portions of the transcript sequence to the 25-mer probes and the hybridized onto Affymetrix oligonucleotide arrays for expression analysis.

Methods follow the *Affymetrix GeneChip Expression Analysis Manual* (© April, 2003, Affymetrix, Inc.). The methods described in this chapter are based on the Affymetrix protocol, with important steps expanded and highlighted and useful procedural variations explained. Although the techniques are not in principle difficult, several important considerations must be explored, including input and maintenance of sample integrity and assurance of quality throughout. Emphasis must be given to issues of sample variability, potential chip variability and sensitivity, number of necessary replicates, experiment thresholds, experiment controls, and particular biological questions to be answered. The limitations, advantages, and rapid evolution of data mining strategies must also be understood, even though such matters are largely beyond the scope of this chapter. With the vast amount of information generated by these experiments, there is little room in the already unwieldy microarray analysis paradigms for more noise introduced by poor sample quality or human error *(23)*.

2. Materials

2.1. Sample Preparation

1. 5 U/mL Heparin in phosphate-buffered saline (PBS; Gibco-BRL).
2. 1 L Cardioplegia solution: 4 g NaCl, 1 g NaHCO₃, 2 g glucose, 3 g 2,3-butanedione monoxime, 3.8 g EGTA, 0.0002 g nifedipine, 10.0 mL Heparin (10,000 U/L), 3.73 g KCl. Adjust pH to 7.2–7.5 with NaOH.

2.2. Sample Homogenization

1. RLT buffer, available in the commercial RNeasy® Mini kit (Qiagen, Valencia, CA).
2. Polytron homogenizer (Brinkmann/Kinematica model PT3100) with 7-mm easy care foam reducing generator with saw teeth (Brinkmann model PT-Da3007/2EC) (*see* **Note 1**).
3. QIAshredder spin column and 2-mL collection tube available in the commercial RNeasy Mini kit.

2.3. RNA Extraction, Quantification, and Optional Precipitation

1. RNeasy Mini kit buffer RLT solution: add 10.0 μL β-mercaptoethanol (β-ME; *see* **Note 2**) for every 1.0 mL RLT buffer\.
2. RNeasy Mini kit buffer RPE solution: add 4 vol of ethanol (96–100%).
3. 96–100% Ethanol.
4. RNase-free water.
5. Sterile RNase-free pipet tips.

6. 3 *M* sodium acetate, pH 5.2.
7. Clones pglbs-lys, pglbs-phe, pglbs-thr, pglbs-trp, and pglbs-dap (American Type Culture Collection [ATCC], Manassas, VA) containing poly-A recombinant plasmids (*see* **Note 3**).

2.4. cDNA Creation

1. High-performance liquid chromatography (HPLC)-purified T7-(dT)$_{24}$ primer (*see* **Note 4**).
2. SSII Reverse transcriptase (200 U/µL; Gibco-BRL/Life Technologies, Burlington, ON; order comes with 5X first-strand cDNA buffer and 0.1 *M* dithiothreitol [DTT]).
3. 10 m*M* dNTP mix, 5X second-strand buffer, 10 U/µL *E. coli* DNA ligase, 10 U/ µL DNA polymerase I, 2 U/µL RNase H, and 10 U/µL T4 DNA polymerase (Gibco-BRL/Life Technologies).
4. 0.5 *M* EDTA disodium salt in diethyl pyrocarbonate (DEPC)-treated H$_2$O.
5. 7.5 *M* Ammonium acetate.
6. 96–100% Ethanol.
7. QIAquick PCR purification kit (QIAGEN Inc).

2.5. In Vitro Transcription

1. Enzo BioArray™ HighYield™ RNA Transcript Labeling Kit (Enzo Life Sciences, Farmingdale, NY).
2. RNeasy Mini kit (Qiagen).
3. 7.5 *M* Ammonium acetate.
4. 96–100% Ethanol.

2.6. Fragmentation

1. 20.0 mL 5X Fragmentation buffer: 4.0 mL Trizma base (Sigma , St. Louis, MO; 1 *M*) adjusted to pH 8.1 with glacial acetic acid, 0.64 g magnesium acetate, 0.98 g potassium acetate.

2.7. Hybridization

1. 1 L 12X MES stock: 1.22 *M* MES, 0.89 *M* [Na^{2+}], 70.4 g MES-free acid monohydrate.
2. GeneChip Eukaryotic Hybridization Control Kit (Affymetrix, Santa Clara, CA) for staggered control of cRNA stock of hybridization controls bioB, bioC, bioD, and Cre (*see* **Note 5**).
3. Acetylated bovine serum albumin (BSA) solution (50 mg/mL).
4. Herring sperm DNA.
5. Control Oligo B2 (Affymetrix).
6. 5 *M* NaCl (RNase-free, DNase-free).
7. MES-free acid monohydrate SigmaUltra (Sigma).
8. MES sodium salt.
9. 0.5 M EDTA disodium salt.
10. GeneChip Hybridization oven, GeneChip Test2 Array, and GeneChip array

(Affymetrix).

2.8. Washing, Staining, and Scanning

1. 50 mg/mL Acetylated BSA solution.
2. R-phycoerythrin streptavidin (Cedar Lane Laboratories, Eugene, OR).
3. 5 *M* NaCl (RNase-free, DNase-free).
4. PBS (Gibco-BRL), pH 7.2.
5. 20X SSPE.
6. Goat IgG, reagent grade (Sigma).
7. Antistreptavidin antibody, biotinylated (Vector, Burlingame, CA).
8. Antifoam 0-30 (Sigma).
9. 10% Tween-20 (Pierce Chemical, Rockford, IL).

3. Methods

The methods outlined below describe (1) the preparation of sample from heart tissue; (2) the homogenization of sample materials; (3) the extraction of RNA; (4) the creation of cDNA; (5) in vitro transcription and (6) fragmentation of cRNA; (7) hybridization; (8) washing, staining, and scanning of probe arrays; and (9) data analysis.

3.1. Sample Preparation

1. Complete *in situ* flushing of blood cells is critical in order to observe gene expression changes in cardiac resident or infiltrating hematopoietic cells, as well as to be able to detect cytokine expression from cardiac myocytes or fibroblasts.
2. Approximately 30 min prior to in situ flushing, the animal should be pre-heparinized using 30–50 U heparin ip per 25 g body weight.
3. Subsequently, snip the abdominal aorta and vena cava, and flush at physiological pressures with three times the blood volume using heparinized PBS via the thoracic vena cava, followed by three times the blood volume, at physiological pressure, of a cardioplegia solution retrograde via the thoracic aorta.
4. Without adequate retrograde aortic flushing, as much as 1/16th of the normal blood volume could contaminate the heart. In such a preparation, circulating white blood cells could account for up to 10% of the total cardiac cell number.

3.2. Sample Homogenization

3.2.1. Homogenization of Cardiac Tissue

The amount of starting sample recommended by Qiagen for total RNA extraction using the RNeasy Mini kit (*see* **Note 6**) of animal tissue is 30 mg (*see* **Note 7**).

1. Add 300 µL RLT buffer to 5-mL sterile, polypropylene tubes for use as a lysis buffer.
2. Take tissue sample from dry ice, and add directly into lysis buffer.
3. Homogenize tissue immediately using a Brinkmann homogenizer until sample is

homogeneous, typically for 30–50 s (*see* **Notes 8** and **9**).

3.2.2. Homogenization of Cardiac Cells From Tissue Culture

The amount of starting sample recommended by Qiagen for total RNA extraction using the RNeasy Mini kit (*see* **Note 6**) of animal cells is 1×10^7 cells.
1. Add 300 μL RLT buffer to the cell sample.
2. Load (up to 700 μL) onto a QIAshredder spin column in a 2-mL collection tube.
3. Spin for 2 min at maximum speed in a microcentrifuge and collect the homogenized lysate.

3.3. RNA Extraction, Quantification, and Optional Precipitation

3.3.1. RNA Extraction From Cardiac Tissue

Heat water bath or heating block to 55°C for proteinase K digestion. Follow the manufacturer's modified protocol for the commercial RNeasy Mini kit for extraction of total RNA from lysate (*see* **Notes 10–12**).

3.3.2. RNA Extraction From Cardiac Tissue Culture

Follow the manufacturer's protocol for the commercial RNeasy Mini kit for extraction of total RNA from lysate. Preparation of RNA processing controls is optional. Clones containing poly-A recombinant plasmids are processed to create bacterial poly-A controls for RNA processing using the technique outlined in the *Affymetrix GeneChip® Expression Analysis Manual* (*see* **Note 3**). Once created, a 2X spike cocktail is made with staggered concentrations of individual poly-A controls (*see* **Note 13**).

3.3.3. RNA Quantification

Quantify RNA yield using a standard spectrophotometric technique (*see* **Note 14**).

3.3.4. RNA Precipitation

Although precipitation is not necessary if elution volumes and extraction yields produce at least 0.45 μg/μL (*see* **Note 15**), if the concentration of the RNA sample falls below this, precipitation is necessary to concentrate the total RNA sample (*see* **Note 16**). Follow the *Affymetrix GeneChip® Expression Analysis Manual* for total RNA precipitation (*see* **Note 17**). Resuspend the pellet in DEPC-treated H_2O (*see* **Note 18**).

3.3.5. Optional

Add a 2X cocktail containing poly-A RNA processing controls following the Affymetrix supplemental protocol (*see* **Note 19**).

Table 2
First-Strand cDNA Synthesis Reaction Amounts
of RNA and SSII Reverse Transcriptase

Total RNA (μg)	SSII reverse transcriptase (Z variable; μL)
5.0–8.0	1.0
8.1–16.0	2.0
16.1–24.0	3.0
24.1–32.0	4.0
32.1–40.0	5.0

Table 3
First-Strand cDNA Synthesis Reaction Contents

Reagents	Volume (μL)
RNA	X (variable; volume of total RNA) + (optional fixed amount 2X poly-A spike; *see* **Note 19**)
DEPC-treated water	Y (variabe; add to make up to final reaction volume of 20 μL)
T7-(dT)$_{24}$ primer (100pmol/μL)	1
5X first-strand cDNA buffer	4
0.1 M DTT	2
10 mM dNTP mix	1
SSII reverse transcriptase (200 U/μL)	Z (variable; volume of enzyme corresponding in **Table 2** to amount of RNA added with addition of RNA volume [X])
Total volume	20 μL

3.4. cDNA Creation

1. Determine amount of starting RNA (*see* **Note 20**).
2. Calculate volumes for first-strand reaction of total RNA and reverse transcriptase based on the sample volume containing the amount of starting RNA given in **Table 2**.
3. Determine the amounts of DEPC-treated H$_2$O based on volumes from **Table 2** added to the reagents in **Table 3** for first-strand cDNA synthesis; total volume should be 20 μL.

Table 4
cDNA Amounts for In Vitro Transcription (IVT)

Total RNA (μg)	Volume of cDNA to use in IVT (assuming 12 μL resuspension vol for DNA)
5.0–8.0	10
8.1–16.0	5
16.1–24.0	3.3
24.1–32.0	2.5
32.1–40.0	2

4. Follow the *Affymetrix GeneChip® Expression Analysis Manual* for first- and second-strand cDNA synthesis (*see* **Note 21**).
5. Once the first and second strands are created, clean up the cDNA sample using a commercial QIAquick kit following the manufacturer's protocol.
6. Precipitate the cDNA sample following the *Affymetrix GeneChip® Expression Analysis Manual* for cDNA precipitation.
7. Resuspend pellet in 12 μL RNase-free water.

3.5. In Vitro Transcription

1. Calculate the volume of cDNA for the IVT reaction based on **Table 4**.
2. Follow the manufacturer's protocol for the Enzo BioArray HighYield RNA Transcript Labeling Kit for creation of biotin-labeled cRNA.
3. Once biotin–cRNA has been created, purify the sample using the commercial RNeasy Mini kit for RNA extraction following the manufacturer's protocol (*see* **Note 22**).
4. Quantify the sample using a standard spectrophotometric technique (*see* **Notes 15**, **23**, and **24**).
5. If the biotin-cRNA sample concentration is less than 0.6 μg/μL, precipitate the sample, and resuspend in 10–20 μL RNase-free water. Follow the *Affymetrix GeneChip® Expression Analysis Manual* for biotin–cRNA precipitation (*see* **Note 25**).

3.6. Fragmentation

1. Follow the Affymetrix GeneChip® Expression Analysis Manual for creation of 5X fragmentation buffer and fragmentation of biotin–cRNA (*see* **Notes 26** and **27**).
2. Aliquot at least 1 μg of the product (required for ethidium bromide visualization) for fragmentation quality assurance by agarose gel electrophoresis.
3. RNA fragment sizes should be 35–200 bases. Store fragmented biotin-cRNA at –20°C until hybridization.

3.7. Hybridization

Create a hybridization cocktail according to the *Affymetrix GeneChip®
Expression Analysis Manual* based on array size. Follow the *Manual* for
hybridization of samples on Test2 and GeneChip arrays.

3.8. Washing, Staining, and Scanning Probe Arrays

Follow the *Manual* for washing, staining, and scanning Test2 and GeneChip
arrays (*see* **Notes 28** and **29**).

3.9. Analysis

3.9.1. Image Scanning

Scanning yields an image of the array (.dat file; traditionally occupying 70
Mb of storage space) in the "tiff" file format on which Affymetrix software
overlays a grid for feature identity and location (.cel file; approximately 10 Mb
of storage space). This information is then processed via the GeneChip software into a numerical format called a .chp file, a tab-delimited text file occupying approx 10 Mb of storage space. It is the .chp file that can be used by many
different analysis software packages for analysis and interpretation.

3.9.2. Data Transfer

After data are generated from the microarray scan, they are transferred to
the first of two relational databases that reside on the Affymetrix Laboratory
Information Management System (LIMS) server. Data are initially passed
through the "process" database and from there published to the GATC™
(Affymetrix; *see* **Note 30**) database. The GATC schema is designed to absorb
the results from the .chp file analysis. After the data are published in a standard
GATC format, they can be exported to various sophisticated analysis applications, either offered by academic institutions or third-party vendors or developed internally by biotechnology/pharmaceutical companies.

3.9.3. Bioinformatical Analysis

There are generally two categories of bioinformatics/analysis software suite
applications, namely client–server and workstation-based. Client–server
applications are used for analysis of gene expression data at the high-throughput, mass-storage, enterprise level, usually with the intention of making results
available via the internet, for example, to external parties outside the in-house
network. These applications will usually incorporate their own unique relational databases that import data directly from the GATC database. Some
examples of these types of applications are Genomax® (Informax Data Systems, Los Angeles, CA) or Resolver® (Rosetta Biosoftware, Houston, TX). In

comparison, workstation-based tools will reside on a single workstation that is in direct linkage to the GATC database. These are usually used for smaller scale analysis of gene expression profiles. An example of this type of application is GeneSpring® (Silicon Genetics, Redwood City, CA).

4. Notes

1. A 7-mm generator is appropriate for volumes up to 300 µL and can be used for homogenization in microcentrifuge tubes.
2. The β-ME/RLT buffer is stable for 1 mo.
3. It is recommended that the poly-A controls dap, thr, trp, phe, and lys, genes from *Bacillus subtilis* be spiked into the total RNA prior to cDNA creation for processing controls. Sense strand poly-A RNAs are prepared from the linearized recombinant plasmids derived from the ATCC clones and are mixed together in staggered concentrations. The mix can be spiked into samples prior to cDNA creation for use as RNA processing controls. The linearized plasmids are prepared using the commercially available *Not*I restriction endonuclease and T3 RNA polymerase (Gibco-BRL/Life Technologies).
4. 5'-GGCCAGTGAATTGTAATACGACTCACTATAGGGAGGCGG-(dT)$_{24}$-3'; it is highly recommended that this primer be HPLC-purified.
5. Hybridization controls are created from commercially available clones for bioB, bioC, and bioD, from the *E. coli* biotin synthesis pathway, and Cre, from the P1 bacteriophage recombinase gene. These are spiked into the hybridization cocktail.
6. The maximum amount of starting material is limited by the binding capacity of the RNeasy Mini spin column (100 µg of RNA) rather than by weight and/or count of cells. Yield of total RNA depends not only on the amount and quality of starting material but also on the degree of disruption and homogenization of tissue/cells as well. If column binding capacity is exceeded, yields will not be consistent, and less than 100 µg may be recovered. The quoted amounts, however, may be insufficient for heart samples as they are difficult to homogenize because of their fibrous nature. If the yield of total RNA from heart tissue is lower than expected, the modified protocol including proteinase K digestion can be used. *See* **Note 13** for the modified protocol. Our recommendation for heart samples is to use 40–50 µg of healthy tissue and more if the sample is fatty or fibrous. Note that fatty samples do not appear to work well with the RNeasy column format and should probably be extracted using a different technique, e.g., Trizol extraction.
7. A 3-mm cube (27 mm^3) of most animal tissues weighs 30–35 mg *(9)*.
8. Keep foaming to a minimum using a foam-reducing generator and an appropriate sized tube and by keeping the tip of the homogenizer submerged and against one side of the tube.
9. Technique and degree of homogenization of tissue is critical for yield and quality of isolated total RNA. A piece of tissue must be kept frozen (kept on dry ice) until just prior to transfer into lysis buffer. The process of homogenization can be improved by fractionating tissue into smaller pieces. Start with low rpm for first 15–20 s, while gently moving the probe up and down within the solution to pre-

vent foaming. Bring the rpm gradually up to maximum, and hold for 5 s. The whole cycle should not exceed 40–45 s. Stop the generator, let the sample cool for a few seconds in an ice-water bath and repeat the cycle two to three times depending on the success of the homogenization. For successive cycles, bring the rpm up to maximum gradually and more quickly than the first cycle (assuming no large chunks of tissue remain) and hold for 10–15 s.

10. After homogenization is complete, all steps should be carried out at room temperature.

11. Advice for increased yield: (1) pass the sample over the column twice before the wash and elution steps, (2) wait 1 min before centrifugation after adding water to the column for elution, and (3) use the Qiagen-modified RNeasy protocol that includes the proteinase K digestion step (*see* **Note 13**).

12. The RNeasy modified protocol is designed by Qiagen for isolation of total RNA from heart, muscle, and skin tissue and includes a proteinase K digestion step. Request the modified protocol from Qiagen. Generally, DNase I treatment is not necessary since RNeasy technology removes most of the DNA from the samples. Therefore, it is questionable whether DNase I treatment is beneficial for the Affymetrix application. Affymetrix does not recommend DNase treatment owing to possible DNase contamination of the sample and possible downstream effects on further sample processing.

13. Request a supplemental protocol for the preparation of the 2X poly-A mix from Affymetrix.

14. 1 OD at 260 nm equals 40.0 µg RNA per ml.

15. To use the poly-A controls, we recommend that the threshold concentration of total RNA be a minimum of 1.0 µg/µL.

16. This ensures that enough total RNA (at least 5.0 µg) is added to the first-strand cDNA creation reaction without exceeding the 20.0 µL fixed reaction volume (**Tables 2** and **3**). We recommend using 30.0 µL for sample elution to prevent the need for sample precipitation. All precipitations cause some sample loss, thus introducing additional experimental noise/error in quantifying the "real" cellular transcriptional profile.

17. Addition of 0.5–1.0 µL of (5.0 mg/mL) glycogen to RNA precipitations is recommended for increased visualization and recovery of the pellet. Ensure dryness of the pellet before proceeding.

18. The H_2O volume should be determined based on projected resulting RNA concentration above 0.45 µg/µL (*see* **Note 15**).

19. We recommend the addition of 5.0 µL of 2X poly-A control cocktail for detection of control transcripts spiked into the sample at low concentration.

20. We recommend starting with 5.0–40.0 µg total RNA.

21. Sample can be stored at –20°C after the addition of 10 µL 0.5 *M* EDTA.

22. We recommend using 30.0 µL for sample elution to prevent the need for sample precipitation. All precipitations cause some sample loss, thus introducing additional experimental noise/error in quantifying the "real" cellular transcriptional profile.

23. Adjusted cRNA yield should be calculated to reflect the carryover of unlabeled total RNA (estimated to be 100%) using the formula:

$$\text{adjusted cRNA yield} = \text{RNA}_m - (\text{total RNA}_i)(y)$$

where RNAm = amount of cRNA measured (μg), RNAi = amount of total RNA starting (μg), and y = fraction of cDNA reaction used in IVT.

24. The cRNA sample can be checked by gel electrophoresis to estimate yield and size partitioning. Analyze 1% of each sample by 1% agarose gel electrophoresis. Use ethidium bromide for visualization. For a more accurate estimation of RNA size distribution, run a denaturing gel.

25. The precipitated sample can be stored at –20°C overnight.

26. Use unadjusted yield for cRNA concentration contributing to fragmentation mix. cRNA must be at a minimum concentration of 0.6 μg/μL to minimize the amount of magnesium in the final hybridization cocktail. The final concentration of cRNA in fragmentation mix should be between 0.5 and 2.0 μg/μL.

27. It is critical to incubate at exactly 94°C for exactly 35 min for optimal fragmentation.

28. We recommend priming the Fluidics Station twice prior to washing and enacting the "shut-down" protocol twice after use to prevent fluid errors with the Affymetrix Fluidics Station.

29. We recommend assaying sample quality using the Test2 array (Affymetrix) prior to sample hybridization on the larger expression array. Analysis of this Test2 array is as follows:
    a. Check the presence and relative abundance of bacterial poly-A controls (Dap, Phe, Thr, Lys, and Trp) if used.
    b. Check the presence of stock cRNA hybridization controls (added with the Eukaryotic Hybridization kit = BioB, BioC, BioD, and Cre).
    c. Check the absence of bacterial poly-A controls not spiked into the cDNA creation reaction.
    d. Check the presence of human transcripts GAPDH, HSAC07, and TFRR. The TFRR transcript will be in low abundance; therefore detection of this transcript indicates high quality in the starting sample with retention of that quality throughout sample processing.
    e. Each of the sets of transcripts outlined above has a 5', 3', and M component, indicating abundance measurement at the 3', middle, and 5' end of the transcript. For a single-transcript measurement, all three should be relatively equivalent, with normal variability approx 20% between the 3' and 5' ends. Unequal intensities across these three measurements indicate problems owing to sample degradation or faulty labeling reaction.
    f. Check percentage of total cells present. This number should be at least 45%. Less indicates poor sample quality or labeling.

30. Genetic Analysis Technology Consortium (Affymetrix) *(1)*.

Acknowledgments

The authors would like to thank the Canadian Institutes of Health Research (B.M.M., D.Y., and B.Y.), the Heart and Stroke Foundation (HSF) of Canada

(B.Y.), the HSF of British Columbia and Yukon (B.M.M. and D.Y.), the Michael Smith Foundation for Health Research (B.Y.), the Natural Sciences and Engineering Research Council of Canada (R.N.), and the Network of Centres of Excellence (R.N.) for funding support.

References

1. Warrington, J. A., Dee, S., and Trulson, M. (2000) Large scale genomic analysis using Affymetrix GeneChip probe arrays, in *Microarray Biochip Technology* (Schena, M., ed.), Eaton, Natick, MA, pp. 119–148.
2. Lockhart, D. J. and Winzeler, E. A. (2000) Genomics, gene expression and DNA arrays. *Nature* **405,** 827–836.
3. Ly, D. H., Lockhart, D. J., Lerner, R. A., and Schultz, P. G. (2000) Mitotic misregulation and human aging. *Science* **287,** 2486–2492.
4. Dobson, J. G. Jr, Fray, J., Leonard, J. L., and Pratt, R. E. (2003) Molecular mechanisms of reduced beta-adrenergic signaling in the aged heart as revealed by genomic profiling. *Physiol. Genomics*. **15,** 142–147.
5. Gariboldi, M., Peissel, B., Fabbri, A., et al. (2003) SCCA2-like serpins mediate genetic predisposition to skin tumors. *Cancer. Res.* **63,** 1871–1875.
6. Warrington, J. A., Nair, A., Mahadevappa, M., and Tsyganskaya, M. (2000) Comparison of human adult and fetal expression and identification of 535 housekeeping/maintenance genes. *Physiol. Genomics*. **2,** 143–147.
7. Teague, T. K., Hildeman, D., Kedl, R. M., et al. (1999) Activation changes the spectrum but not the diversity of genes expressed by T cells. *Proc. Natl. Acad. Sci. USA* **96,** 12,691–12,696.
8. Fodor, S. P., Rava, R. P., Huang, X. C., Pease, A. C., Holmes, C. P., and Adams, C. L. (1993) Multiplexed biochemical assays with biological chips. *Nature* **364,** 555–556.
9. Fodor, S. P., Read, J. L., Pirrung, M. C., Stryer, L., Lu, A. T., and Solas, D. (1991) Light-directed, spatially addressable parallel chemical synthesis. *Science* **251,** 767–773.
10. Lockhart, D. J., Dong, H., Byrne, M. C., et al. (1996) Expression monitoring by hybridization to high-density oligonucleotide arrays. *Nat. Biotechnol.* **14,** 1675–1680.
11. Grist, N. R. and Reid, D. (1993) Epidemiology of viral infections of the heart, in *Viral Infections in the Heart*. (Banatvala, J.E., ed.), Edward Arnold, London, UK, pp. 23–30.
12. Saliba, S. J. (2000) Prevention of coronary artery disease. *Prim. Care*. **27,** 525–540.
13. Luo, H., Yanagawa, B., Zhang, J., et al. (2002) Coxsackievirus B3 replication is reduced by inhibition of the extracellular signal-regulated kinase (ERK) signaling pathway. *J. Virol.* **76,** 3365–3373.
14. Yang, D., Yu, J., Luo, Z., Carthy, C. M., Wilson, J. E., Liu, Z., and McManus, B. M. (1999) Viral myocarditis: Identification of five differentially expressed genes in coxsackievirus B3-infected mouse heart. *Circ. Res.* **84,** 704–712.

15. Zhang, H. M., Yanagawa, B., Cheung, P., et al. (2002) Nip21 gene expression reduces coxsackievirus B3 replication by promoting apoptotic cell death via a mitochondria-dependent pathway. *Circ. Res.* **90,** 1251–1258.

16. Zhang, H. M., Yuan, J., Cheung, P., et al. (2003) Overexpression of interferon-gamma-inducible GTPase inhibits coxsackievirus B3-induced apoptosis through the activation of the phosphatidylinositol 3-kinase/Akt pathway and inhibition of viral replication. *J. Biol. Chem.* **278,** 33,011–33,019.

17. Taylor, L. A., Carthy, C. M., Yang, D., et al. (2000) Host gene regulation during coxsackievirus B3 infection in mice: Assessment by microarrays. *Circ. Res.* **87,** 328–334.

18. Zhang, J., Yu, Z. X., Fujita, S., Yamaguchi, M. L., and Ferrans, V. J. (1993) Interstitial dendritic cells of the rat heart. Quantitative and ultrastructural changes in experimental myocardial infarction. *Circulation* **87,** 909–920.

19. Spencer, S. C. and Fabre, J. W. (1990) Characterization of the tissue macrophage and the interstitial dendritic cell as distinct leukocytes normally resident in the connective tissue of rat heart. *J. Exp. Med.* **171,** 1841–1851.

20. Holzinger, C., Zuckermann, A., Reinwald, C., et al. (1996) Are T cells from healthy heart really only passengers? Characterization of cardiac tissue T cells. *Immunol. Lett.* **53,** 63–67.

21. Reiss, K., Cheng, W., Ferber, A., et al. (1996) Overexpression of insulin-like growth factor-1 in the heart is coupled with myocyte proliferation in transgenic mice. *Proc. Natl. Acad. Sci. USA* **93,** 8630–8635.

22. Inoue, H., Hayase, Y., Imura, A., Iwai, S., Miura, K., and Ohtsuka, E. (1987) Synthesis and hybridization studies on two complementary nona(2'-O-methyl)ribonucleotides. *Nucleic Acids Res.* **15,** 6131–6148.

23. Schena, M. and Davis, R. W. (2000) Technology standards for microarray research, in *Microarray Biochip Technology* (Schena, M., ed.), Eaton, Natick, MA, pp. 1–18.

21

Identification and Validation of Loci and Candidate Genes Linked to Cardiac Hypertrophy

Bastien Llamas and Christian F. Deschepper

Summary

Left ventricular hypertrophy (LVH) is a complex quantitative trait that has a strong prognostic value for cardiovascular mortality and morbidity. Cardiac mass is determined in part by the influence of genetic loci that are known as quantitative trait loci (QTLs), the localization of which can be performed experimentally in genetic animal crosses. The present chapter outlines standard procedures for the selection of appropriate animal strains, for assessment of mode of inheritance, for characterizing the cardiac phenotype, for performing whole-genome scans, and for conducting linkage analyses. Identification of QTLs may lead to the identification of candidate genes whose roles can be further investigated in either transgenic, knockout, or pharmacologically manipulated animal models.

Key Words: Left ventricular hypertrophy; cardiomyocyte; complex trait; quantitative trait locus; inbred mouse strains; inbred rat strains; animal genetic crosses; recombinant inbred strains; recombinant congenic strains; simple sequence length polymorphism; linkage mapping; congenic animals; candidate gene.

1. Introduction

Complex traits (also called quantitative traits) can be defined as phenotypic traits that (unlike mendelian traits) are not linked by a simple one-to-one relationship to variants of one particular gene *(1)*. These traits are characterized by measurable phenotypic variations owing to the combined effects of genetic and environmental influences, the combination of which makes it impossible to predict *a priori* the magnitude or importance of the trait *(2)*. Identification of

From: *Methods in Molecular Medicine, vol. 112: Molecular Cardiology: Methods and Protocols*
Edited by: Z. Sun © Humana Press Inc., Totowa, NJ

gene mutations linked to mendelian traits may be a long and challenging process, but the most limiting factor is the availability of informative pedigrees. Once these have been obtained, identification of the locus is highly feasible, as illustrated by the fact that the links between human syndromes and gene mutations have been established in seveal hundreds of examples *(3)*. In contrast, many cardiovascular traits (including susceptibility to cardiovascular diseases) can be defined as complex traits, so that progress in the identification of genes linked to such traits has been lagging. Nonetheless, there has been in recent years an acceleration in the identification of genes linked to complex traits, in part thanks to the availability of new research tools *(4,5)*.

A locus linked to a complex trait is called a quantitative trait locus (QTL). Since finding a QTL in humans remains a difficult task, a viable alternative is first to map QTLs in animal models with quantitative traits differences and then to use this information to identify candidate genes. The successive steps of this strategy have been outlined in **Fig. 1**. This chapter focuses on how QTL mapping strategies can be used to find QTLs linked to cardiac ventricular mass. In both humans and animals, the latter trait is highly variable, and its variance has been shown to be determined to a large extent by heritable factors *(6,7)*. It is also a trait of clinical significance, because chronic left ventricular hypertrophy (LVH) constitutes one of the most powerful independent risk factors for cardiovascular morbidity and mortality *(8,9)*, and is associated with the development of arrhythmias, heart failure and cardiac sudden death *(10)*.

2. Materials

1. Inbred animal strains (*see* **Subheading 3.1.** and **Note 1**).
2. Progeny of crosses between inbred strains (*see* **Subheading 3.2.** and **Notes 2** and **3**).
3. Top-load balance.
4. Micrometer caliper.
5. DNeasy Tissue extraction kit (Qiagen, Valencia, CA), containing spin columns, 2-mL collection tubes, buffer ATL, a proteinase K solution (20 mg/mL), buffer AL, buffer AW1, and buffer AW2.
6. RNase A solution (100 mg/mL H_2O).
7. 96–100% Ethanol.
8. Microcentrifuge tubes.
9. DNA elution buffer: 10 mM Tris-HCl, pH 8.0, 0.01 mM EDTA.
10. Spectrophotometer.
11. 6.6 µM Unlabeled M13 primer (5'-CACGACGTTGTAAAACGAC-3'), in DNA elution buffer (for analysis of polymerase chain reaction [PCR] products on manual sequencing gels).
12. 3000 Ci/mmole [γ-^{32}P]ATP (Amersham Biosciences, Piscataway, NJ).
13. T4 polynucleotide kinase (10 U/µL) and accompanying 5X stock forward buffer: 350 mM Tris-HCl, pH 7.6, 500 mM KCl, 50 mM $MgCl_2$, 5 mM 2-mercaptoethanol.

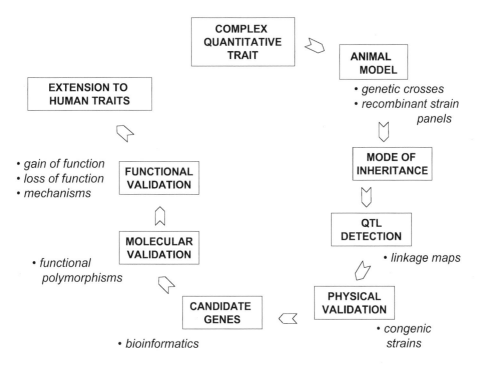

Fig. 1. Diagram of steps required for identification and validation of a quantitative trait locus (QTL) in animal models. Some of the tools and/or techniques required at each step are indicated in italics.

14. SpeedVac lyophylizer.
15. 6.6 μ*M* M13 primer custom-labeled (in the 5' position) with a fluorochrome dye, in DNA elution buffer (for analysis of PCR products with an automated sequencing apparatus).
16. 0.66 μ*M* Forward primer with a 5' M13 tail, in DNA elution buffer.
17. 6.6 μ*M* Reverse primer in DNA elution buffer.
18. dNTP mix: 25 m*M* dATP, 25 m*M* dCTP, 25 m*M* dGTP, 25 m*M* dTTP, in H_2O.
19. 5 U/μL Taq polymerase.
20. 10X PCR buffer: 0.5 *M* KCl, 0.1 *M* Tris-HCl, pH 8.3, 15 m*M* $MgCl_2$, 1 mg/mL gelatin.
21. PCR thermal cycler.
22. DNA sequencing equipment.
23. Personal computer and linkage analysis software (*see* **Subheading 3.7.** and **Note 4**).

3. Methods
3.1. Selection of Parental Strains

Parental inbred strains constitute the starting point for any animal genetic study (*see* **Note 1**). The choice of parental strains should be guided by (1) the presence of quantitative differences for a trait of interest, and (2) the presence of abundant genetic polymorphisms between the two strains. The selection of such strains is greatly facilitated by the availability of several on-line databases. For rats, the main resource is the Rat Genome Database (http:// rgd.mcw.edu/), which makes an inventory of information concerning genetic polymorphisms and phenotypes and maintains up-to-date links to other sites. For mice, the Jackson Laboratories provide comprehensive information on mouse strains via the Mouse Genome Informatics website (http:// www.informatics.jax.org/) as well as the Mouse Phenome Database (http:// aretha.jax.org/pub-cgi/phenome/mpdcgi?rtn=docs/home). An exhaustive list of additional rodent resources is available on the National Institutes of Health website (http://www.nih.gov/science/models/).

3.2. Assessment of Mode of Inheritance in the Progeny of Crosses

When using the progeny of crosses between two parental strains, a phenotypic analysis of the trait of interest (*see* **Subheading 3.4.**) should be performed in the F1 progeny in order to assess the mode of inheritance of the trait of interest. Assuming that the value of a given trait is either low or high in parental strains P1 and P2, respectively, the trait will be either: (1) dominant/recessive (if its value in the F1 progeny is at the same time not statistically different compared with one of the parental strains and statistically different compared with the other parental strain), or (2) codominant (if its value is intermediary between that of the trait in parental strains P1 and P2). Likewise, reciprocal crosses (in which female P1 and male P2 animals are crossed, as well as male P1 and female P2 animals) should be performed to assess whether underlying genetic determinants are on autosomes or sexual chromosomes. If the QTL is on autosomes, the magnitude of a given trait will be similar in crosses performed with either male P1 animals (and female P2 animals) or with male P2 animals (and female P1 animals). If the QTL is on sexual chromosomes, the magnitude of the trait will be different in the F1 progeny according to whether the males used in the cross originated from strain P1 or P2.

3.3. Selection of a Genetic Cross

Genetic studies are performed on animals derived from crosses between parental inbred strains. One classical way of proceeding is to perform an experimental cross between two parental inbred strains, the type of cross being selected on the mode of inheritance of the trait (*see* **Note 2**). Alternative models include that of recombinant inbred (RI) strains and recombinant congenic (RC) panels (*see* **Note 3**). For rats, there is one RI panel that has been derived from an F2 cross between SHR and BN inbred strains *(11)*. This panel comprises 11 BXH (derived from crosses between female BN and male SHR) and 21 HXB strains (derived from the reciprocal cross) and constitutes the only available rat panel with at least 20 different strains. It has been used to elucidate some of the genetic determinants of LVH *(12)*, as well as for other cardiovascular traits (including arterial pressure, dyslipidemia, and glucose metabolism) *(13)*. For mice, several panels of RI mice are available from the Jackson Laboratories. These include 20 AKXD strains (derived from AKR and DBA/2 strains), 29 AXB/BXA strains (derived from A/J and C57Bl/6 strains), and 32 BXD strains (derived from reciprocal crosses between C57Bl/6 and DBA/2 strains). In addition, two informative panels of RC mice strains have been developed. One is composed of 20 CcS (derived from BALB/cHeA and STS/A strains) *(14)*. The other one comprises 37 AcB/BcA (derived from reciprocal crosses between A/J and C57Bl/6 strains) *(15)*. Collectively, these various panels have been used so far for finding QTLs linked to diabetes, susceptibility to cancer and/or infectious agents, and behavioral traits but have not been exploited much for cardiovascular traits. Nonetheless, it has recently been found that A/J and C57Bl6/J mice exhibit differences in LV mass and morphology *(16)* as well as in cardiomyocyte morphology (Llamas and Deschepper, unpublished data). It might therefore be expected that the AXB/BXA RI panel will be useful for finding QTLs linked to LV mass or related traits.

3.4. Phenotypic Characterization

Phenotyping is an important part of a QTL search, and several principles should guide which particular phenotypic measurement should be made (*see* **Note 5**). The present section describes how to measure corrected mass index, arguably the most commonly used phenotype for quantification of cardiac mass (*see* **Note 6**). However, other measurements that should be performed include that of cardiomyocyte morphology (*see* **Note 7**).

1. Weigh the animal to obtain whole body weight.
2. After killing the animal, open the chest and dissect the heart out.
3. With dissection scissors, remove the atria, separate the free wall of the right ventricle (RV) from the LV (which comprises a block of tissue that contains both the septal and the free walls).
4. Dissect out the tibia, and air-dry.
5. Weigh each ventricular sample on a top-load balance.
6. Measure dry tibia length from the tip of the condyles to the tip of the medial malleolus with a micrometer caliper.
7. Divide the weight of each ventricular sample by either BW or by tibia length (*see* **Note 6**).

3.5. Isolation of Genomic DNA

Several considerations should guide the choice of tissue and the type of extraction procedure (*see* **Note 8**). The following protocol describes a standard procedure for isolation of DNA from spleen.

1. Collect the spleen from the animal, snap-freeze the tissue, and powder the tissue with a mortar and pestle under liquid nitrogen.
2. Transfer approx 10 mg of powdered spleen in a chilled microtube.
3. Add 180 μL of ATL buffer and 20 μL of proteinase K solution to the tube, vortex, and incubate at 55°C until complete lysis of the tissue (4–16 h).
4. Add 4 μL of RNase A solution, vortex and incubate for 2 min at room temperature.
5. Vortex for 15 s, add 200 μL of AL buffer, vortex again, and incubate at 70°C for 10 min.
6. Add 200 μL of ethanol, and vortex. A white precipitate should form.
7. Pipet the mixture into a DNeasy spin column, centrifuge for 1 min at 6000g, and discard the flowthrough and collection tube.
8. Place the DNeasy spin column in a new collection tube, add 500 μL of AW1 buffer, centrifuge for 1 min at 6000g, and discard the flowthrough and collection tube.
9. Repeat the same procedure with 500 μL of AW2 buffer, centrifuge for 3 min at full speed (22,000g), and discard flow-through and collection tube.
10. Place the DNeasy spin column in a clean microcentrifuge tube, pipet 100–200 μL of DNA elution buffer onto the membrane at the bottom of the column, incubate for 1 min at room temperature, and recover DNA by centrifugation for 1 min at 6000g.
11. Repeat **step 10** in a new clean microcentrifuge tube, and combine the second eluate with the first one.
12. Quantify DNA by absorbance at 260 nm.
13. Keep stock aliquots of DNA samples in their original concentration (as obtained after elution from the DNeasy columns) at –20°C.
14. Make aliquots of genomic DNA at working dilutions (20 ng/μL of DNA elution buffer).

3.6. Genotyping Procedures

The most common way of genotyping animals is to amplify genomic DNA by PCR, using primers known to flank simple sequence repetitive sequences. Since the length of such sequences is highly polymorphic between strains, their amplification will reveal simple sequence length polymorphisms (SSLPs). Our PCR amplification procedure uses labelled M13 primers (*see* **Note 9**). If the PCR products are to be analyzed manually with a sequencing polyacrylamide gel followed by autoradiography, the M13 primer should first be labeled with [^{32}P], as described below in **Subheading 3.6.2.** If the PCR products are to be analyzed with an automated sequencer, one should custom-order the M13 primer prelabeled in 5' with a fluorochome dye that is compatible with the detection system of the automated sequencer.

3.6.1. Selection of Primer Pairs

Information concerning the nucleotide sequence of primer pairs (along with information concerning the length of the amplified product in several inbred strains and the distribution of each marker on genetic and radiation hybrid maps) can be found in a variety of sites. For mice, the information is provided by the Mouse Genome Informatics website (http://www.informatics.jax.org/). For rats, comparable information can be found on the following websites: MIT (http:/www-genome.wi.mit.edu/rat/public), NIH/Arb (http://www.niams.nih. gov/rtbc/ratgbase/), Wellcome Trust (http://www.well.ox.ac.uk/rat mapping ressources/), Rat Genome Database (http://rgd.mcw.edu/), and RatMap (http:// ratmap.gen.gu.se/). The sequence information obtained on these various sites can be used to order primer pairs from any oligonucleotide provider. Of note, the amplification procedure described below incorporates a labeled M13 primer in the PCR amplification reaction (*see* **Note 9**). This requires the 5'-tailing of all forward primers (whose sequence is defined in the databases described above) with the M13 sequence 5'-CACGACGTTGTAAAACGAC-3' *(17)*.

3.6.2. [^{32}P]-Labeling of M13 Primer (in Case of Manual Sequencing Gels)

1. Add 8 µL of [γ-^{32}P]ATP in a clean microcentrifuge tube, and concentrate in a Speed-Vac lyophylizer (down to ~1 µL).
2. Resuspend concentrated radioisotope in 30 µL of unlabeled M13 primer solution.
3. Add 2 µL of T4 kinase, 8 µL of T4 forward buffer 5X stock, and 4 µL H$_2$O (final volume 46 µL).
4. Mix well, and incubate for 1 h at 37°C.
5. Denature for 10 min at 65°C.

3.6.3. PCR Amplification of Genomic DNA

1. Prepare a PCR/dNTP mix by combining 1 mL of dNTP mix, 10 mL of 10X PCR buffer, and 39 mL H$_2$O.
2. For PCR reactions to be analyzed by manual sequencing gels, prepare a 2X primer mix by combining 10 µL Taq polymerase, 30 µL M13 forward primer, 48 µL of reverse primer, 46 µL of [^{32}P]-labeled M13 primer (as described in **Subheading 3.6.2.**), and adjust up to 1 mL with PCR/dNTP mix. For PCR products to be analyzed by automated sequencing apparati, prepare a 2X primer mix by combining 10 µL Taq polymerase, 30 µL M13 forward primer, 48 µL reverse primer, 24 µL M13 primer custom-labeled with a fluorochrome dye in the 5' position, and adjust up to 1 mL with PCR/dNTP mix (*see* **Note 10**).
3. Add 20–100 ng of genomic DNA in 5 µL of DNA elution buffer in a clean microcentrifuge tube, and mix with 5 µL of 2X primer mix.

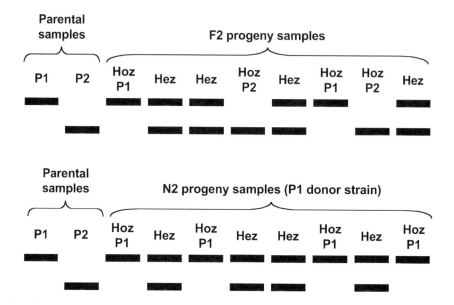

Fig. 2. Examples of electrophoresis migration profiles of an amplified microsatellite marker in F2 or N2 progenies and the relative frequency of allelic occurrence in the same populations. P1, parental 1; P2, parental 2; Hoz, homozygote; Hez, heterozygote.

4. Amplify each sample by cycling in the PCR thermal cycler (*see* **Note 11**).

3.6.4. Analysis of PCR-Amplified Allele Fragments on Sequencing Devices

After amplification, the relative migration profile of each amplified allele fragment is determined by analysis with a sequencing device. Genotyping is performed by comparing the migration position of each amplified allele with that of the allele from each parental strain, as illustrated in **Fig. 2**. Accordingly, each genomic sample will be scored as either homozygous P1, homozygous P2, or heterozygous P1/P2 for a given marker. For each primer pair, the expected size of the corresponding amplified allele can be predicted from the information gathered in the databases given in **Subheading 3.6.1.** If one selects markers whose expected size differs by at least 50 bp, it is then possible to multiplex several PRC reactions and load them together in the same gel lane or capillary (typically three per lane or per capillary). When one is using an automated sequencer, the number of multiplexed reactions can be further multiplied by the number of dyes that can be detected by the corresponding apparatus.

3.7. Coarse Linkage Mapping

After collecting all genotypic and phenotypic data in each animal, QTLs are detected and localized (at low resolution) by statistical calculations. The algorithms used for these calculations *(18,19)* have been implemented in various software applications (*see* **Note 4**). The analysis implies multiple steps: (1) on the basis of the distribution of SSLP markers among the population, one determines the relative position of each marker on each chromosome; the results of this procedure (called linkage mapping) can be fine tuned by comparison with the results of similar linkage maps published for mice and rats on related websites; (2) one calculates the significance of linkage of each genomic locus to the trait of interest and performs interval mapping to construct curves depicting the significance level of linkage at fixed intervals along all chromosomes; (3) one estimates the probability of linkage on the basis of appropriate significance thresholds (*see* **Note 12**); (4) one calculates the confidence interval for the localization of each QTL (*see* **Note 13**); and (5) one performs further calculations to detect possible interactions between each significant QTL (*see* **Note 4**). By proceeding in this manner, linkage of QTLs to heart weight has been reported in genetic populations of normotensive rats *(20,21)* or mice *(22)*.

3.8. Physical Mapping

Since the first step in QTL detection relies on the statistical method, it is important to provide an independent confirmation that the physical region containing the QTL will indeed affect the phenotypic trait under investigation *(2,23)*. This is performed by construction of so-called congenic lines. The procedure involves the transfer of a precise genetic region from one donor inbred strain into the background of another inbred recipient strains. To this end, animals from the F1 progeny are backcrossed to the recipient strain. The resulting progeny is genotyped to identify individuals that have retained the desired genetic region from the donor strain, and these individuals are further backcrossed with the recipient strain. Backcross matings over 10 generations result in animals that are heterozygous for the locus of interest from the donor strain, and approx 99.9% of the remainder of the genome belongs to the recipient strain *(24)*. The introgressed region can then be made homozygous by intercrossing, which generates the congenic strain. The latter is then used to quantitate the phenotypic trait and to confirm that it is influenced by the introgressed genetic material from the donor strain. To speed up the whole process, one can rely on the so-called speed-congenic breeding procedure *(24)*. This procedure implies that, in addition to genotyping the progeny of each backcross for the introgressed region, one also uses additional markers to identify individuals that are most enriched for the background of the recipient strain. By proceeding in this manner, one needs only four cycles of backcrossing to obtain an animal in which the genome outside the introgressed locus is approx 100% that of the recipient strain *(24)*. Congenic rats have previously been generated to confirm physical linkage of a QTL to cardiomyocyte morphology *(25)*.

3.9. Fine Mapping

An additional utility of congenic strains is that they constitute the starting point for fine mapping of a QTL to intervals that range from 1 to 5 cM. Indeed, statistical detection of QTL has limited resolution and is not appropriate to define smaller intervals. Once a congenic strain has been generated, they can be further backcrossed into the recipient strain to generate subcongenics whose differential genetic segments are smaller than in the congenic parent and overlap to different extents. By comparing the phenotypes of several subcongenic strains and the physical boundaries of their respective introgressed region, it is then possible to identify a minimal physical interval that is shared by all subcongenics and that correlates with the trait of interest *(26)*. Although it was usually considered that a QTL should be fine-mapped to an interval no greater than 1 cM in order to be able to identify a candidate gene, the completion of genome sequencing of several model organisms has facilitated the groundwork for identifying candidate genes. Nonetheless, it remains true that the lesser the genes in a given interval, the greater the chances are of identifying the correct causative gene.

3.10. Identification and Validation of Candidate Genes

Causation is an essential concept in the field of genetics, the gold standard being the demonstration that a mutation within a given gene is linked to the trait of interest. In contrast, there is no such gold standard for genes linked to complex traits: instead, one proceeds both by elimination of false links and by accumulation of circumstantial evidence to build a case in favor of the identity of a QTL *(2,3,5)*. To illustrate the approach, others have recently referred to a quotation from the fictional Sherlock Holmes, who stated that: "When you have eliminated all of which is impossible, then whatever remains, however improbable, must be the truth" *(3)*. Suffice it to say, QTL identification requires a combination of flair, experimental evidence, and detective work that is beyond the scope of a simple "methods" chapter. Nonetheless, a classical approach is to test whether: (1) there are variations in the sequences of the alleles of a given gene, (2) whether such changes may lead to either changes in the function and/or the level of expression of the corresponding protein, and (3) whether such changes may cause quantitative changes in the trait of interest. The latter involves the use of animal models in which the gene of interest can be either overexpressed (in transgenic animals), inactivated (by knockout), replaced with a variant allele (by knockin), or modulated by pharmacological means. In the case of LVH, both transgenic and knockout animals strongly support the role of at least one candidate gene whose locus coincides with that of a QTL linked to cardiac mass *(27)*.

4. Notes

1. An inbred strain is isogenic, which implies that all animals from that strain are genetically identical to each other, and all nonsexual genes come in pairs of identical homozygous alleles. In same-sex animals within such a strain, all biological variability is exclusively owing to nongenetic factors (i.e., environment and/or methodology). The genomes of the parental strains are recombined in genetic crosses that are used to identify links between chromosome loci and particular quantitative phenotypes.

2. One can distinguish two basic types of crosses: (1) intercrosses between two F1 animals (which yield F2 progeny), or (2) backcrosses of an F1 animal with one of the initial parents (which yield N2 progeny). Of note, many QTLs are linked to phenotypes in a codominant manner, whereby the quantitative value of the phenotype is linearly related to the number of given alleles of one particular gene. In such cases, intercrosses are advantageous because all combinations of a given genetic locus are present within the F2 progeny in a 1:2:1 distribution (homozygous P1:heterozygous:homozygous P2) (**Fig. 2**). In cases of genes with dominant/recessive effects, N2 populations may be advantageous as they will contain a greater proportion of genes with homozygous combinations in a 1:1 distribution (homozygous P1or P2:heterozygous) (**Fig. 2**).

3. RI strains are produced by inbreeding (by repetitive brother–sister mating) separate pairs of F2 animals. Each animal contains a unique combination of 50% of the genes from each parental strain. Provided there is a sufficient number of these strains (preferably >20), they can be used collectively for QTL detection. Advantages of RI strains include the following: (1) once the genotyping of individuals from each strain is completed, it no longer needs to be repeated; (2) phenotypic traits can be quantitated by averaging the values from several genetically identical animals (which allows for greater precision); (3) phenotypic traits can be quantified at different time-points (i.e., age); and (4) one can quantitate the response of a trait to an environmental stimulus (which is not always possible in individual animals from genetic crosses). One disadvantage is that mapping low-penetrance QTLs might only be possible if sets of several hundred RI strains are used *(28)*. RC strains are derived from two sequential backcrosses (N3) of one donor inbred strain into another recipient inbred strain. In an RC set, each strain contains different combinations of approx 12.5% of the genome of the donor strain within the background of the receiving strain. Although there are caveats about the use of RC strains for mapping studies, they are useful, as the power to detect relevant QTLs may be considerably increased compared with RI strains *(28)*.

4. MAPMAKER/QTL was one of the first software packages developed to construct genetic maps and perform linkage analyses *(37)*. The program was written

for either the DOS or UNIX operating systems. It has been used by many investigators but is no longer used much nowadays, in part because it has not been updated for the last 10 yr, but also because of the development of other applications that have enhanced calculation capabilities and operate in a more user-friendly manner. These new applications can all operate on a personal computer with the Windows and/or Mac operating systems, are regularly updated, are available freely through public distribution programs, allow for importation of data formatted for analysis with MAPMAKER/QTL, perform all the calculations described in the section on coarse linkage mapping, and provide tutorials along with step-by-step examples for uninitiated users. The programs may differ somewhat in terms of which specific algorithms are used for calculations and/or concerning some of the features they offer. One of the most popular packages among investigators is Map Manager QTX (http://www.mapmanager.org), which was developed by Kenneth Manly *(38)*. The program has a user-friendly and flexible interface, allows for the fast and easy construction of framework genetic maps, incorporates algorithms to deal with missing data and genotyping errors, accommodates most possible types of experimental crosses, considers all possible modes of inheritance, performs exhaustive 2D searches for interactions among QTLs, and provides both graphic and tabular text outputs.

Another powerful package (called R/QTL) was developed by Broman et al. *(39)*. It has been implemented as an add-on package for the freely available statistical software called "R" and can be downloaded from the site http://www.biostat.jhsph.edu/~kbroman/qtl/. It is a bit less user-friendly than Map Manager QTX but implements a very comprehensive set of methods, and is written in such a way that the more sophisticated user can readily extend its methods. It has the additional advantages allowing graphic outputs to visualize interactions between QTLs. A third option is the QTL Cartographer program created by Basten and Zeng (http://statgen.ncsu.edu/qtlcart/index.php). It does not construct linkage maps, so these have to be imported from those constructed by one of the above programs. However, it uses a different and perhaps more robust algorithm to calculate possible interactions between QTLs.

5. Since QTL detection relies on statistical procedures, it is preferable to find phenotypic measurements that allow for the greatest possible separation (ideally, >2 standard deviations) between the average values in each parental strain. Although this is determined in part by the choice of parental strains, there are often different techniques to measure one given phenotypic trait, and some techniques may allow for better separation of the trait values than others *(29,30)*. In addition, a detailed phenotypic characterization might define distinct subphenotypes that can each be linked to a different QTL. In the case of cardiac mass, it has been argued that gross heart weight falls short of what is needed to phenotype LVH and that a minimum characterization should also include at least measurements of cardiomyocyte size, characterization of ventricular morphology, and any particular pattern of change in gene expression *(31)*. Other useful variables might include a characterization of heart morphology and function in vivo by echocardiography, as well as measurements of cardiomyocyte contractile function.

6. In young adult animals, body weight is usually appropriate to correct cardiac mass and obtain an indexed value. However, sometimes body weight changes disproportionately as compared with cardiac mass. This may happen, for instance, with senescent animals or in the case of experimental conditions that might either increase (i.e., volume loading, heart failure) or decrease (i.e., muscle wasting) the body weight of the animals in a relatively short period. In such cases, a better reference value is provided by tibia length (which is proportional to the growth status of the animal and is not affected by superimposed rapid changes in body weight) *(32)*. Although this value can be obtained by dissection of the tibia and direct measurement (as described in **Subheading 3.4.**), an alternative method is to obtain an X-ray image of the limbs of the animals and then measure tibia length directly on that image.

7. One common procedure to phenotype hypertrophy at the level of cardiomyocytes themselves is to measure cross-sectional area in sagittal cardiac sections *(33)*. This procedure involves the detection of the external boundaries of cardiomyocytes by labeling them with fluorescein-conjugated wheat germ agglutinin. One can then define the area of the cross-sections of approx 100 cardiomyocytes/heart sections using a digitizer, and calculate the corresponding surface areas with a morphometry computer program. However, some have argued that precise assessments of cardiomyocyte morphology can only be performed on cardiomyocytes isolated from adult hearts *(34)*. The latter procedure requires retrograde aortic perfusion of the hearts with a defined sequence of several warmed and oxygenated solutions. The precise description of that method may constitute a methods chapter by itself and is beyond the scope of the present one. However, several detailed protocols have been published for either rat *(35)* or mouse *(36)* hearts. The particular utility of performing such measurements to phenotype LVH in genetic models has been illustrated previously *(25)*.

8. Genomic DNA can easily be extracted and purified from various tissues and/or plasma. Since a whole-genome scan requires the genotyping of each animal with a large number of markers, spleen is a tissue of choice because it yields relatively high quantities of DNA (5–30 μg) from as little as 10 mg of tissue. Other tissues such as liver or tail clips (when genotyping needs to be performed prior to completion of the phenotypic procedures) can be used as well but require a little more tissue (approx 25 mg). Other considerations concern the quality and stability of the genomic DNA preparation since a QTL mapping project can run over many months (and sometimes years). Although cheaper methods may be available, the genomic DNA one can obtain using the DNeasy kit is both of good quality and particularly stable. Although the DNeasy kit provides its own elution buffer (identified as AE), our protocol uses another DNA elution buffer with a lower EDTA concentration (since higher EDTA concentrations may sometimes interfere with subsequent PCR amplifications). After eluting the DNA from the DNeasy column, it can be conserved at the same concentration to prepare stock aliquots that should be kept at –20°C. Aliquots of genomic DNA at working dilutions (4–20 ng/μL) can be kept at 4°C for as long as satisfactory PCR amplifications can be obtained.

9. The whole-genome scan of the progeny of a genetic cross may typically necessitate the genotyping of approx 200 animals with 150 microsatellite markers, which amounts to at least 30,000 PCR reactions (without even taking in consideration genotyping that needs to be repeated because of technical failures). Cost-effective and high-throughput methods are therefore desirable. Our modification of the standard procedure replaces the forward primer by a mix (in an ~15:1 ratio) of a labeled M 13 primer and a forward primer that is 5'-tailed with the M13 sequence 5'-CACGACGTTGTAAAACGAC-3' *(17)*. This method has several advantages: (1) only one primer needs to be labeled for all primer pairs to be used, which saves time and/or expenses (especially when dye-labeled primers are used); and (2) the reaction products are much cleaner than what is obtained with original nontailed primers, which makes it possible to multiplex at least three SSLP reactions yielding products of different size.

10. The M13 primer (labeled with either $[\gamma\text{-}^{32}P]ATP$ or a fluorochrome dye) is used at the same concentration as the reverse primer. When the M13 primer is combined with an M13-tailed forward primer (in the approximate molar ratio of ~15:1) and the cognate reverse primer, it generates an amplified allele fragment labeled with the tag carried by the M13 primer *(17)*. The 15:1 molar ratio of the labeled M13 primer vs that of the unlabeled M13-tailed forward primer is generally appropriate for most reactions but may vary somewhat according to the true concentration of the M13-tailed forward primer. It is thus recommended to perform preliminary experiments to titrate the relative concentration of M13-tailed forward primer and find its optimal ratio. Each PCR reaction is carried out in a final volume of 10 µL, but it is best to optimize the whole procedure for 96-well PCR plates (or equivalent tube strips), using a multichannel pipetor and a thermal cycler that accommodates 96-well plates. By proceeding in this fashion with a four-block thermal cycler, one can typically generate approx 1500 PCR reactions/day (that need to be further analyzed on a sequencing device).

11. For products ranging from 150 to 300 bp, a typical PCR amplification will comprise one initial denaturation cycle at 94°C for 90 s, followed by 30 alternating cycles of denaturation (30 s at 94°C), annealing (45 s at optimal temperature), and elongation (30 s at 72°C). The procedure is terminated by a final elongation step of 3 min at 72°C. However, some primer pairs may require slightly different conditions.

12. Significance of linkage is calculated by assigning a score to each locus, the most popular one being the log-likelihood ratio of the data under the null hypothesis (i.e., lod score). Great care must be taken in determining which threshold should be used to determine whether a QTL is significantly linked to a given phenotype. Statistical guidelines have been published to determine (on the basis of conservative assumptions) whether linkage results obtained with several types of crosses should be considered either suggestive, significant ($p < 0.05$), or highly significant ($p < 0.001$) *(18)*. More recently, others have proposed the use of permutation tests to actually calculate for the given dataset which threshold should be used to consider data as significant or highly significant *(40)*. Such permutation tests have been implemented in all the recent software applications described above.

13. After determining which QTLs are most significant, one should assign realistic confidence intervals for their localization. One popular method is the *LOD drop-off method*: if one considers the curve that represents graphically the evolution of linkage significance levels (expressed as lod scores) along the chromosome and defines the highest lod score as the peak, the confidence interval is thus defined by the length of chromosome that is covered by significance levels whose values are that of the peak −1 lod score. However, in the case of "weak" QTLs (i.e., those with low linkage probability), this may include most of the chromosome. Bootstrap tests provide more reliable calculations to assign confidence intervals over all QTL strengths and have been implemented in all the software applications described above.

Acknowledgments

This work was supported by grant HL69122 (NIH/NHLBI), by grants MOP-64391 from the Canadian Institutes for Health Research (CIHR), and by a Group Grant of the CIHR to the Multidisciplinary Research Group in Hypertension. We thank Ken Manly, Chris Basten, and Karl Broman for helpful comments concerning the computer applications.

References

1. Lander, E. S. and Schork, N. J. (1994) Genetic dissection of complex traits. *Science* **265**, 2037–2048.
2. Members of the Complex Trait Consortium (2003) The nature and identification of quantitative trait loci: a community's view. *Nature Rev. Genetics* **4**, 911–916.
3. Page, G. P., George, V., Go, R. C., Page, P. Z., and Allison, D. B. (2003) "Are we there yet?": Deciding when one has demonstrated specific genetic causation in complex diseases and quantitative traits. *Am. J. Hum. Genet.* **73**, 711–719.
4. Korstanje, R. and Paigen, B. (2002) From QTL to gene: the harvest begins. *Nature Genet.* **31**, 235,236.
5. Glazier, A. M., Nadeau, J. H., and Aitman, T. J. (2002) Finding genes that underlie complex traits. *Science* **298**, 2345–2349.
6. Tanase, H., Yamori, Y., Hansen, C. T., and Lovenberg, W. (1982) Heart size in inbred strains of rats. Part 1. Genetic determination of the development of cardiovascular enlargement in rats. *Hypertension* **4**, 864–872.
7. Verhaaren, H. A., Schieken, R. M., Mosteller, M., Hewitt, J. K., Eaves, L. J., and Nance, W. E. (1991) Bivariate genetic analysis of left ventricular mass and weight in pubertal twins (the Medical College of Wisconsin twin study). *Am. J. Cardiol.* **68**, 661–668.
8. Levy, D., Garrison, R. J., Savage, D. D., Kannel, W. B., and Castelli, W. P. (1990) Prognostic implications of echocardiographically determined left ventricular mass in the Framingham heart study. *N. Engl. J. Med.* **322**, 1561–1566.
9. Devereux, R. B., de Simone, G., Ganau, A., and Roman, M. J. (1994) Left ventricular hypertrophy and geometric remodeling in hypertension: stimuli, functional consequences and prognostic implications. *J. Hypertens.* **12**, S117–S127.

10. Frey, N. and Olson, E. N. (2003) Cardiac hypertrophy: the good, the bad, and the ugly. *Annu. Rev. Physiol.* **65,** 45–79.

11. Pravenec, M., Klir, P., Kren, V., Zicha, J., and Kunes, J. (1989) An analysis of spontaneous hypertension in spontaneously hypertensive rats by means of new recombinant inbred strains. *J. Hypertens.* **7,** 217–222.

12. Pravenec, M., et al. (1995) Mapping of quantitative trait loci for blood pressure and cardiac mass in the rat by genome scanning of recombinant inbred strains. *J. Clin. Invest.* **96,** 1973–1978.

13. Printz, M. P., Jirout, M., Jaworski, R., Alemayehu, A., and Kren, V. (2003) HXB/BXH rat recombinant inbred strain platform: a newly enhanced tool for cardiovascular, behavioral, and developmental genetics and genomics. *J. Appl. Physiol.* **94,** 2510–2522.

14. Moen, C. J., van der Valk, M. A., Snoek, M., van Zutphen, B. F., von Deimling, O., Hart, A. A., and Demant, P. (1991) The recombinant congenic strains: a novel genetic tool applied to the study of colon tumor development in the mouse. *Mamm. Genome* **1,** 217–227.

15. Fortin, A., Diez, E., Rochefort, D., et al. (2001) Recombinant congenic strains derived from A/J and C57BL/6J: a tool for genetic dissection of complex traits. *Genomics* **74,** 21–35.

16. Hoit, B. D., Kiatchoosakun, S., Restivo, J., et al. (2003) Naturally occurring variation in cardiovascular traits among inbred strains of mice. *Genomics* **79,** 679–685.

17. Boutin-Ganache, I., Raposo, M., Raymond, M., and Deschepper, C. F. (2001) M13-tailed primers improve the readability and usability of microsatellite analyses performed with two different allele-sizing methods. *Biotechniques* **31,** 24–26.

18. Lander, E. S. and Kruglyak, L. (1995) Genetic dissection of compex traits: guidelines for interpreting and reporting linkage results. *Nature Genet.* **11,** 241–247.

19. Sen, S. and Churchill, G. A. (2001) A statistical framework for quantitative trait mapping. *Genetics* **159,** 371–387.

20. Sebkhi, A., Zhao, L., Lu, L., Haley, C. S., Nunez, D. J. R., and Wilkins, M. R. (1999) Genetic determination of cardiac mass in normotensive rats. Results from an F344xWKY cross. *Hypertension* **33,** 949–953.

21. Deschepper, C. F., Masciotra, S., Zahabi, A., Boutin-Ganache, I., Picard, S., and Reudelhuber, T. (2001) Functional alterations of the *Nppa* promoter are linked to cardiac ventricular hypertrophy in WKY/WKHA rat crosses. *Circ. Res.* **88,** 222–227.

22. Sugiyama, F., Churchill, G. A., Li, R., et al. (2002) QTL associated with blood pressure, heart rate, and heart weight in CBA/CaJ and BalB/cJ mice. *Physiol. Genomics* **10,** 5–12.

23. Rapp, J. P. (2000) Genetic analysis of inherited hypertension in the rat. *Physiol. Rev.* **80,** 135–172.

24. Markel, P., Shu, P., Ebeling, C., et al. (1997) Theoretical and empirical issues for marker-assisted breeding of congenic mouse strains. *Nature Genet.* **17,** 280–284.

25. Boutin-Ganache, I., Picard, S., and Deschepper, C. F. (2002) Distinct gene-sex interactions regulate adult rat cardiomyocyte width and length independently. *Physiol. Genomics* **12,** 61–67.

26. Olofsson, P., Holberg, J., Tordson, J., Lu, S., Akerström, B., and Holmdahl, R. (2003) Positional identification of *Ncf1* as a gene that regulates arthritis severity in rats. *Nature Genet.* **33,** 25–32.
27. Zahabi, A., Picard, S., Fortin, N., Reudelhuber, T. L., and Deschepper, C. F. (2003) Expression of constitutively active guanylate cyclase in cardiomyocytes inhibits the hypertrophic effects of isoproterenol and aortic constriction on mouse hearts. *J. Biol. Chem.* **278,** 47,694–47,699.
28. Demant, P. (2003) Cancer susceptibility in the mouse: genetics, biology and implications for human cancer. *Nature Rev. Genetics* **4,** 721–735.
29. Aitman, T. J., et al. (1998) Quantitative trait loci for cellular defects in glucose and fatty acid metabolism in hypertensive rats. *Nature Genet.* **16,** 197–201.
30. Deschepper, C. F., Boutin-Ganache, I., Zahabi, A., and Jiang, Z. (2002) In search of cardiovascular genes. Interactions between phenotypes and genotypes. *Hypertension* **39,** 332–336.
31. Dorn, G. W. I., Robbins, J., and Sugden, P. H. (2003) Phenotyping hypertrophy. Eschew obfuscation. *Circ. Res.* **92,** 1171–1175.
32. Yin, F. C. P., Spurgeon, H. A., Weisfeldt, M. L., and Lakatta, E. G. (1980) Mechanical properties of myocardium from hypertrophied rat hearts. *Circ. Res.* **46,** 292–300.
33. Milano, C. A., Dolber, P. C., Rockman, H. A., et al. (1994) Myocardial expression of a constitutively active a_{1B}-adrenergic receptor in transgenic mice induces cardiac hypertrophy. *Proc. Natl. Acad. Sci. USA* **91,** 10,109–10,113.
34. Gerdes, A. M. (1992) The use of isolated myocytes to evaluate myocardial remodeling. *Trends Cardiovasc. Med.* **2,** 152–155.
35. Mitcheson, J. S., Hancox, J. C., and Levi, A. J. (1998) Cultured adult myocytes: future applications, culture methods, morphological and electrophysiological properties. *Cardiovasc. Res.* **39,** 280–300.
36. Zhou ,Y.-Y., et al. (2000) Culture and adenoviral infection of adult mouse cardiac myocytes: methods for cellular genetic physiology. *Am. J. Physiol.* **279,** H429–H436.
37. Lander, E. S., Green, P., Abrahamson, J., et al. (1987) MAPMAKER: an interactive computer package for constructing primary genetic linkage maps of experimental and natural poulations. *Genomics* **1,** 174–181.
38. Manly, K. F. and Olson, J. M. (1999) Overview of QTL mapping software and introduction to Map Manager QT. *Mamm. Genome* **10,** 327–334.
39. Broman, K. W., Wu, H., Sen, S., and Churchill, G. A. (2003) R/qtl: QTL mapping in experimental crosses. *Bioinformatics* **19,** 889,890.
40. Doerge, R. W. and Churchill, G. A. (1996) Permutation tests for multiple loci affecting a quantitative character. *Genetics* **142,** 285–294.

22

Induction and Analysis of Cardiac Hypertrophy in Transgenic Animal Models

Marcos E. Barbosa, Natalia Alenina, and Michael Bader

Summary

Myocardial hypertrophy is an adaptational process of the heart to increased workload caused by mechanical stress, growth factors, cytokines, catecholamines, or primary genetic abnormalities. Chronic induction of hypertrophy leads to the gradual deterioration of ventricular function and is an independent risk factor for cardiac-related morbidity and mortality in patients with hypertension and ventricular arrythmias. Transgenic animals are very useful models to study the factors involved in the pathogenesis of cardiac hypertrophy. To achieve this goal, rodents lacking or overexpressing a specific gene are subjected to banding of the abdominal aorta, an experimental model of cardiac hypertrophy that leads to pressure overload on the heart. After periods between 3 and 21 d, parameters such as cardiac hemodynamics, morphologic alterations, and expression of marker genes (e.g., the gene for atrial natriuretic peptide) are analyzed in genetically modified animals and compared with controls elucidating a possible implication of the modified gene in the pathogenic process leading to myocardial hypertrophy. This article summarizes the techniques necessary to induce left ventricular hypertrophy by aortic banding and to analyze the effects of this experimental model on hemodynamics, cardiac morphology, and gene expression of transgenic and control animals.

Key Words: Cardiac hypertrophy; fibrosis; pressure overload; aortic banding; transgenic rat; transgenic mouse; knockout mouse; heart failure; atrial natriuretic peptide; RNase protection assay; Masson's trichrome stain.

From: *Methods in Molecular Medicine, vol. 112: Molecular Cardiology: Methods and Protocols*
Edited by: Z. Sun © Humana Press Inc., Totowa, NJ

1. Introduction

Myocardial hypertrophy is an adaptational response of the heart to increased workload and is associated with many cardiovascular disorders leading to the gradual deterioration of ventricular function (for recent reviews, *see* **refs.** *1* and *2*). It is recognized as an independent risk factor for cardiac-related morbidity and mortality including heart failure and coronary diseases and also for sudden death in patients with hypertension and ventricular arrhythmias. Left ventricular hypertrophy (LVH) arises from diverse causes, including mechanical stress, growth factors, cytokines, catecholamines, and primary genetic abnormalities.

Macroscopically, LVH is characterized by an increase in the thickness of the ventricular septum and the free wall of the cardiac left ventricle and is frequently associated with reduction in the lumen of the left ventricle. Microscopically, an increase in cardiomyocyte size is observed. Large-scale expression analyses have identified numerous genes, which are upregulated in hypertrophied hearts including fetal and immediate-early genes encoding proteins involved in signaling pathways, contraction, extracellular matrix, and energy metabolism (for recent reviews, *see* **refs.** *3* and *4*).

Transgenic and knockout techniques are powerful tools for studying cardiovascular diseases (for recent reviews, *see* **refs.** *5* and *6*). With these animal models, the role of a specific gene in pathophysiological processes such as the development of LVH can be studied on the whole-organism level. However, many of the phenotypes resulting from genetic manipulation are slight, and the animals can often compensate, maintaining blood pressure and cardiac output on normal levels. In these cases, interventions must be performed to reveal phenotypic differences in the response to cardiovascular stress. To induce LVH in rodents, different experimental models have been shown to be effective. Among them are exercise, induction of pressure or volume overload or myocardial ischemia, treatment with thyroid hormone or isoproterenol, and renal hypertension. The most frequently used method is the induction of pressure overload by abdominal aortic banding.

2. Materials

1. Standard surgical instruments.
2. Standard surgical suture.
3. 9-0 Nylon suture.
4. 18-Gage needle.
5. Aluminum foil.
6. Rodent ventilator.
7. Commercial polyethylene catheter.
8. Transducer and appropriate software for measurements and analyses.

9. Microwave oven.
10. Light microscope.
11. Glass slides for microscopy.
12. Glass cover slips.
13. Glass cubes for staining.
14. Agarose gel electrophoresis apparatus.
15. PhosphoImager BAS 2000 (FUJIX Tokyo, Japan).
16. Centrifuge.
17. Hybridization oven.
18. Glass–Teflon homogenizer.
19. Liquid scintillation system.
20. Power supply for the gel chamber.
21. Quartz cuvets.
22. Slab gel dryer.
23. Speed Vac.
24. Thermomixer.
25. UV/visible spectrophotometer.
26. Vortex.
27. Vertical polyacrylamide gel electrophoresis apparatus.
28. Whatman 3MM paper.
29. Sodium pentobarbital.
30. Xylazine.
31. Ketamine.
32. Ethanol.
33. Xylene.
34. 60 mM KCl.
35. Saline: 0.9% NaCl.
36. 10% Sucrose.
37. 0.1% acetic acid.
38. Phosphate buffer solution (PBS): 0.02 M potassium phosphate, 0.15 M NaCl, pH 7.2.
39. 10% Formaldehyde.
40. Tissue Tek®.
41. Weigert's iron hematoxylin:
    a. Solution A: 1% hematoxylin in 95% ethanol.
    b. Solution B: 1% ferric chloride in 5% hydrochloric acid solution.
42. Biebrich scarlet: 0.9% Biebrich scarlet and 0.1% acid fuchsin in 1% acetic acid solution.
43. Phosphotungstic/phosphomolybdic acid solution: 25 g phosphotungstic acid and 25 g phosphomolybdic acid in 1 L distilled water.
44. Aniline blue: 2.5% anilin blue in 2% acetic acid solution.
45. 40% Acrylamide/bis-acrylamide (20:1).
46. Isopropanol.
47. TEMED.
48. Chloroform.

49. 5X TBE buffer: 445 m*M* Tris, pH 8.0, 445 m*M* boric acid, 10 m*M* EDTA.
50. 10% Ammonium persulfate (APS) in dH$_2$O.
51. 9 *M* Urea.
52. 75% Ethanol.
53. DNase I (RNase-free; Roche Basel, Switzerland).
54. RNasin (Promega, Madison, WI).
55. 800 Ci/mmol [α-^{32}P]gUTP (Amersham, Freiburg, Germany).
56. TRIzol reagent (Gibco, Bethesda, MD).
57. Ambion RPA II Kit (AMS Biotechnology, Whitney, UK).
58. QIAquick Gel Extract Kit (Qiagen, Hilden, Germany).
59. Riboprobe System (Promega, Madison, WI).
60. Quickspin™ columns, Sephadex G-50 (Boehringer Mannheim, Germany).
61. DEPC-H$_2$O: 0.1% diethyl pyrocarbonate in H$_2$O bidest; keep at 37°C overnight
    and autoclave.

3. Methods

The following sections summarize methods for (1) banding of the abdominal aorta, (2) measurement of hemodynamic parameters, (3) tissue collection and storage, (4) cardiac morphology and fibrosis, and (5) molecular biological methods.

3.1. Aortic Banding

The coarctation of the ascending aorta (aortic banding) is a surgical method commonly used to induce pressure-overload hypertrophy (*see* **Fig. 1**). It is a model for characterizing the development of LVH caused by hemodynamic stress with subsequent development of heart failure.

1. Select male transgenic rats with weights between 180 and 230 g and respective control animals.
2. Follow institutional guidelines to perform animal handling, surgery, and postoperative care.
3. Aseptic procedures should be adopted for surgical operation.
4. Inject 50 mg/kg sodium pentobarbital ip and begin surgery under full anesthesia.
5. Shave abdominal area of the rat.
6. Make an incision in the abdominal midline, and expose a 5-mm segment of the aorta.
7. Place an 18-gage needle parallel to the abdominal aorta.
8. Ligate by tying a 9-0 nylon suture around the aorta and the needle.
9. Remove the needle, maintaining the ligation.
10. To perform sham operations, use identical procedures, but do not tie the nylon suture around the vessel.
11. Surgically close the abdomen.
12. Analysis of LVH is done between 3 and 21 d after the operation.

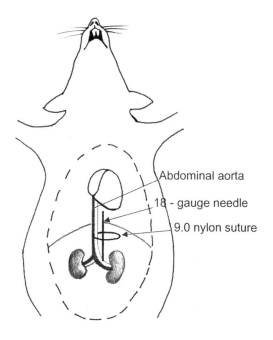

Fig. 1. Surgical schema for aortic banding. Aortic banding is used to induce pressure-overload hypertrophy and is a model to characterize the development of left ventricular hypertrophy, caused by hemodynamic stress. A ligation is produced by tying a 9-0 nylon suture around the aorta and a 18-gage needle, after which the needle is removed to create a coarctation of defined diameter.

3.2. Hemodynamic Measurements

For analysis, the rats are anesthetized, ventilated, and then instrumented for the assessment of systemic and left ventricular hemodynamics such as systolic and diastolic pressure (*see* **Fig. 2**).

1. Anesthetize the rat with 10 mg/kg xylazine and 50 mg/kg ketamine ip.
2. Fix the animal in the supine position.
3. Retract the tongue of the rat, cannulate the trachea, and connect a rodent ventilator.
4. Isolate and expose the carotid artery through a midline incision over the trachea and throat of the rat.
5. Advance a polyethylene catheter coupled to a transducer through the carotid into the left ventricle to assess cardiac parameters.

3.3. Tissue Collection and Storage

After concluding hemodynamic measurements, the polyethylene catheter is removed, and the heart is arrested in diastole (injection of KCl) for histological

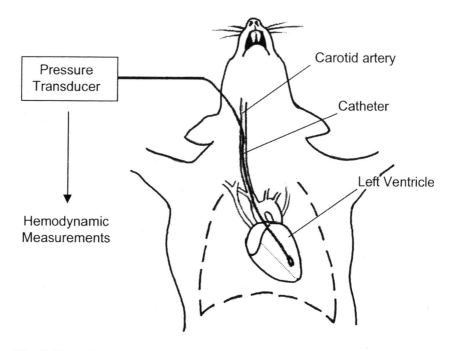

Fig. 2. Hemodynamic measurements. In anesthetised and ventilated rats, systemic and left ventricular hemodynamics and parameters such as systolic and diastolic pressure are assessed by the introduction of a polyethylene catheter through the carotid artery into the left ventricle.

and molecular biological analysis. The tissues of the different parts of the heart are separated, weighed, and prepared in different ways, for different kind of analyses.

1. After the hemodynamic measurements, inject 1 mL 60 m*M* KCl iv in the animal.
2. Rapidly excise the heart, and place it in ice-cold saline. Wash to remove blood, blot dry, and weigh the organ (*see* **Note 1**).
3. Quickly trim away the atria and great vessels, and weigh the isolated ventricles.
4. Separate and weigh the right ventricle, septum, and left ventricle.
5. From this moment, tissues used for different purposes have to be treated differently. For histology and immunohistochemistry, tissues must be placed in specific fixative solutions (*see* **Subheading 3.4.**).
6. For gene expression analysis the tissue is snap-frozen as follows:
   a. Pack the tissues in previously labeled aluminum foil.
   b. Freeze in liquid nitrogen, and store at –80°C until further use (*see* **Note 2**).

3.4. Cardiac Morphology and Fibrosis

Histopathologically, cardiac remodeling is characterized by a structural re-arrangement of components of the normal chamber wall from the heart. In addition to cardiomyocyte hypertrophy, such rearranging involves cardiac fibroblast proliferation, fibrosis, and cell death. Disproportionate accumulation of fibrillar collagen is a feature of the remodeling characteristic of the failing heart. Accumulation of collagen, especially type I, stiffens the ventricles and impedes both contraction and relaxation. Furthermore, fibrosis can also impair the electrical coupling of cardiomyocytes by separating myocytes owing to extracellular protein accumulation.

The following Masson's trichrome staining allows one to assess changes in the size and shape of cardiomyocytes and to identify and quantify collagen in cardiac tissues:

1. After isolation of the left ventricle, put the tissue in PBS with 10% formaldehyde for about 3 h.
2. Transfer the tissue to a 10% sucrose solution, and incubate for 4 h.
3. Place the tissue in a TissueTek block, and store at −80°C until use.
4. In a refrigerated microtome, make 5–8-μm slices, and place them on glass slides.
5. Incubate slides in PBS with 10% formaldehyde and put into the microwave oven (maximum power) for 1 min.
6. Allow to stand for 15 min.
7. Incubate in Weigert's hematoxylin (1:1 solutions A and B) for 10 min.
8. Wash in running tap water for 5 min, and rinse in distilled water.
9. Put in Biebrich scarlet for 5 min.
10. Rinse in distilled water.
11. Incubate in phosphotungstic/phosphomolybdic acid for 10 min, and discard solution.
12. Transfer directly to Aniline blue for 5 min.
13. Rinse in distilled water.
14. Incubate for 1 min in 1% acetic acid, and rinse in distilled water.
15. Rinse three times for 3 min in 95% ethanol.
16. Rinse three times for 3 min in 100% ethanol.
17. Rinse three times for 5 min in xylene.
18. Analyze under a light microscope.

3.5. Molecular Biology Methods

In LVH, upregulation of several genes is observed. The gene most used as a marker for upregulation in LVH is the gene encoding the atrial natriuretic peptide (ANP). ANP mRNA levels can be quantified in hearts after aortic banding by ribonuclease protection assay (RPA). RPA is a sensitive method for the detection and quantitation of mRNA using a labeled radioactive RNA probe complementary to a part of the target mRNA. The antisense radiolabeled probe is hybridized in excess to the target mRNA, and then the mixture is treated with single-strand specific ribonucleases to degrade unbound probe and other single-stranded RNA (*see* **Fig. 3**). The remaining RNase-resistant double-stranded RNA can be separated on a polyacrylamide gel and quantified by autoradiography or phosphoimaging. The intensity of the protected fragment will be directly proportional to the amount of target mRNA in the original RNA sample (*see* **Note 3**).

3.5.1. Design of the Probe

The probe for RPA is a labeled RNA complementary to a short region (~200–400 bp) of the mRNA to be analyzed. (Optimally it should cover more than one exon of the corresponding gene; *see* **Note 4**.) To generate this probe, a cDNA fragment is cloned into a vector containing RNA-polymerase promoters (from bacteriophage T3, T7, or SP6). The construct can then be used as a template for in vitro synthesis of radiolabeled antisense RNA probe by the T3, T7, or SP6 RNA polymerase after linearization at the 5'end (*see* **Note 5**).

1. Use the total RNA of a tissue in which the gene of interest is highly expressed to generate the cDNA.
2. Design primers in two neighboring exons, so the amplified fragment will be around 200–400 bp long.
3. Generate and purify the polymerase chain reaction (PCR) fragment, and subclone it into a plasmid containing bacteriophage RNA polymerase promoters (e.g., pGEM [Promega] or pBluescript [Stratagene] vectors).
4. Sequence the insert to determine the integrity and orientation of the cloned fragment (*see* **Note 6**).
5. Choose a restriction site upstream of the 5' end of the insert. Prove by both analysis of the sequence and digestion that this enzyme is not cutting elsewhere in the insert. The vector linearized with this enzyme is used for in vitro transcription from the bacteriophage promoter at the 3' end of the insertion.

3.5.2. Probe Labeling

1. Linearize 10–20 μg of the vector containing the cloned probe by digestion with the chosen restriction enzyme at the 5' end of the insertion in a whole volume of 50–100 μL (*see* **Note 5**).

Fig. 3. (*opposite page*) Detection and quantitation of mRNA using the RNase protection assay. Asterisks indicate the incorporated [α-^{32}P]rUTP; solid arrows indicate the orientation of the mRNAs (the arrowhead represents the 3' end of the mRNA); small arrows show the position of the primers used to generate the probe by polymerase chain reaction (PCR); the vertical arrow indicates the unique restriction site used for linearization of the plasmid. For further explanations, *see* text.

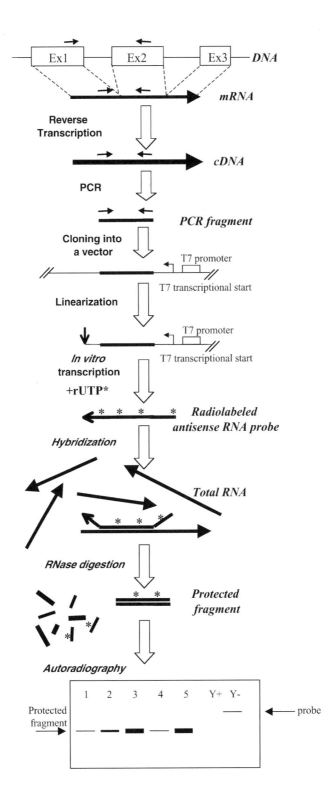

2. Analyze 2 µL of the digestion on a 1% agarose gel to confirm that the digestion is complete.
3. Load the rest of the digestion, purify the fragment from 1% agarose gel using the QIAquick Gel Extract Kit, and dissolve it in DEPC H_2O.
4. The labeled antisense RNA probe is synthesized by T7, or T3, or SP6 RNA polymerase in the presence of $[\alpha\text{-}^{32}P]$rUTP using Riboprobe System. To perform in vitro transcription, mix on ice 0.5 µg of linearized DNA, 1 µL 10 mM rATP, 1 µL 10 mM rCTP, 1 µL 10 mM rGTP, 5 µL 5X transcription buffer, 1 µL RNasin, 1 µL 0.2 M dithreitol (DTT), 3 µL $[\alpha\text{-}^{32}P]$rUTP (800 Ci/mM), and 1 µL of T7, or T3, or SP6- polymerase in a final volume of 25 µL (DEPC H_2O).
5. Incubate at 37°C for 1 h.
6. Add 1 µL of RNase-free DNase I to digest the DNA template. Incubate at 37°C for 15 min.
7. Use Quick-Spin-column Sephadex G50 to clean the probe from free unincorporated nucleotides. Centrifuge the column at 770g for 2 min. Add 25 µL DEPC H_2O to the reaction mix, and spin the final 50 µL through a Sephadex G-50 column at 770g for 2 min.
8. Measure the activity of the probe by a scintillation counter. Usually the activity is between 1×10^5 and 2×10^6 cpm/µL. If it is less than 10^5 cpm/µL labeling was not effective and should be repeated. The probe may be stored 2–3 wk at –20°C.

3.5.3. Isolation of Total RNA From Rat Tissue

Total tissue RNA can be isolated using the TRIzol reagent (Gibco) with sufficient purity to perform the RPA (*see* **Note 7**).

1. Kill animals by cervical dislocation; collect the tissues, and freeze them immediately in liquid nitrogen (*see* **Subheading 3.3.**). The tissues may be stored at least for 1 yr at –80° (*see* **Note 2**).
2. Weigh the organ, and add 1 mL of TRIzol reagent per 100–200 mg of tissue.
3. Homogenize the tissue by using a glass–Teflon homogenizer.
4. Incubate the homogenate at room temperature (RT) for 5 min to permit complete dissociation of nucleoprotein complexes.
5. Add 0.2 mL of chloroform per 1 mL of TRIzol, vortex vigorously, and incubate the homogenate at RT for another 5 min.
6. Spin the samples at 12,000g for 15 min at 4°C, and transfer the colorless upper aqueous phase containing RNA into a new tube.
7. Precipitate the RNA by adding 0.5 mL of isopropanol per 1 mL of TRIzol used. Mix by inversion.
8. Let stand at RT for 5 min (or overnight at –20°C if a small yield is expected).
9. Spin at 12,000g for 15 min at 4°C, and gently pour off the supernatant.
10. Add 1 mL of 75% ethanol, and mix gently by inversion. Spin at 7500g for 15 min at 4°C.
11. Discard the supernatant, and air-dry the RNA pellet.

12. Dissolve the RNAs in 100–200 μL of DEPC H_2O per 1 mL of TRIzol used by shaking for 10–30 min at 60°C. Be sure that the RNA is completely dissolved. If not, add more DEPC H_2O, and let it shake for an additional 10 min.
13. Measure the concentration of extracted RNA using a 10-mm light-path quartz cuvet and a UV-spectrophotometer. Dilute 2 μL of RNA in 200 μL of DEPC H_2O, place in a quartz cuvet, and measure the absorption of the samples at 260 and 280 nm. At this dilution the RNA concentration may be estimated by the following relationships:

$$C = A260 \times 4$$

where C = concentration of sample (μg/μL).

$$A260 = \text{absorption at 260 nm}$$

The ratio A260:A280, which is an indication of the purity of the RNA (i.e., contamination with salt and protein) should be between 1.8 and 2.0. However, even if the ratio is less than 1.8, the RNA quality may be acceptable. Alternatively, the quality and quantity of RNA may be assessed on an ethidium bromide-stained agarose gel.
14. Isolated RNA may be stored at –80°C for several months.

3.5.4. RNase Protection Assay

RPA may be performed using commercially available Ambion RPA II kits according to the protocol described below.

1. Pipet the desired amount of the RNAs into an Eppendorf tube (*see* **Notes 3** and **4**). Set up two control tubes with the same amount of yeast RNA (supplied in the kit).
2. Vacuum-dry the RNAs in a Speed Vac.
3. Prepare the master mix (*see* **Note 8**): 20 μL hybridization buffer (supplied by kit), 20,000 cpm of radiolabeled probes for gene of interest, and 40,000 cpm for the housekeeping gene per one RNA sample.
   The volume of the probes should not exceed 2 μL per sample. If the probe has a very high activity, it can be diluted first with DEPC H_2O.
4. Resuspend the vacuum-dried RNA in 20 μL of master mix, vortex each tube for about 5–10 s, and spin briefly to collect the liquid at the bottom of the tube.
5. Incubate for 3 min at 95°C to solubilize and to denature the RNA.
6. Vortex again for 5–10 s, and spin briefly.
7. Incubate overnight at 42°C
8. Dilute the RNase A/RNase T1 (supplied in the kit) with RNase Digestion Buffer (supplied in the kit) in proportion 1:100. Vortex the RNase mixture, and add 200 μL of diluted RNase solution to each sample RNA tube and to one of each pair of yeast RNA controls (Y+). Vortex, and spin tubes briefly.
9. Add 200 μL RNase digestion buffer *without* RNase to the remaining yeast RNA control tube (Y–).

10. Incubate for 45 min at 37°C to digest the unprotected single-stranded RNA.
11. Add to each tube 1 μL of GlycoBlue™ (supplied in the kit) and 300 μL of RNase inactivation/precipitation solution, vortex, and spin briefly.
12. Incubate at –20°C for at least 15 min.
13. Microfuge probes for 15 min at 12,000*g*, 4°C to precipitate the protected RNAs.
14. Carefully remove the supernatant from the tubes, spin briefly, and aspirate the rest of supernatant with a Pasteur pipet.
15. Resuspend the pellets in 8 μL of the gel loading buffer (supplied in the kit). Add 24 μL of loading buffer to the (Y–) tube.
16. Incubate for 3 min at 95°C to solubilize and to denature the RNAs. Vortex, microfuge briefly, and store the tubes on ice before loading the content on the gel.
17. Prepare a denaturing 5% polyacrylamide gel by mixing: 46 mL 9 *M* urea, 6 mL 5X TBE, 7.6 mL 40% acrylamide/bis-acrylamide (20:1), 480 μL 10% APS, 64 μL TEMED. Filter the solution through a 45-μm filter, and fill up the gel; 60 ml of the solution is enough to fill up a 1-mm-thick gel 20 × 20 cm with 18 or 24 wells (equipment from Biometra).
18. Prerun the gel for 30 min at 250 V constant voltage, rinse the urea out of the wells and immediately load the samples. Load only 2 μL of the (Y–) control. Run the gel until the leading dye band (bromophenol blue) is near the bottom of the gel.
19. Transfer the gel to the Whatman 3MM paper, cover with plastic wrap, and let the gel vacuum-dry for 1.5 h at 90°C.
20. Expose the dried gel to an autoradiography film or a PhosphoImager plate for 1–15 d. Analyze the data using a computer or a PhosphoImager system. The Y– lane shows gel migration of the full-length undigested probe (*see* **Note 9**). This lane should show a single band migrating at the expected probe size. Lane Y+ serves as positive control for the function of the RNases, and there should be no signal at all in this lane. The RNA expression level in the samples can be calculated by comparison of the intensity of the band for the gene of interest with the one of the housekeeping gene.

4. Notes

1. Instruments should be cleaned between tissues and animals by dipping in 70% ethanol. Wipe the instruments with a clean tissue paper before using them again.
2. The tissue samples are stored at –80°C. Most RNA isolation kits guarantee to extract high-quality RNA from tissue samples that have been stored for 1 yr at –70°C. If you plan on long-term storage of your samples, store them at –192°C (in liquid nitrogen). Do not allow the samples to thaw during the transfer to the freezer. The vials can be removed from the liquid nitrogen container, placed on dry ice, organized, and then placed in the –80°C freezer again.
3. The first step in RPA is hybridization of total RNA with the radiolabeled antisense RNA probe. The amount of sample RNA required depends on the abundance of the mRNA being detected. Approximately 10–50 μg of total RNA can be used in the assay. In most cases, 20–50,000 cpm of the probe with high specific activity is sufficient to achieve molar excess of the probe over target mRNA. Several radiola-

beled probes may be hybridized simultaneously with the same RNA sample. For quantification of mRNA expression level, detection of the mRNA for a housekeeping genes (e.g., for the ribosomal protein L32) in the same sample is necessary.

4. RNAs isolated from animal tissues are often contaminated with genomic DNA. These DNA may serve as a source of additional bands, or altered intensity of the bands of interest. This problem may be solved by digestion of RNA with RNase-free DNase I before the hybridization procedure. Even better is the inclusion of several exons in the radiolabeled probe since genomic DNA will only be partially complementary to the probe and will thus generate short protected fragments, if any.

5. Linearization of the vector is important to stop the transcription at a certain point. Incomplete linearization may lead to ineffective labeling.

6. Sequencing of the probe before in vitro transcription is important not only to clarify the orientation of the fragment but also to be sure that no mutation was inserted by Taq-polymerase during PCR. Since RPA is highly specific owing to the RNase sensitivity for mismatched base pairs, even one mismatch may lead to the appearance of additional bands.

7. One of the major difficulties in working with RNA is its susceptibility to hydrolytic cleavage by ribonucleases. To avoid RNA degradation, always use gloves, RNase-free chemicals and reagents, and DEPC-treated water (DEPC H_2O). For RPA, all solutions that are not heat sensitive are sterilized at 121°C, 105 Pa for 60 min in an autoclave. Heat-sensitive solutions are filtered through a disposable sterile filter (0.22–0.45-μm pore size). Plasticware is autoclaved as above, and glassware is sterilized overnight in an oven at 220°C.

8. Since housekeeping genes are usually expressed at very high levels, the amount of the corresponding mRNA molecules may exceed the amount of labeled probe molecules, resulting in an underestimation of the expression level of the housekeeping gene. In this case, a low-labeling protocol for the housekeeping gene, which includes the use of both [α-^{32}P]rUTP and cold rUTP in the in vitro transcription reaction, may be useful. Since incorporation rate of labeled rUTP will be decreased owing to the competition with cold ribonucleotides, even a low amount of the radiolabeled probe (around 5000 cpm per RNA sample) will be sufficient to reach molar excess over the target mRNA in the hybridization reaction. To perform low labeling of the probe for the housekeeping gene, mix on ice: 0.5 μg of linearized DNA, 1 μL 10 mM rATP, 1 μL 10 mM rCTP, 1 μL 10 mM rGTP, 1 μL 0.1 mM rUTP, 5 μL 5X transcription buffer, 1 μL RNasin, 1 μL 0.2 M DTT, 3 μL [α-^{32}P]gUTP (800 Ci/mM), and 1 μL of T7, or T3, or SP6- polymerase in a final volume of 25 μL (DEPC H_2O). Continue with **Subheading 3.5.4., step 5** of the probe labeling protocol.

9. The probe is always longer than the protected fragment. Thus, if there is a band of the probe size in any lane, the RNase digestion was not complete.

References

1. Frey, N. and Olson, E. N. (2003) Cardiac hypertrophy: the good, the bad, and the ugly. *Annu. Rev. Physiol.* **65,** 45–79.

2. Hunter, J. J. and Chien, K. R. (1999) Signaling pathways for cardiac hypertrophy and failure. *N. Engl. J. Med.* **341,** 1276–1283.
3. Manabe, I., Shindo, T., and Nagai, R. (2002) Gene expression in fibroblasts and fibrosis: involvement in cardiac hypertrophy. *Circ. Res.* **91,** 1103–1113.
4. Akazawa, H. and Komuro, I. (2003) Roles of cardiac transcription factors in cardiac hypertrophy. *Circ. Res.* **92,** 1079–1088.
5. Bader, M. (2002) Role of the local renin-angiotensin system in cardiac damage: a minireview focussing on transgenic animal models. *J Mol. Cell. Cardiol.* **34,** 1455–1462.
6. Bader, M., Bohnemeier, H., Zollmann, F. S., Lockley-Jones, O. E., and Ganten, D. (2000) Transgenic animals in cardiovascular disease research. *Exp. Physiol;* **85,** 713–731.

23

Methods for the Detection of Altered β-Adrenergic Receptor Signaling Pathways in Hypertrophied Hearts

Matthew J. Wolf, Hideo Tachibana, and Howard A. Rockman

Summary

β-Adrenergic receptor signaling, desensitization, and downregualtion are fundamental mechanisms that contribute to both normal and altered myocardial function. The development of pharmacological and biochemical assays has provided the ability to measure alterations both in adrenergic receptor density and the subsequent coupling of adrenergic receptors downstream effectors, namely, adenylyl cyclase. Furthermore, transthoracic echocardiography of the murine heart has provided insight into changes in cardiac physiology that accompany altered adrenergic receptor signaling. The protocols described within this chapter provide the means to quantify β-adrenergic density, measure adenylyl cyclase activity, and evaluate cardiac hypertrophy to better understand the mechanisms responsible for cardiac hypertrophy and heart failure.

Key Words: β-adrenergic receptors; adenylyl cyclase; myocardial membranes; transthoracic echocardiography.

1. Introduction

Recent advances in gene targeting, transgene overexpression, and mapping of quantitative trait loci in genetic mouse models of cardiovascular disease have shown that a number of molecular mechanisms are involved in the transition from normal cardiac function to the hypertrophied state and ultimately heart failure (1–4). β-adrenergic receptor signaling, receptor desensitization, and receptor downregulation are fundamental mechanisms that contribute to both normal and altered myocardial function (5–7). The ability to quantify β-

From: *Methods in Molecular Medicine, vol. 112: Molecular Cardiology: Methods and Protocols*
Edited by: Z. Sun © Humana Press Inc., Totowa, NJ

adrenergic receptor density through competitive ligand binding and to examine second-messenger activation through adenylyl cyclase activity is critical for understanding alterations in myocardial β-adrenergic function *(8,9)*. Moreover, the ability to measure the hemodynamic effects of altered β-adrenergic function in mouse models of hypertrophy and heart failure has provided a means to correlate the biochemical effects observed in vitro with the physiologic phenotype observed in vivo. This chapter outlines the methods necessary to detect alterations in the key components of receptor signaling: ligand binding to the β-adrenergic receptor; the resultant activation of second-messenger molecules in myocardial membrane preparations; and hemodynamic measurements of the β-adrenergic receptor system in hypertrophied myocardium.

2. Materials

2.1. Myocardial Membrane Preparation

1. Mouse left ventricle, flash frozen in liquid nitrogen.
2. Polytron PT1200 (Brinkman Instruments, Westbury, NY).
3. Homogenization buffer: 25 mM Tris-HCl, pH 7.4, 5 mM EDTA, 2 mg/mL leupeptin, 2 mg/mL aprotinin; should be made on the same day as needed and stored at 4°C (all reagents from Sigma).
4. Centrifuge (Sorvall or equivalent) and centrifuge tubes.
5. Membrane resuspension buffer: 75 mM Tris-HCl, pH 7.4, 4 mM EDTA, 12.5 mM MgCl$_2$; should be made on the same day as needed and stored at 4°C (all reagents from Sigma).
6. Protein quantification assay (Bio-Rad Dye-Binding Reagent).
7. Spectrophotometer.

2.2. β-Adrenergic Receptor Quantification

1. Myocardial membranes (*see* **Subheading 2.1.**), either prepared on the same day as assayed or from a –80°C sample (i.e., can use frozen membrane preparations).
2. Membrane resuspension buffer: 75 mM Tris-HCl, pH 7.4, 4 mM EDTA, 12.5 mM MgCl$_2$; store at 4°C (all reagents from Sigma).
3. [^{125}I]cyanopindolol ([^{125}I]CYP) (NEN).
4. Alprenolol stock: 1 mM in membrane resuspension buffer; prepare immediately prior to use (Sigma).
5. Propranolol stock: 1 mM in membrane resuspension buffer; prepare immediately prior to use (Sigma).
6. Glass fiber (GF/C) filters (Whatman International, Maidstone, UK).
7. Brandel Generic Rack, Semi-Automated 48 Sample Cell Harvester (Brandel, Gaithersburg, MD).
8. Binding buffer: 10 mM Tris-HCl, pH 7.4, 5 mM EDTA; store at 4°C (all reagents from Sigma).
9. γ-Counter (Packard, Downers Grove, IL).

2.3. Adenylyl Cyclase Assay

1. Myocardial membranes (*see* **Subheading 2.1.**): must be prepared fresh on the same day as assayed, cannot use frozen membrane preparations.
2. Poly-prep polypropylene chromatography columns (Bio-Rad).
3. Aluminum oxide resin (Sigma).
4. Membrane resuspension buffer: 75 mM Tris-HCl, pH 7.4, 4 mM EDTA, 12.5 mM MgCl$_2$; should be made on the same day as needed and stored at 4°C (all reagents from Sigma).
5. Cyclase mix: (per 10 mL vol in distilled H2O) 32.3 mg phospho(enol)pyruvate trisodium salt, 0.8 mg GTP, 2.5 mL of 1 mM cAMP, 20 µL of 150 mM ATP, 500 IU myokinase, 100 IU pyruvate kinase; aliquot cyclase mix into 0.5- and 1.0-mL samples and store at –80°C (all reagents from Sigma).
6. 50 µCi [α-^{32}P]ATP (Amersham).
7. Tracer stop solution: (per 1 L vol in distilled H2O) 200 mg ATP, 100 mg cAMP, 25 µCi [^{3}H]cAMP; this solution can be stored a 4°C for several weeks (ATP, cAMP from Sigma; [^{3}H]cAMP from Amersham).
8. 0.2 mg/mL Ascorbic acid (Sigma).
9. 500 µM Isoproterenol (this must be made immediately prior to use) (Sigma).
10. 50 mM Sodium fluoride (Sigma).
11. 100 mM Ammonium acetate, pH 7.0.: can be stored at room temperature for several weeks (Sigma).
12. Scintillation fluid (Lefkofluor, Research Products, Mount Prospect, IL).
13. Scintillation counter (Packard 1900TR liquid scintillation analyzer).
14. 2-mL Scintillation vials (VWR).
15. Water bath at 37°C with shaking.

2.4. Hemodynamic Measurements in Mice

1. Echocardiograph with high frequency transducer (available from several vendors, for example, Philips, Siemens, Visual Sonics).
2. Transgenic or wild-type mice.
3. 100 mg/kg Ketamine.
4. 2.5 mg/kg Xylazine.
5. Dissecting microscope (TZ 240, Nissho Optical, Tokyo, Japan) equipped with 150-W fiber-optic illuminator (Techni-Quip Corp, El Segundo, CA).
6. Rodent micro ventilator-minivent type 845 (Hugo Sachs Elect., March/ Hughsteten, Germany).
7. 1.4-Fr High-fidelity micromanometer catheter (Millar Instruments, Houston, TX).
8. PE50 catheter-fluid filled Statham pressure transducer and PC for digital recording.
9. Eight-channel chart recorder (Gould/Brush).
10. Isoproterenol (Sigma).

3. Methods

3.1. Preparation of Myocardial Membranes

Preparation of myocardial membranes is necessary for all the assays described in this chapter. All steps should be carried out in a 4°C cold room or with samples on ice unless otherwise indicated.

1. Place the left ventricle from a mouse (either freshly obtained or a frozen sample from a –80°C freezer) in a 14-mL disposable polypropylene tube (Falcon), and add ice-cold homogenization buffer (*see* **Subheading 2.1., item 3**) in a ratio of 1.5 mL buffer to 120–180 mg tissue.
2. Immediately homogenize the tissue on ice using a polytron tissue homogenizer (Brinkman, model PT1200, power level 5, continuous) until the tissue completely disappears. This step usually requires 1–3 min of homogenization on ice.
3. Incubate the sample on ice for 20 min.
4. Centrifuge the sample at $750g_{max}$ (2500 rpm in a Sorvall SS-34 rotor) for 5 min at 4°C.
5. Immediately remove the supernatant, and place it in a clean, ice-cold centrifugation tube and then centrifuge at $36,600g_{max}$ (17,500 rpm in a Sorvall SS-34 rotor) for 30 min at 4°C (*see* **Note 1**). After this step, a membrane pellet should be visible in the centrifugation tube.
6. Carefully decant the supernatant, and gently resuspend the pellet in approx 500 µL of membrane resuspension buffer (*see* **Subheading 2.1., item 5**) by repeated pipeting.
7. Once the pellet is resuspended, quantify the protein content using the Bio-Rad dye binding method (*see* **Subheading 2.1., item 6**).

The membrane preparation is diluted into membrane resuspension buffer to the desired protein concentration for enzymatic assays (*see* **Subheadings 3.2. and 3.3.**). If adenylyl cyclase assays are desired, then the freshly made myocardial membrane preparation must be used (*see* **Note 2**). β-Adrenergic receptor quantification can be performed with either fresh or frozen myocardial membrane preparations. The myocardial membranes can be stored at –80°C for future use.

3.2. β-Adrenergic Receptor Quantification Via Radioligand Binding Assays

The quantification of β-adrenergic receptor binding is based on the difference between the measurements of total membrane binding and nonspecific ligand binding (*see* **Note 3**). The assay can be conducted utilizing either freshly prepared or frozen membranes (*see* **Subheading 3.1.**).

1. Dilute the membrane preparation to a protein concentration of 1 mg/mL in membrane resuspension buffer (*see* **Subheading 2.2., item 2.**), and keep on ice until the assay is performed.
2. Label 12 × 75-mm polystyrene test tubes in triplicate for (1) total membrane binding, (2) nonspecific membrane binding, and (3) blank assay tubes; place on ice.

3. Add 360 µL of membrane binding buffer (*see* **Subheading 2.2., item 8**) to each total membrane binding assay tube, 340 µL of membrane binding buffer to each nonspecific binding tube, and 380 µL to each blank assay tube.
4. Add 20 µL of the membrane preparation to each total membrane binding and nonspecific binding assay tube. The blank tubes do not contain membrane preparations.
5. Next, add 20 µL of a 200 µM stock of alprenolol to the nonspecific binding assay tubes.
6. Finally, add 20 µL of radiolabeled [^{125}I]CYP (final concentration of 200 pM) to each tube.
7. Remove the tubes from the ice, and incubate in a 37°C water for 1 h.
8. After incubation, remove the tube from the 37°C water bath, and place on ice.
9. Quantification of [^{125}I]CYP bound to the membrane fractions is performed by measuring radioactivity retained on the glass fiber (GF/C) filter. A clean GF/C filter is placed in the Brandel sample harvester and then moistened with sterile water. The assay contents are applied to the filter, and unbound [^{125}I]CYP is removed by washing the filter with three applications of 5 mL of binding buffer (*see* **Subheading 2.2., item 8**). The GC/F filter is then removed and placed in an appropriate vial, and [^{125}I] is measured in a γ-counter (Packard or equivalent).

Receptor density is calculated based on the amount of radioactivity detected on the filter paper, the specific activity of the radiolabeled ligand (i.e., [^{125}I]CYP), and the amount of protein used in the assay. Typically, this is expressed as fmol/mg protein.

Table 1 lists the contents of the assay tubes

β-Adrenergic receptors are further quantified through the use of competitive binding assays to determine populations of receptors with high- and low-affinity binding. This is conducted in a similar manner as just described except different concentrations of isoproterenol are added to each binding assay. The final isoproterenol concentrations range from $10^{-12}\,M$ to $10^{-3}\,M$. The order of reagents added to each assay tube is important:

1. First, prepare the buffers as just described.
2. Label 12 × 75-mm polystyrene test tubes in triplicate for (1) total membrane binding, (2) nonspecific membrane binding, and (3) blank assay tubes; place on ice.
3. Add 140 µL of binding buffer to each assay tube.
4. Prepare isoproterenol concentrations in ascorbic acid by serially diluting to provide a final concentration range of $10^{-12}\,M$ to $10^{-3}\,M$.
5. Add 20 µL of the diluted isoproterenol concentration to each assay tube.
6. Add 20 µL of [^{125}I]CYP to all assay tubes to provide a final concentration of 80 pM.
7. Finally, add 20 µL of the membrane preparation to each assay tube.
8. Place the tubes in a 37°C water bath for 1 h.
9. After the reaction is complete, remove the tubes from the 37°C water bath, and place the tubes on ice.
10. Filter and quantify the reaction contents as just described using glass fiber (GF/C) filter via a Brandel sample harvester.

Table 1
Assay Contents for β-Adrenergic Receptor Binding

	Blank (μL)	Total membrane binding (μL)	Nonspecific membrane binding (μL)
Binding buffer	380	360	340
Membrane preparation	—	20	20
Alprenolol	—	—	20
[^{125}I]CYP	20	20	20

Table 2
Assay Contents for Adenylyl Cyclase Assays

	Baseline (μL)	Basal (μL)	Isoproterenol (10 μM final) (μL)	Sodium fluoride (10 mM final) (μL)
Ascorbic acid (0.2 mg/mL)	30	10	—	—
Cyclase mix ([α-^{32}P]ATP)	20	20	20	20
Myocardial membranes	—	20	20	20
500 μM Isoproterenol	—	—	10	—
50 mM Sodium fluoride	—	—	—	10

3.3. Measurement of Adenylyl Cyclase Activity in Myocardial Membranes

The measurement of adenylyl cyclase activity requires freshly prepared myocardial membranes. Several of the reagents must be prepared or dissolved in buffer immediately prior to use and as indicated below (*see* **Notes 4** and **5**). Myocardial membranes are assayed for basal adenylyl cyclase activity, isoproterenol-induced adenylyl cyclase activity, and sodium fluoride-induced adenylyl cyclase activity. The assay is conducted in triplicate in 12 × 75-mm borosilicate test tubes for each sample; therefore, for one myocardial membrane preparation there are triplicate assay tubes for basal, and isoproterenol-, and sodium fluoride-treated samples. Additionally, there are triplicate control assays in which no membranes are added so that a baseline level of radioactivity is obtained from the column (*see* **Note 6**).

The following is a sample of the assay tubes required for the measurement of adenylyl cyclase (*see* **Table 2**).

1. Prepare the aluminum columns by adding approx 760 mg of aluminum oxide to each Bio-Rad Poly-Prep column (or the equivalent). Place the columns in a plexiglas stand with a scintillation vial below each column to collect the eluant.

2. Thaw the cyclase mix either on ice or at 4°C. The cyclase mix is prepared prior to starting the assay, and aliquots of 0.5 and 1.0 mL are prepared and stored at −80°C prior to use.

3. Label the assay tubes for each membrane preparation as well as for a single triplicate set of assays conducted without the addition of membranes.

4. Prepare the following buffers:
   a. A 0.2 mg/mL solution of ascorbic acid (9.9 mg per 50 mL distilled water) is prepared and placed on ice.
   b. Isoproterenol and sodium fluoride are measured and placed into separate tubes.
   c. The isoproterenol (500 μM stock that provides a final concentration of 100 μM) and sodium fluoride (50 mM stock that provides a final concentration of 10 mM) are reconstituted in the ascorbic acid buffer immediately prior to use.

5. Thaw the [α-^{32}P]ATP, and add 50 μCi to 1 mL of cyclase mix.

6. Once all the buffers are prepared, place the assay tubes on ice, and add 20 μL of the membrane preparation to the basal, isoproterenol, and sodium fluoride assay tubes. The membrane preparation is sensitive to the shearing forces of pipeting; therefore, the ends of the pipet tips are cut prior to their use when one is pipeting the membrane fraction.

7. Add 20 μL of the ascorbic acid stock solution to the control tubes.

8. Add 20 μL of the cyclase mix that contains [α-^{32}P]ATP.

9. Add 10 μL of the ascorbic acid stock solution to the basal assay tube, 10 μL of the 500 μM isoproterenol stock solution to the isoproterenol assay tubes, and 10 μL of the 50 mM sodium fluoride stock solution to the sodium fluoride tubes.

10. Remove the tubes from the ice and place in a 37°C water bath with shaking for exactly 10 min.

11. Place the tubes on ice, and add 1 mL of the tracer stop solution to each tube (*see* **Note 7**).

12. Pour the contents of each assay tube onto individual aluminum columns, and allow the solution to drain from the resin into individual scintillation vials. This usually takes 10–15 min.

13. After the solution has drained from the column, add 4 mL of 100 mM ammonium acetate, pH 7.0, to each column, and collect the eluant in the same scintillation vial. This step usually takes 20–30 min.

14. After the resin has drained, properly discard the columns, and add 15 mL of Lefkofluor scintillation fluid to each scintillation vial, and cap tightly.

15. Label the vials, and place in a scintillation counter (Packard 1900TR liquid scintillation analyzer) for measurement of radioactivity.

Once the samples have been read by the scintillation counter, the baseline activity should be subtracted from the sample values, and the basal, isoproterenol-induced, and sodium fluoride-induced adenylyl cyclase activity can be calculated. Typically, the above membrane preparation and assay produces 30–40 pmol/mg/min activity in the basal samples, 60–80 pmol/mg/min activity in the isoproterenol-induced samples, and 180–240 pmol/mg/min in the sodium fluoride-induced samples. In other words, isoproterenol typically produces a

2.5-fold increase in adenylyl cyclase activity over basal levels, and sodium fluoride typically produces a five- to sixfold increase in adenylyl cyclase activity over basal levels.

3.4. Hemodynamic Measurements in Mice

3.4.1. Transthoracic Echocardiography

Transthoracic echocardiography is used to evaluate cardiac function in mice. We perform 2D guided M-mode echocardiography using an HDI 5000 echocardiograph (ATL, Bothell, WA). A number of echocardiograph machines from different manufacturers are now available providing excellent resolution of high-quality echocardiograms. A high frequency transducer with a wide bandwidth that can be shifted to carry frequencies of 9.0, 7.5, and 5.0 MHz is typically used. Optimal resolution and penetration with 2D and M-mode imaging is achieved with at least a 15-MHz frequency.

We study mice in the conscious state using gentle manual restraint following a period of acclimation. We place the mouse in a supine position and position the transducer on the left hemithorax. It is important to avoid excessive pressure when applying the transducer probe since excess pressure can induce bradycardia. First, we obtain a 2D parasternal short-axis imaging plane as a guide to assist in obtaining further images, and then we obtain a left-ventricular M-mode tracing close to the papillary muscle level using a sweep speed of 50 or 100 mm/s (**Fig. 1**).

We determine the heart rate from at least three consecutive RR intervals on the left-ventricular M-mode. The left ventricular end-diastolic diameter, left ventricular end systolic diameter, left ventricular posterior wall thickness, and intraventricular septal thickness are also calculated from the M-mode recording. We define end diastole as the maximal left ventricular diastolic dimension and end systole as the most anterior systolic excursion of the left ventricular posterior wall. All left ventricular dimension data are based on the average of three consecutive selected heart beats. We also define the fractional shortening of the left ventricle as a percentage change in left ventricular size:

Fractional shortening = 100 × [(left ventricular end-diastolic dimension] – [left ventricular end-systolic dimension])/(left ventricular end-diastolic dimension)

3.4.2. Invasive Hemodynamic Monitoring

Hemodynamic measurements in closed chest mice provide insight into the mechanisms of altered β-adrenergic signaling pathways.

1. In general, mice are anesthetized with a mixture of 100 mg/kg ketamine and 2.5 mg/kg xylazine ip.
2. Next, the mice undergo endotracheal intubation and are connected to a rodent ventilator.

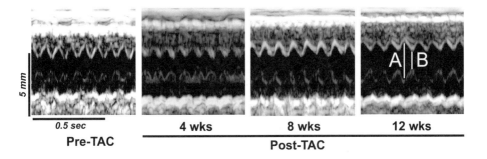

Fig. 1. Representative transthoracic echocardiograms from wild-type mouse after transverse aortic constriction (TAC). Left ventricular end-diastolic dimension (**A**) and left ventricular systolic dimension (**B**) are represented by arrows. (Adapted from **ref. *10*.**)

3. The mice are placed under a dissecting microscope, thoracetomy and bilateral vagotomy are performed.
4. A 1.4-Fr high-fidelity micromanometer catheter (Millar Instruments, Houston, TX) is inserted into the right carotid artery, advanced retrograde through the aortic valve, and secured in the left ventricle for continuous measurement of high-fidelity left ventricular pressure.
5. A flame-stretched PE50 fluid-filled catheter is placed in the left carotid artery or axillary artery for recording of blood pressure and into the right external jugular vein for injection of drugs.
6. The left ventricular pressure and fluid-filled (heparinized saline) aortic pressure are simultaneously recorded in a chart recorder and in digitized form at 2000 Hz for later analysis.
7. A PE50 catheter is inserted into the external jugular vein for drug infusion.
8. Hemodynamic measurements are recorded at baseline and 45–60 s after injection of incremental doses of agonist (usually 50–5000 pg of isoprotenol). Doses of isoproterenol are specifically chosen to maximize the contractile response but limit the increase in heart rate. Parameters that are measured consist of the heart rate, the left ventricular systolic and end-diastolic pressure, and the maximal and minimal first derivative of left ventricular pressure (LV dP/dt_{max} and LV dP/dt_{min}). Ten sequential beats should be averaged for each measurement.

4. Notes

1. The supernatant should be transferred by pipeting, not directly decanting, to minimize transfer of cellular debris from the $2500g_{max}$ pelleted material.
2. Freshly prepared myocardial membranes are required for the adenylyl cyclase activity assays. Membranes that have been prepared and flash frozen for storage cannot be used for measurements of adenylyl cyclase.
3. Binding assays are based on measurements of total radiolabeled ligand binding (i.e., [^{125}I]CYP binding alone) vs nonspecific radiolabeled ligand binding (i.e.,

[^{125}I]CYP in the presence of either alprenolol or propranolol) to myocardial membranes. The amount of β-adrenergic receptor binding is calculated by subtracting the measured nonspecific binding from the measured total binding.

4. Isoproterenol needs to be reconstituted in the ascorbic acid solution immediately prior to use and stored on ice. Additionally, the order of addition of the reagents to the assay is important. The ligands are added to the assay tubes first, and the myocardial membrane preparation should be added last.

5. We find it useful to prepare a stock of cyclase mix and store aliquots of the solution at –80°C for future use.

6. An orderly method to setup the cyclase assay is important. We always prepare the aluminum columns and assay tubes first. Then we prepare the myocardial membranes and thaw/prepare all assay buffers. The isoproterenol is reconstituted in ascorbic acid immediately prior to use.

7. The stop solution contains [^{3}H]cAMP and serves as a control for the separation of the cAMP product from the ATP starting material. A column efficiency value can be calculated by measuring tritium values in 1 mL of stop solution and comparing this value with the amount of tritium in each sample from the column elution. A typical ratio is 60–80% when the assay is performed correctly.

References

1. Lin, M. C., Rockman, H. A., and Chien, K. R. (1995) Heart and lung disease in engineered mice. *Nat. Med.* **8,** 749–751.

2. Prasad, S. V., Nienaber, J. and Rockman, H. A. (2002) G-protein-coupled receptor function in heart failure. *Cold Spring Harb. Symp. Quant. Biol.* **67,** 439–444.

3. Prasad, S. V., Perrino, C. and Rockman, H. A. (2003) Role of phosphoinositol 3-kinase in cardiac function and heart failure. *Trends Cardiovasc. Med.* **13,** 206–212.

4. LeCorvoisier, P., Park, H. Y., Carlson, K. M., Marchuk, D. A., and Rockman, H. A. (2003) Multiple quantitative trait loci modify the heart failure phenotype in murine cardiomyopathy. *Hum. Mol. Genet.* **12,** 3097–3107.

5. Cho, M. C., Rapacciuolo, A., Koch, W. J., Kobayashi, Y., Jones, L. R., and Rockman, H. A. (1999) Defective β-adrenergic receptor signaling precedes the development of dilated cardiomyopathy in transgenic mice with calsequestrin overexpression. *J. Biol. Chem.* **274,** 22,251–22,260.

6. Koch, W. J., Lefkowitz, R. J., and Rockman, H. A. (2002) Functional consequences of altered myocardial adrenergic signaling. *Annu. Rev. Physiol.* **62,** 237–260.

7. Rockman, H. A., Koch, W. J., and Lefkowitz R. J. (2002) Seven-transmembrane-spanning receptors and heart failure. *Nature* **415,** 206–212.

8. Salomon, Y., Londos, C., and Rodbell, M. (1974) A highly sensitive adenylate cyclase assay. *Anal. Biochem.* **58,** 541–548.

9. Johnson, R. A. and Solomon, Y. (1991) Assay of adenylyl cyclase catalytic activity. *Methods Enzymol.* **195,** 3–21.

10. Nienaber, J. J., Tachibana, H., Prasad, S. V., et al. (2003) Inhibition of receptor-localized PI3K preserves cardiac beta-adrenergic receptor function and ameliorates pressure overload heart failure. *J. Clin. Invest.* **112,** 1067–1079.

V

TRANSGENES IN CARDIOVASCULAR RESEARCH

24

Transgenic Mouse Models for Cardiac Dysfunction by a Specific Gene Manipulation

Gopal J. Babu and Muthu Periasamy

Summary

The sarcoplasmic reticulum Ca^{2+} ATPase (SERCA) plays a pivotal role in calcium cycling and the beat-to-beat function of the heart. Recent studies have shown that decreased expression and activity of SERCA are associated with end-stage heart failure in humans and in experimental animal models of heart failure. There has been considerable controversy over whether a decrease in SERCA level is a cause or effect of hypertrophy. To address directly whether alterations in SERCA levels modify calcium homeostasis and heart function, we have chosen to alter the SERCA protein expression genetically using transgenic and gene-targeted knockout mouse technology. This chapter describes the methodology for generation of mouse models that overexpress different SERCA isoforms and a SERCA2 knockout mouse model with decreased SERCA levels.

Key Words: SR Ca^{2+} ATPase; α-MHC promoter; transgenic; knockout; mouse; heart.

1. Introduction

The sarcoplasmic reticulum (SR) membrane network plays a central role in the beat-to-beat function of the heart by regulating the intracellular Ca^{2+} concentration (1–4). Release of Ca^{2+} from the SR initiates muscle contraction, whereas reuptake of Ca^{2+} by the SR results in muscle relaxation. The rate of muscle relaxation is primarily determined by the Ca^{2+} uptake function of a Ca^{2+} transport pump, the sarco(endo)plasmic reticulum Ca^{2+} ATPase (SERCA) (1–4). SERCA is a transmembrane protein of approx 110 kDa and belongs to a family of P-type ion pumps (2,5). SERCA protein isoforms are encoded by a

From: *Methods in Molecular Medicine, vol. 112: Molecular Cardiology: Methods and Protocols*
Edited by: Z. Sun © Humana Press Inc., Totowa, NJ

highly conserved family of genes; SERCA1, SERCA2, and SERCA3 *(6,7)*. The SERCA1 gene encodes two alternatively spliced transcripts, SERCA1a and SERCA1b, and is exclusively expressed in fast skeletal muscle. The SERCA2 gene encodes SERCA2a and SERCA2b isoforms, which differ only in the carboxyl terminus. SERCA2a has a short carboxyl terminus with four unique amino acids, whereas SERCA2b has 49 amino acids at the carboxyl terminus *(6,7)*. SERCA2a is the primary isoform expressed in the adult atria and ventricle *(8,9)*. SERCA3 is expressed in many tissues, but its cell-type distribution is quite limited *(7)*.

Studies have shown that alterations in SR function, including decreased SR Ca^{2+} store, slower Ca^{2+} release, elevated diastolic Ca^{2+}, and reduced rate of Ca^{2+} removal are hallmarks of the failing heart *(10,11)*. It has been documented that these changes are caused by reduced expression and activity of the SERCA pump. This phenomenon could account for diastolic dysfunction (increased diastolic calcium levels) and systolic dysfunction (decreased availability of SR calcium) and thereby contribute to the progression of heart failure *(10,11)*. To establish the role of SERCA unequivocally in cardiac dysfunction and heart failure, we chose to alter its expression (increased as well as decreased levels of SERCA pump) using transgenic mouse models. In this chapter, we describe the methods we have used to generate transgenic mouse models with altered SERCA pump levels.

2. Materials

1. α-Myosin heavy chain (α-MHC) vector *(12)*.
2. DH5α competent cells.
3. cDNAs for rat SERCA1a (Gene Bank accession no. M99223), rat SERCA2a (Gene Bank accession no. NM017290) and mouse SERCA2b (Gene Bank accession no. AJ131821).
4. Relevant restriction enzymes, ligase, and buffers (New England Biolabs).
5. Antibodies specific for SERCA1a, SERCA2a, and SERCA2b (gift from Dr. Frank Wuytack) and sarcomeric α-actin (Sigma).
6. Antirabbit and antimouse horseradish peroxidase (HRP)-conjugated secondary antibody.
7. QIAEX II gel extraction kit (Qiagen, cat. no. 20021).
8. Titanium Taq DNA polymerase (Clontech, cat. no. 8424).
9. RPA III kit (Ambion).
10. DNA elution buffer: 5 mM Tris-HCl, 0.1 mM EDTA, pH 7.4.
11. DNA extraction buffer: 50 mM Tris-HCl, 1.0 mM EDTA, pH 8.0, 0.5% Tween-20, and 20 μL of 10 mg/mL proteinase K.
12. Homogenizing buffer: 10 mM imidazole, pH 7.0, 300 mM sucrose, 1 mM dithiothretiol (DTT), 1 mM sodium metabisufite.
13. Tris-buffered saline (TBS): 50 mM Tris-HCl, pH 7.5, 0.3% NaCl.

14. Protein extraction buffer: 50 m*M* KPi, 10 m*M* NaF, 1 m*M* EDTA, 300 m*M* sucrose, 0.5 m*M* DTT, and 0.3 m*M* phenylmethylsulfonyl fluoride (PMSF).
15. Calcium uptake medium: 40 m*M* imidazole, pH 7.0, 100 m*M* KCl, 5 m*M* MgCl$_2$, 5m*M* NaN$_3$, 5 m*M* potassium oxalate, 0.5 m*M* EGTA.
16. SuperSignal West Dura substrate (Pierce, cat. no. 34075).
17. Nitrocellulose membrane.
18. Radioactive nucleotides.
19. Thermal cycler.
20. Core facilities to generate transgenic and knockout mice.
21. Equipment necessary for working heart preparations.

3. Methods
3.1. Generation of α-MHC–SERCA2 Gene Construct

1. The cardiac α-MHC promoter-based vector system, which has been used by several investigators *(12–17)*, was used to target the ectopic expression of SERCA isoforms in the heart muscle (*see* **Notes 1–4**).
2. DNA manipulations were performed by standard recombinant DNA techniques. The transgene construct is shown in **Fig. 1**.
3. cDNA specific for rat SERCA2a, mouse SERCA2b, or rat SERCA1a containing the entire coding sequence and the complete 3' untranslated region (UTR) was used to generate the transgene construct. The 5' UTR sequences were removed to provide efficient mRNA translation.
4. *Sal*I and *Hin*dIII linkers were added to 5' and 3' ends of the cDNA, respectively, to facilitate cloning into the a-MHC gene promoter at the *Sal*I and *Hin*dIII sites.
5. The ligated transgene construct (α-MHC–SERCA) was transformed into DH5α bacterial competent cells, and the colonies were selected on LB-ampicillin agar plates.
6. The recombinant transgene constructs were checked for the presence of the insert and for the correct orientation by DNA sequencing.

3.2. Generation of Transgenic Mice

1. The recombinant transgene (α-MHC–SERCA) construct was digested with *Not*I restriction enzyme to release the transgene from the plasmid vector.
2. The recombinant transgene construct was purified by the gel extraction method, using the QIAEX II gel purification kit, and eluted in DNA elution buffer. The final concentration of the purified fragment should be at least 5 ng/μL.
3. The purified recombinant transgene construct was injected into the male pronucleus of fertilized mouse oocytes derived from superovulated FVB/N females *(18)*.
4. The surviving embryos were implanted into the oviduct of pseudopregnant FVB/N females for the production of transgenic mice (*see* **Note 5**).
5. Transgenic founder mice were identified by polymerase chain reaction (PCR; *see* **Subheading 3.4.**) by screening 3-wk-old pups.
6. Transgenic colonies were expanded by breeding the transgenic males with FVB/N wild-type females (*see* **Notes 6** and **7**).

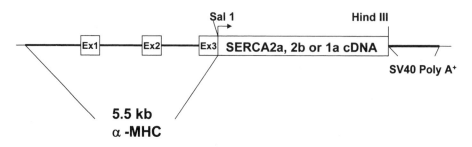

Fig. 1. Schematic representation of the α-MHC/SERCA transgene construct.

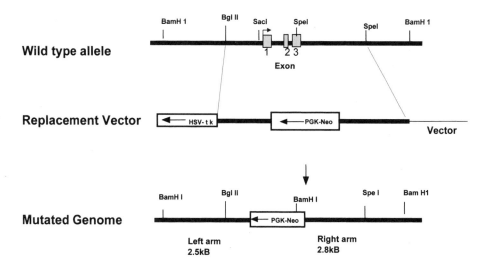

Fig. 2. Gene targeting strategy for the generation of SERCA2 knockout mice.

3.3. Generation of Knockout Animals

1. A genomic clone containing the 5' end of the SERCA2 gene was isolated from a phage library containing the 129/SvJ mouse genome and characterized by restriction mapping and sequence analysis *(19)*.
2. The plasmid vector pMJKO was used to generate the SERCA2 gene knockout targeting vector *(19)*.
3. To disrupt the SERCA2 gene, two restriction fragments, a *Bgl*II–*Sac*I fragment containing 2.5 kb of the 5' flanking sequence and terminating 53 bp 5' of the transcription start site and a 2.8-kb *Spe*I restriction fragment beginning in exon 3 and terminating in intron 3, were inserted on either side of the neomycin gene in the pMJKO vector by standard cloning techniques. The orientation of the neomycin gene was opposite that of the SERCA2 gene (*see* **Fig. 2** and **ref.** *19*).

4. The linearized construct was electroporated into mouse SvJ/129 embryonic stem cells and selected for neomycin resistance.

5. DNA from targeted ES cells were analyzed by Southern blot hybridization using probes from outside the region used to prepare the construct. The 3' probe was a 2.4-kb *Eco*RV–*Spe*I fragment from intron 3 that began 3.3 kb downstream from exon 3. The 5' probe was a 360-bp *Pst*I–*Eco*RI fragment beginning approx 3.6 kb upstream of the transcription initiation site.

6. Targeted clones were injected into blastocysts from C57BL/6 mice, and chimeric mice were identified by coat color.

7. Chimeric males were then mated to wild-type B6 females.

8. Germline transmission of the targeted allele to the pups was detected by Southern blot analysis as described above in **step 5** as well as by PCR analysis (*see* **Subheading 3.4.**).

9. The heterozygous mice identified by PCR were bred together to generate SERCA2 knockout animals

3.4. Genotyping

1. Transgenic mice were identified by PCR. Primers derived from the second intron of the α-MHC promoter (5'-GCCCACACCAGAAATGACAGA-3') and mouse SERCA2a cDNA exon (5'-TCACCTTCTTCGAACCAAGC-3') were used for SERCA2a or SERCA2b transgenic mice; primers derived from the second intron of the α-MHC promoter (5'-GCCCACACCAGA AATGACAGA-3') and primer complementary to rat SERCA1 cDNA (5'-TCGATGGCATTCTCTGCATTCC-3') were used for SERCA1a transgenic mouse.

2. SERCA2 knockout animals were identified by PCR analysis using a combination of three primers that amplify both wild-type and mutant alleles in the same reaction. The following primers were used:
   a. Primer 1 (5'-CGGCCTTCTAGAATTGCCGGCTG-3'), corresponding to genomic sequences near the 3' end of the *Sac*I–*Spe*I fragment that was deleted in the targeted allele.
   b. Primer 2 (5'-CTTACTAAAGATATACATGCTGCCAGCAG-3'), complementary to sequences just 3' to the *Spe*I site in exon 3 that was used to prepare the construct.
   c. Primer 3 (5'-CTGACTAGGGGAGGAGTAGAAGG-3'), corresponding to sequences in the promoter region of the neocassette.

3. Genomic DNA was extracted from tail biopsies by digesting the tail biopsies in DNA extraction buffer overnight at 55°C. Proteinase K was inactivated at 99°C for 5 min, and the samples were centrifuged at 10,000*g* for 5 min.

4. The supernatant was used for PCR assays. the PCR reaction was carried out in a 50 μL reaction vol containing 1 μL of tail DNA using Titanium Taq polymerase. PCR conditions used were: 35 cycles of denaturation at 94°C for 30 s, annealing for 30 s at 55°C, and extension for 1 min at 72°C.

3.5. Determination of Transgene Copy Numbers

1. The copy number of the transgene in each transgenic line was determined by Southern blot analysis.
2. About 10 μg of genomic DNA prepared from tail biopsies was digested with *Eco*RI, electrophoresed on a 0.7% agarose gel, and transferred to a nitrocellulose membrane using a standard Southern blot technique.
3. The blots were hybridized with the [α-^{32}P]dCTP-labeled *Nde*I-to-*Sal*I fragment of the mouse α-MHC promoter.
4. DNA from nontransgenic tails gave a 3.0-kb endogenous band, whereas transgenic samples gave 3.0- and 2.7-kb bands.
5. Intensities of the transgene band were compared with the endogenous band to determine copy number.

3.6. RNAse Protection Analysis

1. RNAse protection analysis was carried out to quantitate the transgene expression (*see* **Note 8**).
2. The mouse SERCA2 riboprobe consisted of a 451-bp genomic *Not*I–*Xho*I fragment containing 278 bp of exon 1 and 173 bp of intron 1 that can differentiate endogenous SERCA2, and a rat SERCA2a transgene was used for SERCA2a transgenic mice (**Fig. 3**).
3. The SERCA2b-specific riboprobe contains the last 45 bp of exon 22 and 123 bp of exon 23, and the SERCA1 riboprobe spanned from +16 bp to +162 bp relative to the start codon of SERCA1a cDNA. The mouse glyceraldehyde-3-phosphate dehydrogenase (GAPDH) riboprobe corresponds to –46 bp to +179 bp relative to the start codon.
4. To synthesize RNA probes specific for mouse SERCA2, SERCA2b or SERCA1a DNA were cloned into pBluescript SK$^+$II. [^{32}P]UTP-labeled riboprobes were synthesized from linearized recombinant plasmid using T7 RNA polymerase (Maxiscript, Ambion).
5. Total RNA (5 μg) purified from the ventricles of transgenic and nontransgenic littermate mice was hybridized simultaneously with RNA probes specific for SERCA2, SERCA2b, or SERCA1a and GAPDH.
6. After digestion with RNAse T1 and RNAse A (RPA III, Ambion), the protected fragments were separated by electrophoresis on a 5% denaturing polyacrylamide gel and analyzed by autoradiography.

3.7. Western Blot Analysis

1. Whole mouse heart homogenates were used to determine SERCA protein levels in the transgenic and knockout hearts.
2. Tissues were excised, placed in liquid N_2, and powdered. The powdered samples were resuspended in 8 vol of homogenization buffer, homogenized using a blender, and incubated on ice for 30 min. Protein concentrations were determined by the Bradford method using bovine serum albumin as standard.

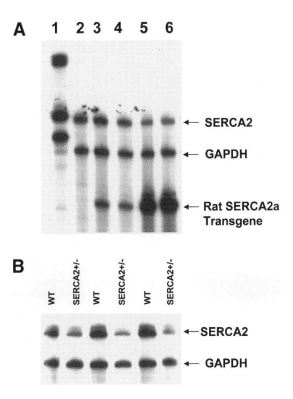

Fig. 3. RNAse protection analysis. **(A)** RNAse protection analysis of SERCA2 mRNA expression in SERCA2a transgenic hearts. Lane 1, mRNA marker; lane 2, RNA from nontransgenic mouse heart; lanes 3–6, RNA from SERCA2a Transgenic mice hearts. Lane 3 and 4 indicate the low-copy numbers, and lanes 5 and 6 indicate the high-copy numbers. **(B)** RNAse protection analysis of SERCA2 mRNA expression in SERCA2$^{+/-}$ knockout hearts. Note that RNA levels for SERCA2 are reduced to approx 50% in the heterozygous (SERCA2$^{+/-}$) knockout mice hearts.

3. Three different concentrations (1, 2, and 3 µg) of the total homogenate from control and transgenic hearts were separated on 8% sodium dodecyl sulfate (SDS)-polyacrylamide gel and blotted on to 0.22-µm nitrocellulose membrane by standard Western blot techniques.

4. The filters were blocked with 5% milk powder in TBS for 2 h and probed with rabbit antibody specific for SERCA2a, SERCA2b, or SERCA1 (**Fig. 4**) and mouse monoclonal sarcomeric α-actin antibody (1:5000 dilutions). After incubation with primary antibody for 2 h, the membranes were washed thoroughly with TBS containing 0.05% Tween-20 and then incubated with HRP-conjugated secondary antibody for 30 min.

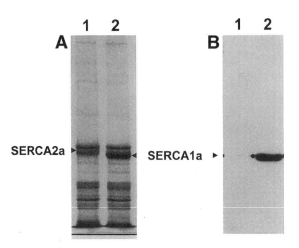

Fig. 4. Western blot analysis of SERCA1a expression. Equal amounts of total protein isolated from nontransgenic and SERCA1a transgenic hearts were resolved on an 8% SDS-PAGE and stained with Coomassie blue **(A)** or transferred to nitrocellulose membrane and immunoblotted with SERCA1a-specific antibody **(B)**. Lane 1, nontransgenic heart; lane 2, SERCA1a transgenic heart.

5. The membranes were washed for 1 h with TBS containing 0.05% Tween-20 and developed using SuperSignal West Dura substrate. The signals were captured using the UV-P Biochemi system and quantitated. The values were normalized to sarcomeric α-actin levels (*see* **Note 8**).

3.8. Calcium Uptake Assays

1. Whole heart tissues were homogenized in 8 vol of protein extraction buffer, and calcium uptake was measured by a Millipore filtration technique.
2. Cardiac homogenates (150 μg) from control and transgenic animals were incubated at 37°C in a 1.5-mL calcium uptake medium and various concentrations of $CaCl_2$ to yield 0.03–3 μmol/L free Ca^{2+} (containing 1 μCi/μmol $^{45}Ca^{2+}$).
3. To obtain the maximal stimulation of SR Ca^{2+} uptake, 1 μ*M* of ruthenium red was added immediately prior to the addition of the substrates to begin the calcium uptake.
4. The reaction was initiated by the addition of 5 m*M* ATP and terminated at 0.5, 1.0, and 1.5 min by filtration. The rate of Ca^{2+} uptake was calculated from linear regression analysis of Ca^{2+} uptake values determined at 30, 60, and 90 s. The results were analyzed using the MicroCal Origin Software.

3.9. Measurements of Cardiac Contractile Parameters (Work-Performing Heart Preparations)

1. The work-performing heart preparations have been described in detail in our previous publications (*20–22*). Age-matched transgenic and nontransgenic mice (12-

to 16-wk-old) were used. ECG and heart rates were recorded before opening of the chest and removal of the heart. The optimal venous return and the afterload required to maintain constant function of the hearts were 5 mL/min cardiac output and 50 mmHg aortic pressure, respectively, providing a basal workload of 250 mL × mmHg/min.

2. Heart rate, aortic pressure, left intraventricular pressure (IVP; systolic, diastolic, and end-diastolic), and atrial pressure were monitored continuously. The first derivative of IVP (+dP/dt and -dP/dt), the time to peak pressure (TPP)/mmHg, and the time to half-relaxation $(RT_{1/2})$/mmHg were calculated with a custom-designed computer program.

3. Venous return (equal to cardiac output) and aortic flows were measured continuously with a Dual Channel Transonic Flowmeter. Coronary flow was computer calculated as venous return–aortic flow.

3.10. Highlights of the Results Obtained With the SERCA Transgenic and Knockout Mouse Models

1. We have successfully generated transgenic mouse models that overexpress SERCA2a, SERCA2b, or SERCA1a isoforms in the heart muscle *(20,23,24)*.

2. For SERCA2a overexpression, we have obtained two independent lines that showed a four- to eightfold increase in SERCA2a mRNA levels; the protein level was increased to 30–50%. Maximal velocity of SR Ca^{2+} uptake was increased by approx 37%. Studies using isolated work-performing hearts showed increased rates of contraction and relaxation *(20)*.

3. In the SERCA2b-overexpressing mice, the SERCA2b mRNA level was approx 20-fold higher than the control animals, and the protein was increased 8- to 10-fold. The maximal velocity of SR Ca^{2+} uptake was not changed, but the apparent pump affinity for Ca^{2+} was increased. Work-performing heart preparations showed that SERCA2b transgenic hearts had higher rates of contraction–relaxation and shorter time to peak pressure and half-time for relaxation than control hearts *(23)*.

4. Overexpression of SERCA1a in the hearts resulted in an approx 2.5-fold increase in SERCA protein levels. Interestingly, SERCA2a levels decreased to approx 50% in the SERCA1a transgenic hearts. The maximal velocity of Ca^{2+} uptake and the steady-state level of SERCA phosphoenzyme intermediate were significantly higher in the transgenic hearts. Functional analysis revealed that rates of contraction–relaxation were significantly higher. Our studies also demonstrate that SERCA1a can functionally substitute for endogenous SERCA2a *(21,24,25)*.

5. Disruption of both copies of the SERCA2 gene is lethal, whereas heterozygous mice with one functional allele are alive and reproduce well. SERCA2a protein levels and the maximal velocity of SR Ca^{2+} uptake were reduced by approx 35%. Measurements of in vivo cardiac function revealed reductions in heart rate, mean arterial pressure, systolic ventricular pressure, and maximal rates ofboth contraction and relaxation. However, SERCA2 heterozygous mice did not develop cardiac pathology, contrary to expectations *(19,22,26)*.

6. Studies using these transgenic animal models suggest that there is a clear correlation between SERCA pump level and the contractile state of the heart.

4. Notes

1. The α-MHC promoter construct has been proved highly effective in cardiac-specific expression of genes. However, other promoter constructs like the ventricular-specific myosin light chain 2 promoter can also be used to generate transgenic mice *(27–29)*.

2. The temporal regulation of transgene expression might prevent investigation of a number of important questions because of a lack of its expression during development and other compensatory alterations. These limitations can be overcome by *conditional* transgenic systems that allow control of the timing as well as the spatial pattern of gene expression. Transgenic mice models with tetracycline-controlled cardiac-specific gene expression using the α-MHC promoter *(30,31)* can also be utilized to overexpress SERCA isoforms.

3. Recently Molkentin and his group developed a MerCreMer transgenic mouse model *(32)* that will permit temporally regulated activation of a properly designed transgene or inactivation of a loxP-targeted genetic locus within the heart. Generation of conditional gene overexpression *(33)* or a knockout mouse model for SERCA will further dissect the function of SERCA within either the developing or adult heart.

4. Alternatively, recombinant adenoviral vectors can also be effectively used to express SERCA pumps in the heart *(34–37)*.

5. Transgenic and knockout mice were generated with the help of the transgenic and gene targeting core facilities at the University of Cincinnati College of Medicine.

6. FVB/N is the murine strain of choice for the generation of transgenic animals; the B6D2/F1 strain has also been used.

7. It is better to avoid crossbreeding the littermates. The transgenic mice should be regularly crossed with outbred wild-type mice to avoid genetic drift, which may cause many compensatory alterations.

8. Some of the techniques like Western blotting and RNAse protection analysis have to be standardized for each antibody and riboprobe.

Acknowledgment

This work was supported by NIH grant HL 64140.

References

1. Bers, D. M. and Perez-Reyes, E. (1999) Ca channels in cardiac myocytes: structure and function in Ca influx and intracellular Ca release. *Cardiovasc. Res.* **42,** 339–360.

2. Stokes, D. L. and Wagenknecht, T. (2000) Calcium transport across the sarcoplasmic reticulum: structure and function of Ca2+-ATPase and the ryanodine receptor. *Eur. J. Biochem.* **267,** 5274–5279.

3. Periasamy, M. and Huke, S. (2001) SERCA pump level is a critical determinant of Ca(2+)homeostasis and cardiac contractility. *J. Mol. Cell. Cardiol.* **33,** 1053–1063.

4. Frank, K. F., Bolck. B., Erdmann, E., and Schwinger R. H (2003) Sarcoplasmic reticulum Ca2+-ATPase modulates cardiac contraction and relaxation. *Cardiovasc. Res.* **57**, 20–27.

5. MacLennan, D. H., Abu-Abed, M., and Kang, C. (2002) Structure-function relationships in Ca(2+) cycling proteins. *J. Mol. Cell. Cardiol.* **34**, 897–918.

6. Loukianov, E., Ji, Y., Baker, D. L., et al. (1998) Sarco(endo)plasmic reticulum Ca2+ ATPase isoforms and their role in muscle physiology and pathology. *Ann. NY Acad. Sci.* **853**, 251–259.

7. Shull, G. E. (2000) Gene knockout studies of Ca2+-transporting ATPases. *Eur. J. Biochem.* **267**, 5284–5290.

8. Luss, I., Boknik, P., Jones, L. R., et al. (1999) Expression of cardiac calcium regulatory proteins in atrium v ventricle in different species. *J. Mol. Cell. Cardiol.* **31**, 1299–1314.

9. Reed, T. D., Babu, G. J., Ji, Y., et al. (2000) The expression of SR calcium transport ATPase and the Na(+)/Ca(2+)exchanger are antithetically regulated during mouse cardiac development and in hypo/hyperthyroidism. *J. Mol. Cell. Cardiol.* **32**, 453–464.

10. Arai, M., Matsui, H., and Periasamy, M. (1994) Sarcoplasmic reticulum gene expression in cardiac hypertrophy and heart failure. *Circ. Res.* **74**, 555–564.

11. Houser, S. R., Piacentino, V. 3rd, and Weisser, J. (2000) Abnormalities of calcium cycling in the hypertrophied and failing heart. *J. Mol. Cell. Cardiol.* **32**, 1595–1607.

12. Subramaniam, A., Jones, W. K., Gulick, J., Wert, S., Neumann, J., and Robbins, J. (1991) Tissue-specific regulation of the alpha-myosin heavy chain gene promoter in transgenic mice. *J. Biol. Chem.* **266**, 24,613–24,620.

13. Chu, G., Dorn, G. W. 2nd, Luo, W., et al. (1997) Monomeric phospholamban overexpression in transgenic mouse hearts. *Circ. Res.* **81**, 485–492.

14. James, J., Zhang, Y., Osinska, H., et al. (2000) Transgenic modeling of a cardiac troponin I mutation linked to familial hypertrophic cardiomyopathy. *Circ. Res.* **87**, 805–811.

15. Bueno, O. F., De Windt, L. J., Tymitz, K. M., et al. (2000) The MEK1-ERK1/2 signaling pathway promotes compensated cardiac hypertrophy in transgenic mice. *EMBO J.* **19**, 6341–6350.

16. Yang, Q., Osinska, H., Klevitsky, R., and Robbins, J. (2001) Phenotypic deficits in mice expressing a myosin binding protein C lacking the titin and myosin binding domains. *J. Mol. Cell. Cardiol.* **33**, 1649–1658.

17. Prabhakar, R., Boivin, G. P., Grupp, I. L., et al. (2001) A familial hypertrophic cardiomyopathy alpha-tropomyosin mutation causes severe cardiac hypertrophy and death in mice. *J. Mol. Cell. Cardiol.* **33**, 1815–1828.

18. Hogan, B., Constantini, F., and Lacy, E. (1986) *Manipulating the Mouse Embryo: A Laboratory Manual*, Cold Spring Harbor laboratory, Cold Spring Harbor, NY, pp. 79–173.

19. Periasamy, M., Reed, T. D., Liu, L. H., et al. (1999) Impaired cardiac performance in heterozygous mice with a null mutation in the sarco(endo)plasmic reticulum Ca2+-ATPase isoform 2 (SERCA2) gene. *J. Biol. Chem.* **274**, 2556–2562.

20. Baker, D. L., Hashimoto, K., Grupp, I. L., et al. (1998) Targeted overexpression of the sarcoplasmic reticulum Ca2+-ATPase increases cardiac contractility in transgenic mouse hearts. *Circ. Res.* **83,** 1205–1214.

21. Huke, S., Prasad, V., Nieman, M. L., et al. (2002) Altered dose response to beta-agonists in SERCA1a-expressing hearts ex vivo and in vivo. *Am. J. Physiol. Heart Circ. Physiol.* 283, H958–H965.

22. Huke, S., Liu, L. H., Biniakiewicz, D., Abraham, W. T., and Periasamy, M. (2003) Altered force-frequency response in non-failing hearts with decreased SERCA pump-level. *Cardiovas. Res.* **59,** 668–677.

23. Greene, A. L., Lalli, M. J., Ji, Y., Babu, G. J., Grupp, I., Sussman, M., and Periasamy M. (2000) Overexpression of SERCA2b in the heart leads to an increase in sarcoplasmic reticulum calcium transport function and increased cardiac contractility. *J. Biol. Chem.* **275,** 24,722–24,727.

24. Loukianov, E., Ji, Y., Grupp, I. L., Kirkpatrick, D. L., et al. (1998) Enhanced myocardial contractility and increased Ca2+ transport function in transgenic hearts expressing the fast-twitch skeletal muscle sarcoplasmic reticulum Ca2+-ATPase. *Circ. Res.* **83,** 889–897.

25. Ji, Y., Loukianov, E., Loukianova, T., Jones, L. R., and Periasamy, M. (1999) SERCA1a can functionally substitute for SERCA2a in the heart. *Am. J. Physiol* **276,** H89–H97.

26. Ji, Y., Lalli, M. J., Babu, G. J., et al. (2000) Disruption of a single copy of the SERCA2 gene results in altered Ca2+ homeostasis and cardiomyocyte function. *J. Biol. Chem.* **275,** 38,073–38,080.

27. Franz, W. M., Breves, D., Klingel, K., Brem, G., Hofschneider, P. H., and Kandolf, R. (1993) Heart-specific targeting of firefly luciferase by the myosin light chain-2 promoter and developmental regulation in transgenic mice. *Circ. Res.* **73,** 629–638.

28. Wessely, R., Klingel, K., Santana, L. F., et al. (1998) Transgenic expression of replication-restricted enteroviral genomes in heart muscle induces defective excitation-contraction coupling and dilated cardiomyopathy. *J. Clin. Invest.* **102,** 1444–1453.

29. Yan, X., Price, R. L., Nakayama, M., et al. (2003) Ventricular-specific expression of angiotensin II type 2 receptor causes dilated cardiomyopathy and heart failure in transgenic mice. *Am. J. Physiol. Heart. Circ. Physiol.* **285,** H2179–H2187.

30. Passman, R. S. and Fishman, G. I. (1994) Regulated expression of foreign genes in vivo after germline transfer. *J. Clin. Invest.* **94,** 2421–2425.

31. Sanbe, A., Gulick, J., Hanks, M. C., Liang, Q., Osinska, H., and Robbins, J. (2003) Reengineering inducible cardiac-specific transgenesis with an attenuated myosin heavy chain promoter. *Circ. Res.* **92,** 609–616.

32. Sohal, D. S., Nghiem, M., Crackower, M. A., et al. (2001) Temporally regulated and tissue-specific gene manipulations in the adult and embryonic heart using a tamoxifen-inducible Cre protein. *Circ. Res.* **89,** 20–25.

33. Petrich, B. G., Molkentin, J. D., and Wang, Y. (2003) Temporal activation of c-Jun N-terminal kinase in adult transgenic heart via cre-loxP-mediated DNA recombination. *FASEB J.* **17,** 749–751.

34. Hajjar, R. J., Kang, J. X., Gwathmey, J. K., and Rosenzweig, A. (1997) Physiological effects of adenoviral gene transfer of sarcoplasmic reticulum calcium ATPase in isolated rat myocytes. *Circulation.* **95,** 423–429.

35. Hajjar, R. J., Schmidt, U., Kang, J. X., Matsui, T., and Rosenzweig, A. (1997) Adenoviral gene transfer of phospholamban in isolated rat cardiomyocytes. Rescue effects by concomitant gene transfer of sarcoplasmic reticulum Ca(2+)-ATPase. *Circ. Res.* **81,** 145–153.

36. Chossat, N., Griscelli, F., Jourdon, P., et al. (2001) Adenoviral SERCA1a gene transfer to adult rat ventricular myocytes induces physiological changes in calcium handling. *Cardiovasc. Res.* **49,** 288–297.

37. Periasamy, M. (2001) Adenoviral-mediated serca gene transfer into cardiac myocytes: how much is too much? *Circ. Res* **88,** 373–375.

25

Cardiomyocyte Defects in Diabetic Models and Protection With Cardiac-Targeted Transgenes

Xia Shen, Gang Ye, Naira S. Metreveli, and Paul N. Epstein

Summary

Diabetic cardiomyopathy is a common chronic complication leading to heightened risk of heart failure among diabetic patients. In this chapter, we describe the methods for maintenance and breeding of two diabetic animal models, OVE26 and Agouti mice, for type 1 and type 2 diabetes, respectively. To understand the pathological mechanism, antioxidants such as manganese superoxide dismutase are overexpressed specifically in hearts of diabetic mice. Methods utilized to produce cardiac-targeted transgenic mice are presented in this chapter. Diabetic cardiomyopathy is evaluated in control, diabetic and transgene-protected diabetic animals by measuring contractility of isolated cardiomyocytes. Preparation and contractile analysis of cardiac myocytes are described in detail. Diabetic cardiomyocytes exhibit impaired contractility as well as delayed relaxation, and cardiac-overexpressed antioxidant transgenes are shown to reverse this damage.

Key Words: Diabetes; diabetic cardiomyopathy; transgenic mouse; cardiac-specific transgene; cardiomyocyte; contractility.

1. Introduction

The risk of heart failure is increased twofold among diabetic men and fivefold among diabetic women *(1)*. This heart failure is caused at least partly to a cardiomyopathy affecting diabetic cardiomyocytes. Diabetic cardiomyopathy, like other diabetic complications, develops after months to years of diabetes. To study this disease process in animal models, it is necessary to maintain animals with long-term diabetes. We use inbred strains of mice with transgenic or natural genetic mutations that cause type 1 or type 2 diabetes. This provides early-onset, severe, and consistent diabetes free from the toxic side effects that

From: *Methods in Molecular Medicine, vol. 112: Molecular Cardiology: Methods and Protocols*
Edited by: Z. Sun © Humana Press Inc., Totowa, NJ

occur when toxins such as streptozotocin are used to induce diabetes. To develop treatments that can prevent diabetic cardiomyopathy, it is essential to provide protective methods that are permanent, stable, and reproducible. Transgenic mice are an optimal means to this goal. Transgenes are active from an early age. They can produce high-level expression, and their activities are stable and almost identical from animal to animal in the same line. It is also important to target transgene expression to cardiomyocytes. Otherwise it is impossible to discern whether favorable treatment outcomes are owing to alterations in the cardiovascular system that originate outside of the heart. Fortunately, cardiac-specific promoters such as the α-myosin heavy chain (α-MHC) promoter make it easy to produce cardiac-specific expression.

Evaluation of diabetic cardiomyopathy and the protective effects of treatment is performed on cardiomyocytes isolated from diabetic mice. Diabetic cardiomyocytes exhibit impaired contractility and delayed relaxation. Overexpression of antioxidants in the diabetic heart was able to prevent this damage. We have found that isolated myocytes provide a more sensitive indication of diabetic damage than whole heart assays.

2. Materials

2.1. Genetic Models of Diabetes

1. Heterozygous OVE26 mice on the FVB background (*see* **Note 1**).
2. Heterozygous agouti mice on the KK background (Jackson Laboratories; *see* **Notes 2** and **3**).
3. Fast Take Glucometer (Lifescan).

2.2. Genetic Models Potentially Protective From Diabetic Cardiomyopathy

In our laboratory we use MyMT, MyMC, MySOD, and MyHX transgenic mice on the FVB background that overexpress metallothionein, catalase, manganese superoxide dismutase (MnSOD), or hexokinase, respectively. Each transgene uses the α-MHC promoter to produce cardiomyocyte-specific high-level expression (*see* **Note 4**).

2.3. Production of Cardiac-Specific Transgenic Mice

1. cDNA or gene of choice.
2. MyADH or other plasmid containing mouse α-MHC promoter.
3. Primers for polymerase chain reaction (PCR) amplification of cDNA or gene.
4. Restriction enzymes *Eco*RI, *Hin*dIII, *Sal*I, and *Not*I.
5. Agarose gels in Tris/acetate/EDTA buffer containing 0.5 µg/mL ethidium bromide.
6. StrataPrep DNA gel extraction kit (Stratagene).
7. Bio-spin 6 spin chromatography columns (Bio-Rad).

8. Molecular mass markers (Gibco-BRL).
9. Minigel apparatus.
10. LB agar and LB media containing 100 μg/mL ampicillin.
11. Epicurian Coli XL1-blue competent cells (Stratagene).
12. DNeasy tissue kit (Qiagen).

2.4. Preparation and Culture of Cardiac Myocytes

1. Basic buffer: 135 mM NaCl, 4 mM KCl, 1 mM MgCl$_2$, 10 mM HEPES, 0.33 mM NaH$_2$PO$_4$, pH 7.4.
2. Perfusion buffer: 10 mM glucose, 20 mM butanedione monoxime (BDM), pH 7.4, in basic buffer (glucose and BDM added on the day of use), bubbled with 95% O$_2$ and 5% CO$_2$.
3. Digestion buffer: 0.5 mL of 10 mg/mL liberase blendzyme 4 (Roche, Indianapolis, IN) in 15 mL perfusion buffer.
4. Ketamine HCl/xylazine HCl solution (Sigma).
5. Water bath heating circulator.
6. Water-jacketed heat exchange glass coil.
7. Peristaltic pump.
8. Fine scissors.
9. Two fine forceps.
10. 6-0 Silk thread.
11. 95% O$_2$ and 5% CO$_2$.

2.5. Contractile Analysis of Cardiac Myocytes

1. Contractility buffer: 135 mM NaCl, 4 mM KCl, 1 mM MgCl$_2$, 10 mM HEPES, 0.33 mM NaH$_2$PO$_4$, 10 mM glucose, 10 mM 2,3 butanedione monoxime (BDM), 1.2 mM CaCl$_2$.
2. Teflon glass cover slip plate (Harvard Apparatus, Holliston, MA).
3. Platinum electrodes.
4. Myopacer field stimulator (Ionoptix, Milton, MA).
5. Inverted microscope (Olympus, IX-70) equipped with 10× and 40× objectives.
6. MyoCam camera (Ionoptix) connected to computer.
7. Computer running Soft-Edge software (Ionoptix).

3. Methods

The following sections describe: (1) maintaining diabetic lines of mice, (2) production of a cardiac-specific protective transgene, (3) breeding of diabetic mice to cardiac transgenic mice, (4) isolation of mouse cardiac myocytes, and (5) analysis of myocyte contractility in control, diabetic, and transgene protected mice.

3.1. Maintaining Diabetic Lines of Mice

We maintain all our diabetic strains in force-ventilated HEPA filtered racks, usually one breeding pair per cage. Bedding for diabetic cages should be changed daily. Animals have continuous access to water and standard rodent Lab Chow. Heterozygous OVE26 diabetic mice are maintained by continuous breeding of female FVB mice to male OVE26 mice (*see* **Note 5**). The OVE26 male mice are most fertile from 45 to 130 d of age but may maintain fertility for up to 200 d of age. OVE26 positive offspring are recognized by the presence of small eyes owing to the cointegration of the GR19 gene *(2)*, which is expressed in the eye. Agouti mice are maintained on the KK background by breeding male agouti mice to nondiabetic KK females. Agouti-positive mice are readily recognized by their obvious brownish coat color.

No attempt is made to time estrus during breeding. Since females generally reenter estrus immediately after giving birth, it is advantageous to keep males and females together for maximal production of offspring. It is essential to wean the older litter before the birth of a second litter.

3.2. Production of a Cardiac-Specific Protective Transgene

3.2.1. Production of Cardiac-Specific MnSOD Transgene

As an example of transgene construction, we show our methods for developing the MnSOD cardiac-specific transgene (**Fig. 1**) regulated by the mouse α-MHC promoter (kindly provided to us by Dr. Jeff Robbins). This method is similar to what we have used successfully for seven other transgenes derived from cDNA or genomic sequences of yeast and mammalian origin. It can be readily applied to any gene of interest.

1. Human MnSOD sequences were obtained from the plasmid InSOD (manuscript in preparation) that we used for expression of MnSOD in pancreatic β-cells. The 830 bp of MnSOD coding sequences were originally derived from plasmid phMnSOD4 (from American Type Culture Collection) *(3)*.
2. The MnSOD cDNA was inserted between the α-MHC fragment, containing the promoter and parts of the first three exons, and the polyadenylation region of the rat insulin II gene (**Fig. 1**). Construction was accomplished by removal of the insert of MyADH *(4)* with *Sal*I and *Hin*dIII, followed by blunt-ending these termini with the Klenow fragment of DNA polymerase I.
3. Excess nucleotides were removed on a Bio-spin 6 chromatography column followed by treatment with calf intestinal phosphatase (CIP) to eliminate terminal phosphates. Then 1 µg of this fragment was purified on a 0.7% agarose gel.
4. Next, 1 µg of the blunt-ended MnSOD cDNA fragment was obtained by cleavage of InSOD with *Eco*RI and treatment with the Klenow fragment of DNA polymerase I. This fragment was purified on a 0.7% agarose gel.
5. Fifty nanograms each of the vector and insert were ligated at 15°C for 16 h in a total volume of 10 µL with 2000 U of T4 DNA ligase.
6. Then 2 µL of the ligation reaction were used to transform 50 µL of Epicurian Coli XL1-blue competent cells and plated on LB agar plates containing 100 µg/mL ampicillin. Plasmids were isolated from single colonies.

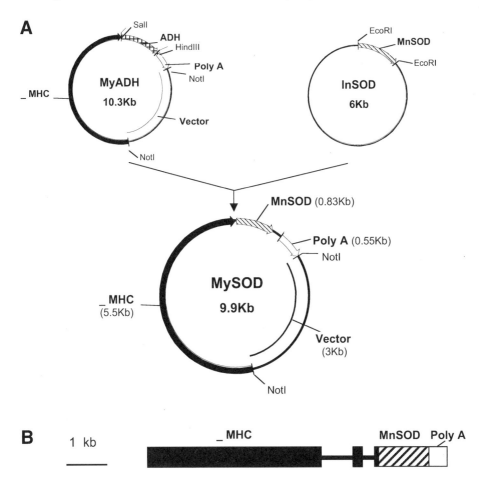

Fig. 1. Construction of the MySOD transgene. (**A**) Preparation of plasmid MySOD from fragments of plasmids MyADH and InSOD, by procedures described in the text. Relevant DNA fragments and restriction sites are shown. (**B**) Map of MySOD transgene. The black boxes on the left indicate 5.5 kb of the murine α-MHC promoter and all of the noncoding portions of the first three exons of the α-MHC gene. The polyadenylation portion of the rat insulin II gene is indicated by the open box at the right. The MnSOD cDNA is indicated by the hatched box.

7. Correct construction and orientation of the MnSOD clone with the myosin promoter was determined by restriction enzyme digestion and verified by sequencing across the ligated regions.

3.2.2. Production of MnSOD Transgenic Mouse

Before embryo microinjection, 20 µg of MySOD was digested with *Not*I, and the plasmid-free transgene was purified on a 0.5% Seakem Gold agarose gel.

The fragment was purified with the StrataPrep DNA gel extraction kit and then passed through a Bio-spin 6 chromatography column prior to microinjection.

The procedures we use for embryo microinjection and embryo implantation are standard for production of transgenic mice *(5)* and are widely performed in commercial facilities or university core facilities.

3.3. Breeding of Diabetic Mice to Cardiac Transgenic Mice

Female transgenic mice on the FVB background are bred to male agouti-positive mice on the KK background or to male OVE26 mice on the FVB background. The same housing and breeding conditions used to maintain the diabetic lines as described in **Subheading 3.1.** are used for crosses of different strains. Each litter will yield approximately equal numbers of four types of offspring: mice positive for the diabetogenic agouti or OVE26 gene, mice positive for the cardiac transgene, mice with both cardiac and diabetes genes, and mice with neither gene. Mice carrying the OVE26 or agouti genes are recognized by the phenotypic markers described in **Subheading 3.1.** To determine the presence of cardiac transgenes, PCRs of tail DNA are carried out. DNA is isolated using a Qiagen DNeasy tissue kit from a 1–3-mm slice of tail. Approximately 50 ng of DNA is subject to standard PCR conditions using one oligonucleotide complementary to the mouse α-MHC promoter and another oligonucleotide complimentary to the coding strand of the transgene.

3.4. Isolation of Mouse Cardiac Myocytes

1. On the morning of the isolation, fresh perfusion buffer is prepared from basic buffer by adding glucose and BDM.
2. The perfusion system is prepared as follows:
   a. The temperature of the circulation water bath is set so that the temperature of the outflow liquid at the tip of the cannula (20-gage needle with the nub filed flat and smooth) is 37°C.
   b. Flow rate is set at 1.2 mL/min.
   c. Prior to the cardiomyocyte isolation, about 100 mL of distilled water is run through the system.
   d. Then the system is perfused with oxygenated (5% CO_2/95% O_2) perfusion buffer for at least 5 min.
3. A mouse of at least 20 g is injected with heparin (1000 U/kg, ip). Then the mouse is anesthetized with a cocktail of ketamine/xylazine (150 mg/kg and 22.5 mg/kg, respectively, ip).
4. Dissection.
   a. The chest is wiped with 70% ethanol.
   b. A skin incision is made revealing the xiphoid process.
   c. The rib cage is completely cut starting at the xiphoid process running up the chest cavity.

d. To avoid heart damage, the diaphragm is cut as well.

e. The heart is secured with forceps, and all vessels are cut.

f. The aorta is cut so as to leave the maximal length, which is important for rapid cannulation.

5. The dissected heart is immediately placed in a Petri dish containing ice-cold calcium-free perfusion buffer, pH 7.4. To expose the aorta, all the remaining excess tissue is removed and discarded.

6. The aorta is held with two fine forceps and slid onto the vertically mounted cannula until the tip of the needle reaches the aortic valve. The heart is secured on the cannula with a small brass clip and immediately perfused with oxygenated (5% CO_2/95% O_2) perfusion buffer at a flow rate of 1.2 mL/min. The aorta is tied to the cannula with silk thread. The time from heart dissection to start of perfusion should not exceed 1 min.

7. The heart is perfused with perfusion buffer for 4 min, or until the outflow from apex is clear from blood. Then the perfusion with digestion buffer consisting of 15 mL perfusion buffer and 0.5 mL 10mg/mL liberase blendzyme 4 (Roche) is continued for 10–12 min, with constant oxygenation. At the end of perfusion the tissue becomes soft, swollen, and light pink.

8. After perfusion, the heart is cut from the cannula just below the atria using sterile fine scissors and placed in a Petri dish with 5 mL room temperature perfusion buffer. The heart is cut in half, and the tissue is gently teased into small pieces with fine forceps. The obtained suspension of cardiomyocytes is gently pipeted up and down with a plastic pipet (2-mm tip) several times.

9. Then the cells are transferred to a 15-mL sterile polypropylene conical tube, and 10, 20, 30, 40, and 100 µL of a 30 mM $CaCl_2$ solution is added at 5-min intervals. The final concentration of calcium is 1.2 mM.

10. Five minutes after the final addition of calcium, myocytes are filtered through three layers of gauze. Isolated myocytes are maintained at room temperature in this buffer (*see* **Note 6**).

3.5. Analysis of Myocyte Contractility

Cardiomyocyte contractility is controlled by electrical stimulation. Mechanical properties of isolated ventricular myocytes are assessed by video-based edge detection. An inverted microscope, a low-light-level video camera, and a computer-based motion analyzer are used to track the movement of cell edges (*6*).

1. The isolated myocytes are diluted approx 10-fold with contractility buffer (135 mM NaCl, 4 mM KCl, 1 mM $MgCl_2$, 10 mM HEPES, 0.33 mM NaH_2PO_4, 10 mM glucose, 10 mM BDM, 1.2 mM $CaCl_2$) and placed on a Teflon glass cover slip dish mounted on the stage of an inverted microscope (Olympus, IX-70).

2. The cells are field-stimulated to contract by the MyoPacer field stimulator through a pair of platinum electrodes at a frequency of 1.0 Hz, pulse duration of 4 ms, and amplitude of 10 V (*see* **Note 7**).

3. The image of the myocyte is obtained with an IonOptix MyoCam camera side-

mounted onto the microscope and displayed on a computer monitor using the Soft-Edge software (*see* **Note 8**). Twenty myocytes are recorded for each heart.

4. The cells being studied are scanned every 8.3 ms so that the amplitude and velocity of shortening and lengthening can be recorded with good fidelity. The displacements of cell edges at both ends of the myocyte are detected and converted to an analog voltage signal, which is then digitized and stored for off-line analysis.

5. Steady-state twitches *(8–10)* are analyzed for cell length changes using the Soft-Edge software and averaged for each myocyte. Cell shortening and relengthening are assessed by percentage of peak shortening (%PS), time to 90% peak shortening (TPS$_{90}$), time to 90% relengthening (TR$_{90}$), and maximal velocities of shortening and relengthening (±dL/dt) (**Fig. 2**). The data in **Table 1** indicate how these parameters reveal impaired function in diabetic cardiomyocytes and protection of function by an antioxidant transgene.

4. Notes

1. The OVE26 diabetic line *(2)* has maintained a consistent phenotype of severe, early-onset, type 1-like diabetes for the past 15 yr. The onset of diabetes is caused by a transgene that overexpresses calmodulin exclusively in pancreatic β-cells, leading to markedly diminished islet insulin content and secretion. Unlike streptozotocin-treated mice, these animals require no special treatment and will survive with diabetes for over a year.

2. Agouti mice are a spontaneous genetic model of type 2 diabetes that carry the agouti mutation, A^y. This dominant mutation results in obesity, hyperlipidemia, insulin resistance, hyperinsulinemia, and hyperglycemia, especially when on the KK background strain. The degree of diabetes is dependent on the background strain *(7)*. Because of this background dependence, it was uncertain whether F1 offspring from KK agouti mice and our transgenic FVB mice would demonstrate type 2 diabetes. We have found that agouti-positive F1 offspring have blood glucose levels 100 mg/dL higher than control mice and that they are 30% heavier than their non-agouti siblings at 90 d of age (not shown).

3. For our studies, a major advantage of the agouti mouse over other models of type 2 diabetes is that the agouti mutation is dominant. Mice of the F1 generation from two inbred strains, but not subsequent backcrosses, are genetically homogeneous. Therefore we do not have to deal with the variations in phenotypes caused by different genetic backgrounds. All other natural models of type 2 diabetes are polygenic or require that the mutation be homozygous. For those models, approx 10 generations of backcrossing are required to produce new lines of diabetic mice that are genetically homogenous.

4. Over the past 5 yr we have produced more than 70 lines of transgenic mice using the α-MHC promoter with no examples failing to express.

5. For study of diabetic cardiomyopathy, it is especially important to breed females that are not diabetic since diabetes during gestation can have an adverse impact on cardiovascular development, even if the offspring are not diabetic *(8)*.

6. Mouse myocytes are used within 6 h after isolation. Longer periods lead to reduced contractility.

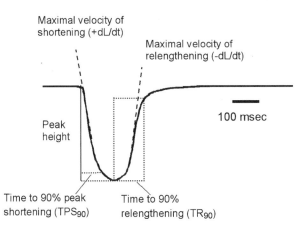

Fig. 2. Representative cell contractile trace. Transient characteristics of myocyte are determined as shown. Percentage of peak shortening (%PS) = (peak height/cell length × 100%).

Table 1
Typical Contractility Parameters for Control, Diabetic, and Transgene-Protected Diabetic Cardiomyocytes[a]

	$+dL/dt$ (µm/s)	$-dL/dt$ (µm/s)	TPS_{90} (ms)	TR_{90} (ms)	%PS
Control	174.59	162.62	0.109	0.121	10.63
OVE26	135.41	127.91	0.117	0.138	7.72
OVE26-MT	168.26	165.78	0.108	0.119	9.06

Abbreviations: PS, peak shortening; TPS_{90}, time to 90% PS; TR_{90}, time to 90% relengthening.

[a]Typical contractility parameters for control, OVE26 and OVE26, mice overexpressing metallothionein in the heart (OVE26-MT) demonstrating impaired contractility in diabetic OVE26 mice and normal contractility in diabetic OVE26-MT mice. Values are the mean obtained from 10 to 20 myocytes isolated from one mouse.

7. The polarities of the stimulatory electrodes are reversed periodically to avoid possible accumulation of electrolyte byproducts while one is measuring myocytes contractility.
8. Typically five individual myocytes are recorded before replacing the myocytes with a fresh dilution of unstimulated myocytes. This prevents exhaustion of the myocytes owing to prolonged stimulation.

References

1. Kannel, W. B., Hjortland, M., and Castelli, W. P. (1974). Role of diabetes in congestive heart failure: the Framingham study. *Am. J. Cardiol.* **34,** 29–34.
2. Epstein, P. N., Overbeek, P. A., and Means, A. R. (1989). Calmodulin-induced early-onset diabetes in transgenic mice. *Cell* **58,** 1067–1073.

3. Xiang, K., Cox, N. J., Hallewell, R. A., and Bell, G. I. (1987). Multiple Taq I RFLPs at the human manganese superoxide dismutase (SOD2) locus on chromosome 6. *Nucleic Acids Res.* **15**, 7654.

4. Liang, Q., Carlson, E. C., Borgerding, A. J., and Epstein, P. N. (1999). A transgenic model of acetaldehyde overproduction accelerates alcohol cardiomyopathy. *J. Pharmacol. Exp. Ther.* **291**, 766–772.

5. Palmiter, R. D. and Brinster, R. L. (1986). Germ-line transformation of mice. *Annu. Rev. Genet.* **20**, 465–499.

6. Ye, G., Metreveli, N. S., Ren, J., and Epstein, P. N. (2003). Metallothionein prevents diabetes-induced deficits in cardiomyocytes by inhibiting reactive oxygen species production. *Diabetes* **52,** 777–783.

7. Herberg, L. and Coleman, D. L. (1977). Laboratory animals exhibiting obesity and diabetes syndromes. *Metabolism* **26,** 59–99.

8. Eriksson, U. J. and Borg, L. A. (1993). Diabetes and embryonic malformations. Role of substrate-induced free-oxygen radical production for dysmorphogenesis in cultured rat embryos. *Diabetes* **42,** 411–419.

26

Cardiac-Specific Overexpression of Angiotensin II Type 1 Receptor in Transgenic Rats

Sigrid Hoffmann

Summary

This chapter describes the methods required for overexpression of the angiotensin II type I receptor (AT_1) in cardiomyocytes of transgenic rats. This includes cloning of the transgenic construct consisting of the α-myosin heavy chain (MHC) promoter, the human AT_1 cDNA and SV40 T-antigen splicing and polyadenylation sites, and purification of the transgenic DNA for microinjection by electroelution. The individual steps for the introduction of the transgene into the germline of rats by pronuclear microinjection are described, with special emphasis on the adaptation made to the standard procedure in mice. The identification of transgenic rats by PCR and Southern blot and the principles of establishing transgenic lines as well as characterizing transgene expression by Northern blot and RT-PCR are outlined.

Key Words: Angiotensin II; AT_1 receptor; transgenic rats; cardiac-specific expression; PCR for human AT_1 receptor; pronuclear microinjection.

1. Introduction

Angiotensin II (Ang II) is a key regulator of cardiovascular homeostasis. It elicits most of its known cardiovascular effects via the angiotensin II type 1 receptor (AT_1) *(1,2)*. Besides acting as a circulating hormone, locally produced Ang II contributes to regulation via paracrine and autocrine effects in tissues such as heart, kidney, and brain *(3–7)*. Transgenic technology provides a powerful tool enabling the complex pattern of Ang II action to be differentiated and the AT_1-transmitted Ang II effects in a specific tissue to be studied in the context of the whole animal *(7)*. For many years, the rat was the most appropriate

From: *Methods in Molecular Medicine, vol. 112: Molecular Cardiology: Methods and Protocols*
Edited by: Z. Sun © Humana Press Inc., Totowa, NJ

model in fields such as cardiovascular research. Therefore, the transgenic rat is more suitable than the mouse for studying AT_1 in respect to cardiac function *(8)*. To overexpress the transgene in the heart, regulatory elements are required for direct cardiac-specific gene expression at high levels. In the past, a number of cardiac-specific promoters were described and used to induce specific overexpression of distinct genes in transgenic mice. These include the promoters of the genes for α-myosin heavy chain (α-MHC) *(9,10)*, atrial natriuretic factor *(11,12)*, and myosin light chain *(13)*. It has been shown that these promoters also drive a cardiac-specific gene expression pattern in transgenic rats *(14,15)*. In this chapter, we briefly delineate the methods required for generating transgenic rats overexpressing the human AT_1 (hAT_1) specifically in the heart.

2. Materials
2.1. Cloning

1. Plasmid vector pBluescript SKII (+/–) (pBSKII[+/–]) and cDNAs of hAT_1, α-MHC promoter and intron and polyadenylation signal of the SV40 T antigen (SV40 intron + polyA).
2. *E. coli* strain DH5α, restriction enzymes, T4 DNA ligase, and ampicillin.
3. Agarose gel equipment, agarose (molecular genetic grade), and ethidium bromide.
4. Standard TAE buffer (50X): 2 *M* Tris-HCl, 1 *M* aceto-acetate, and 50 m*M* EDTA; prior to use add 980 mL H_2O to 20 mL of 50X TAE.
5. LB medium and agar: 10 g tryptone and 5 g yeast extract.

2.2. Purification of the Transgene

1. Dialysis tubing and dialysis membrane (Millipore [Bedford, MA] VSWP04700, 0.025 μm, white 47 mm.
2. Phenol, chloroform/isoamylalkohol, and 3 *M* sodium acetate.
3. Microinjection buffer: 8 m*M* Tris-HCl, 0.15 m*M* EDTA, pH 7.4, filtered through a 0.22-μm filter.
4. 0.22-μm Filter unit (Ultrafree-MC-Millipore 0.2-cm^2 membranes, Millipore).

2.3. Generation of Transgenic Rats

1. Pregnant mare serum gonadotropin (PMSG; Intergonan, 1000 IU/vial, Intervet, Germany); stock: 100 IU/mL 0.9% NaCl; aliquot and store at –20°C for up to 6 mo.
2. Alternatively: follicle-stimulating hormone (FSH) from porcine pituitary (ICN, cat. no. 101727)/choriogonadotropin from human pregnancy urine (HCG) freshly prepared. Solubilize 1 vial (50 U FSH) in 1150 μL 0.9% NaCl, add 100 μL HCG stock solution (100 IU/mL; *see* **item 3**). Place 200 μL of this solution into an Alzet mini-osmotic pump 2001 (pumping rate 1 μL/h) the day prior to implantation into the rat, and incubate the pump in 0.9% NaCl in a 2-mL Eppendorf tube

overnight at room temperature.

3. 5000 IU/vial HCG (Sigma, cat. no. CG5), stock: 100 IU/mL 0.9% NaCl; aliquot and store at –20°C for up to 6 mo.
4. des Gly^{10}[D-Ala^{6}]-luteinizing hormone releasing hormone ethylamine (LHRH-a; Sigma, cat. no. L-4513).
5. 100,000 U Hyaluronidase100 (Calbiochem), stock: 100 U/µL 0.9% NaCl. Aliquot and store at –20°C for up to 6 mo.
6. Pipets for transfer, microinjection, and holding of eggs.
7. Eppendorf Microloader (Eppendorf, Hamburg).
8. M2 and M16 media, and mineral oil, embryo tested (Sigma).
9. Suprarenin® (Höchst, Frankfurt, Germany).
10. Stereo microscope with understage illumination, stereo microscope for operation, and inverse microscope with micromanipulators.

2.4. Identification of the Transgene

1. Specific primers for the hAT₁ cDNA:
   a. sense 5'-TGC AGA TAT TGT GGA CAC GG-3' corresponding to sequence 1183–2002 in the coding region.
   b. Reverse 5'-ACA TTG TTC TTC GAG CAG CC-3' corresponding to the sequence 1657–1676 in the 3' untranslated region of the hAT₁ c DNA (Gene Bank no. NM 004835).
2. Blotting membrane (Stratagene).
3. Taq polymerase, 10X polymerase chain reaction (PCR) buffer and d NTP.
4. Thermal cycler (Perkin Elmer Gene Amp PCR System 2400).
5. ^{32}P-dCTP.
6. Prime It Random Primer Labeling Kit (Stratagene).

3. Methods

The methods described below outline (1) the design and construction of the transgene, (2) purification of the transgenic fragment for microinjection, (3) generation of transgenic rats, (4) the identification of the transgenic founders, (5) establishment of transgenic lines, and (6) characterization of the transgene expression.

3.1. Design and Construction of the Transgene

The hAT₁ cDNA is under the control of the α-MHC promoter. Introns have been shown to improve the efficiency of overall transgene activity even if they derive from foreign sources. Thus, the transgene is terminated by the SV40 intron + polyA sequences *(14)*. The structure of the transgene is delineated in **Subheading 3.1.1.–3.1.5.** This includes a description of the promoter, the hAT₁ cDNA, the cloning vector, and the cloning procedure.

3.1.1. The α-Myosin Heavy Chain Promoter

The α-MHC promoter specifically elicits expression of the hAT$_1$ gene in the heart. The 1.03-kb *Eco*RI/*Hin*dIII fragment of the α-MHC promoter (cloned between the *Pst*I and *Hin*dIII polylinker region of the vector pGCATC) contains 612 bp of the 5'-regulatory region including the CCAAATTT and TATAAA sequences and 420 bp of the 5'-untranslated region of the α-MHC gene *(16)*. For cloning, the promoter was excised out of the vector as an *Xba*I/*Hin*dIII fragment.

3.1.2. Human AT$_1$ Receptor cDNA

A 2.19-kb fragment of the hAT$_1$ cDNA containing the entire coding region as well as 260 bp of the 5'- and 854 bp of the 3'-untranslated regions was kindly donated by T. Inagami *(17)*. For cloning, it was excised out of the vector as an *Eco*RI/*Xho*I fragment (*see* **Note 1**).

3.1.3. SV 40 Intron and PolyA Sequences

SV40 T-antigen splicing and polyadenylation sites were obtained from the pMAM expression vector (Clontech) as an *Xho*I/*Kpn*I fragment.

3.1.4. Cloning Vector

We used pBSKII(+/–) as a vector to subclone the transgenic construct, which is composed of a polylinker with 21 unique restriction sites and an ampicillin resistance gene.

3.1.5. Cloning

The different DNA fragments were cloned into the vector plasmid in such a way that the final transgenic construct was terminated by single restriction sites (**Fig. 1**). This enables the intact transgene to be cut out without including any plasmid sequences that might inhibit the expression of the transgene. DNA manipulations were performed using standard recombinant DNA methods *(18)* and are not described in detail here.

1. Digest pMAM (SV40 intron + polyA) and pBSKII(+/–) with *Xho*I and *Kpn*I, and fractionate the DNA together with a DNA marker on a preparative 0.8% agarose gel containing 0.5 µg/mL ethidium bromide in TAE buffer.
2. Excise the two bands of interest using a long-wave UV lamp (*see* **Note 2**), and extract the DNA using a QIAquick® spin column (Quiagen) according to the manufacturer's instructions.
3. Ligate the SV40 *Xho*I/*Kpn*I fragment between the *Xho*I and *Kpn*I sites of the pBSKII(+/–) vector, and transform *E. coli* DH5α cells with the DNA using standard methods *(18)*.

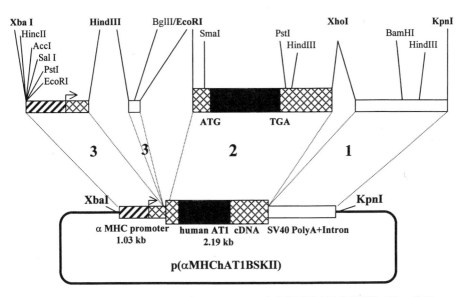

Fig. 1. Cloning of the transgenic construct p(αMHC-hAT₁BSKII). The different cloning steps are indicated by 1, 2, and 3. For microinjection the transgene is excised by *Xba*I and *Kpn*I digestion.

4. Plate the cells on LB plates containing ampicillin (50 μg/mL), and incubate overnight at 37°C. Select single colonies, and grow overnight in LB medium with ampicillin (50 μg/mL) at 37°C.

5. Isolate the plasmid DNA *(18)*, and check for the presence of the transgene and for correct orientation (pSV40BSKII[+/–]) using restriction enzyme digestions.

6. Next, excise the hAT₁ cDNA from the vector with *Eco*RI and *Xho*I. After gel separation and DNA extraction as described in **steps 1** and **2**, ligate the DNA between the *Eco*RI and *Xho*I sites of the plasmid pSV40BSKII(+/–) directly upstream of the SV40 sequences to generate the phAT₁SV40pBSKII. Amplify and purify the plasmid as described in **steps 3–5**.

7. Finally, ligate the α-MHC promoter *Xba*I/*Hind*III fragment and an *Hind*III/*Bgl*II/ *Eco*RI linker simultaneously between the *Xba*I and *Eco*RI sites of the phAT₁SV40BSKII to generate p(αMHChAT₁BSKII).

8. Check the correct orientation and integrity of the different fragments in the transgenic construct using restriction enzyme digestions and DNA sequencing *(18)*.

3.2. Purification of the Transgenic Construct for Microinjection

The purity of the transgenic DNA may have profound consequences for the survival of zygotes after microinjection.

1. Excise the transgenic fragment from the vector with *Xba*I and *Kpn*I (*see* **Note 3**), and fractionate the digested DNA on a preparative 0.8% agarose gel in TAE buffer and 0.5 µg/mL ethidium bromide using a wide slot (4–5 cm) in conjunction with an appropriate DNA size marker and an uncut sample of the clone (*see* **Note 4**). On completion of the run, excise the fragment of interest using a long-wave UV light transilluminator (*see* **Note 2**).

2. Extract the transgenic fragment from the gel by electroelution. Place the agarose slice into dialysis tubing with TAE buffer, and subject the sealed tubing to electrophoresis again at a constant voltage of 2 V/cm for 3 h. The DNA migrates out of the gel slice into the buffer. After the electroelution is complete, reverse the polarity of the electrodes, and turn up the voltage to 100 V for 30 s to free any DNA that has adhered to the dialysis tubing (*see* **Note 5**).

3. Aliquot the DNA-containing buffer to 400 µL into an Eppendorf tube. Extract the DNA with phenol/chloroform. Perform the chloroform extraction twice. Precipitate the DNA with sodium acetate and ethanol, and wash twice with 80% ethanol. Solubilize the DNA pellet in a small quantity of microinjection buffer, and measure the DNA concentration photometrically.

4. Dilute the DNA to 2 ng/µL in microinjection buffer. Check the concentration of the diluted DNA again on an agarose gel using 1, 2, 5, and 10 µL of the diluted DNA, and compare with serial dilutions of a known concentration (*see* **Note 3**).

5. Finally, dialyze the DNA against 30 mL of microinjection buffer for 3 h by placing a drop of DNA on a dialysis membrane (Millipore VSWP04700) and floating on the buffer in a tissue culture dish. Then centrifuge the DNA through a 0.22-µm filter unit prior to use.

3.3. Generation of Transgenic Rats

The techniques for generation of transgenic rats by microinjection of the DNA into fertilized one-cell eggs are essentially the same as for mice. The reader is referred to various excellent manuals that describe the different steps of the standard technique in detail *(19,20)*. Some adaptations to the rat were required and are outlined in more detail in **Subheadings 3.3.1.– 3.3.6.** These include induction of superovulation, production of pseudopregnant foster mothers, recovery of fertilized eggs, microinjection of the transgene, and embryo transfer. One microinjection experiment (lasting 1 d) is sufficient to produce at least one transgenic founder rat (*see* **Note 6**). For one experiment, 8 female rats (28–29 d old) as donors, 8 stud males to mate with the donors, 15 vasectomized males, and 35–40 female rats (8- to 12-wk-old) as foster mothers are required when the outbred strain Sprague-Dawley is used (*see* **Note 7**). With the exception of the donor females and the females used as embryo recipients, the rats can be used repeatedly for further experiments. The rats should be maintained on a controlled light and dark period of 12 h each.

3.3.1. Induction of Superovulation in "Donor" Females

In order to obtain a sufficiently large number of fertilized eggs, superovulation is induced by treating immature females with gonadotropins.

1. Eight 28- to 29-d-old female Sprague-Dawley rats are injected ip with 25 IU PMSG at 11 AM followed by an injection of 30 IU of HCG 48 h later (*see* **Note 8**).
2. Then females are individually placed with a stud male that had not copulated for at least 5 d.
3. In all, 80–90% of the superovulated females should mate successfully and can be identified by copulatory plugs next morning. Superovulation will yield 42.7 ± 19.3 eggs per donor.

3.3.2. Vasectomized Males

Male Sprague-Dawley rats are sterilized by vasectomy, i.e., interruption of the Vas deferens using standard methods (*19*). They should have a rest of 2 wk before first mating. One male can be placed with three females. Therefore, 15 vasectomized males are necessary. They can be used up to an age of 1 yr.

3.3.3. Production of Pseudopregnant Foster Mothers

Mate 35–40 female Sprague-Dawley rats with 15 vasectomized males in the evening prior to the embryo transfer, and check for copulatory plugs early the next morning (*see* **Note 9**).

3.3.4. Recovery of Fertilized One-Cell Eggs

Fertilized eggs are harvested from donor females on the day following mating between 10 and 12 AM using standard methods (*19*).

1. Sacrifice copulation-positive donors by cervical dislocation, and open the abdominal cavity.
2. Dissect the oviducts, and transfer them into a drop of M2 medium + hyaluronidase (5000 IU/mL M2 medium; *see* **Note 10**).
3. View the oviducts under a stereomicroscope, and rupture the swollen ampulla with a small incision using a microscalpel to pour out the eggs, which will be surrounded by cumulus cells. The individual zygotes are released from the cumulus cells within a few minutes.
4. Collect the zygotes by using a general embryo transfer pipet, and rinse twice in M2 medium.
5. Transfer the eggs to an M16 media microdrop culture covered by mineral oil, and keep it in a 37°C incubator gassed with 5% (v/v) CO_2 to await microinjection.

3.3.5. Microinjection of the Transgene Into the Pronucleus

The transgenic DNA is injected into the pronucleus using standard protocols (*19,20*). Pronuclei are visible after 3 PM, and injection can be performed between 3 and 6 PM the same day.

1. Fill the injection pipet with the transgenic DNA solution (2 ng/µL) through the back end of the capillary using an Eppendorf microloader.
2. Place a drop of M2 medium into the well of a siliconized glass depression slide, cover with mineral oil, and transfer 20 eggs into the M2 medium drop.
3. Start the injection using an inverse microscope and micromanipulators. The eggs are kept in position with a glass pipet under vacuum, and the DNA is injected with the injection pipet under controlled pressure. The rat egg membrane is considerably more elastic than the mouse egg membrane. This makes it more difficult to penetrate the egg and requires injection pipets with an optimal shape (*see* **Note 11**). Pronuclei in rat eggs are sometimes difficult to view, since the rat egg cytoplasm is very granular. The fertilized rat egg can have a very irregular shape.
4. Store the microinjected zygotes in an M16 medium microdrop culture dish in the incubator until to transfer into foster mothers.

3.3.6. Embryo Transfer Into Pseudopregnant Foster Mothers

We prefer to transfer the microinjected eggs into the oviduct of foster mothers immediately after finishing the microinjection. However, they can also be transferred the next morning into pseudopregnant females that were mated the night prior to the transfer.

1. Anesthetize the pseudopregnant recipient females with a combination of 11.5 mg ketamine hydrochloride and 0.1 mg xylazine per 100 g body weight, shave and disinfect the lower back of the rat, and place it on its belly on a sterile tissue.
2. Make a longitudinal skin incision about 1 cm in length above the lumbar spine, and dissect the skin from the body wall around the incision with a pair of scissors. After an incision through the left body wall about 1 cm to the left of the spinal cord, exteriorize the fat pad that is connected to the ovary, and fix it with an artery clip in such a way that the oviduct is displayed in the uppermost position and the infundibulum points caudally. Add two drops of Suprarenin to the bursa ovarica to prevent excessive bleeding when it is dissected.
3. Wash the eggs in M2 medium; load the transfer pipet with a small amount of M2 medium followed by air bubble, some more medium, and another air bubble. Then take up 15 eggs in the smallest possible volume of M2 medium.
4. Now open the transparent bursa membrane at the point between the ovary and oviduct where the infundibulum is located using microscissors and microforceps; correct the rat's position so that the opening of the infundibulum is immediately in front of you.
5. Pick up the bursa ovarica at the end of the incision so that you can easily insert the transfer pipet into the infundibulum until the tip reaches the first coil of the oviduct. Deposit the embryos by gently blowing into the pipet, thereby controlling the movement of the air bubbles behind the embryos. Withdraw the transfer pipet, and view it under the stereo microscope to make sure that all embryos were released.

6. Return the ovary and oviduct to the abdominal cavity cautiously without touching them, and close the body wall and skin.
7. Repeat the procedure on the other oviduct with 15 more embryos.

About 80–90% of the recipients become pregnant (*see* **Note 9**). The pups should be born approx 23 d after the transfer.

3.4. Genotyping

Transgenic founders are identified by PCR using genomic DNA isolated from tail DNA by standard protocols *(18,20)*. PCR can detect low-copy-number and mosaic transgenics that may not be clearly identifiable by Southern blotting. However, the transgenic founders and F1 rats should always be screened by Southern blotting in addition to PCR. PCR alone is insufficient to provide direct information on transgene copy number, transgene integrity, and the number of independent transgene integration sites.

3.4.1. PCR

1. Prepare the PCR reaction as follows: 5 µL 10X PCR buffer, 4 µL (200 µ*M* each dNTP) 2.5 m*M* dNTP mix, 2.5 µL (500 n*M* each primer) specific PCR primers for the hAT1 cDNA (10 µ*M*), 0.5 µL (0.25 U) AmpliTaq polymerase, and 2.5 µL (100 ng/µL) genomic DNA sample. Add sterile water to a final volume of 50 µL. Use the plasmid harboring the transgene as a positive control (*see* **Note 12**).
2. Amplify the PCR in a thermal cycler using the following cycling parameters: initial denaturation: 5 min at 94°C; then 35 three-step cycles: denaturation: 45 s at 94°C, annealing: 45 s at 58°C and extension: 1.5 min at 72°C; final extension for 10 min at 72°C.
3. To assess the PCR, the amplification product (493 bp in size) can be visualized by UV illumination following electrophoresis on a 1.5% agarose gel (**Fig. 2**).

3.4.2. Southern Blotting

Southern blot is performed using standard molecular genetic methods *(21)*. As a probe, we use a ³²P–dCTP labeled 1.5-kb *Hind*III fragment corresponding to the 5'-untranslated region, the total coding region, and 160 bp of 3'-untranslated region of the hAT₁ cDNA. To check the number of transgene integration sites, the genomic DNA is restricted by an enzyme that does not cut the transgenic construct, e.g., *Pvu*II. The number of bands specific to the transgene corresponds to the number of independent transgene integration sites (**Fig. 3**). To check the integrity of the transgene, the genomic DNA is digested with *Bam*H1, which cuts the transgene once. Since the transgene is generally integrated as multicopy tandem repeats, the resulting primary band corresponds to the size of the transgene.

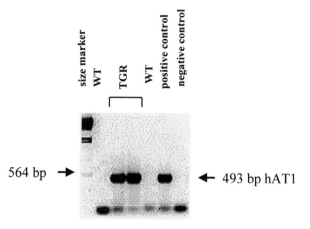

Fig. 2. Genotyping for the human AT$_1$ receptor (hAT$_1$) by PCR. Visualization of the 493-bp PCR product on a 1.5% agarose gel. Water is used as a negative control. TGR, transgenic rat; WT, wild-type rats.

3.5. Establishing a Transgenic Line

Each founder is unique and is used to establish a separate transgenic line by mating with a nontransgenic rat from the background strain (*see* **Note 6**). The transgene is transmitted to 50% of the progeny. All the transgenic F1 animals harvest the transgene in the same chromosomal position and can be mated with each other to produce homozygous progeny and establish a line. Some founders transmit the transgene to less than 50% of their progeny. Such founders are chimeric and may comprise a mixed population of transgene-bearing and non-transgene-bearing germ cells. This happens when the DNA integrates after the first embryo cleavage. However, their transgenic progeny is hemizygous and can be mated with each other. Some founders may have more than one transgene integration site, which segregate independently among their off-spring. F1 progeny with a single transgene integration site are mated with nontransgenic rats to establish separate transgenic lines. Therefore, two or more distinct lines may diverge from such founders. The integration sites can be determined by Southern blotting (*see* **Subheading 3.4.2.**).

3.6. Expression Analysis of the Transgene

Expression of hAT$_1$ should be determined at the RNA and protein level. Despite the use of a tissue-specific promoter to overexpress the hAT$_1$, all tissues should be checked for transgene expression by reverse transcriptase (RT)-PCR, since the specific integration site can cause an aberrant transgene expression. RNA isolation from tissue is performed using standard methods

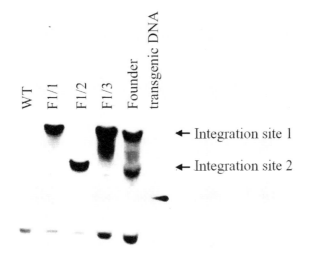

Fig. 3. Southern blot for determination of the number of integration sites for the transgene. Genomic DNA was restricted by *Pvu*II, which does not cut within the transgene. The transgenic founder has integrated the human AT₁ receptor in two chromosomal positions and transmits them independently to the progeny. F1/1–F1/3, individual transgenic offspring in the F1 generation; WT, wild-type rats.

(21). Tissue screening for transgene expression is performed by RT-PCR using the same primer as described in **Subheading 3.4.1.** In addition, RNA from transgene-positive tissues, e.g., the heart, is analyzed using standard Northern blot protocols *(18)*. We used a ^{32}P-labeled 1.5-kb *Hin*dIII fragment of the hAT₁ cDNA as a probe that is specific for the transgenic mRNA. To quantify the transgenic mRNA level, the same Northern blot was probed with a GAPDH probe, and the ratios between the individual hAT₁ and GAPDH levels were calculated (**Fig. 4**). Transgene expression at the RNA level does not necessarily result in increased Ang II binding to the tissue. Therefore, it is necessary to determine the binding properties (B_{max}, K_D) of ^{125}I Ang II to cardiac membrane proteins. The description of these methods is beyond the scope of this chapter.

4. Notes

1. The 3'- and 5'-untranslated regions of the hAT₁ cDNA contain sequences that decrease the stability of the mRNA as well as the translation efficiency. Removal of these sequences might therefore increase the transgene expression level.
2. Minimize the exposure of the DNA to the UV light as much as possible, since UV light can damage the DNA. Alternatively, you can cut off a gel slice containing the marker and a small part of the fractionated DNA; mark the position of the

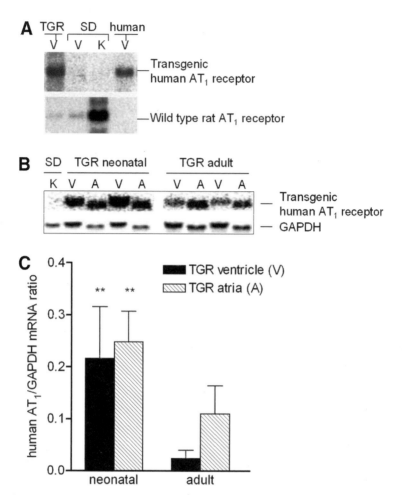

Fig. 4. Northern blot analysis. (**A**) Specificity of the human AT$_1$ receptor (hAT$_1$) probe. RNA (20 μg/lane) from ventricles (V) of transgenic (TGR) and Sprague-Dawley (SD) rats and of humans as well as from SD rat kidney (K) were hybridized with the 1497-bp *Hin*dIII hAT$_1$ cDNA probe and subsequently with a probe corresponding to the wild-type rat AT$_1$. (**B**) Typical autoradiographs of h AT$_1$ and glyceraldehyde-3-phosphate dehydrogenase (GAPDH) mRNA (20 μg/lane) from TGR hearts. Kidney from SD rats (K) serves as negative control, since it exhibits high levels of wild-type rat AT$_1$ receptor expression in contrast to the cardiac tissue. (**C**) Bar graphs of the h AT$_1$ mRNA values normalized to GAPDH expression in atria and ventricles.

band of interest using a UV light illuminator, and take this gel slice to identify the position of band containing the transgenic DNA in the remaining gel; cut out this band without using UV light.

3. We prefer to digest an excess of plasmid DNA (20 μg) to ensure that enough transgenic DNA is left after purification to enable the DNA concentration to be measured accurately in the photometer. The concentration of the injected DNA can have profound effects on the success of microinjection. Injection of too little DNA reduces the frequency of transgenic founders, whereas too much DNA is harmful for embryos and may seriously reduce survival after microinjection.

4. If there are minor differences in size between the transgenic fragment and the remaining plasmid sequences or uncut plasmid DNA, use a large gel and let it run for 5–6 h until the bands are clearly separated; avoid overloading the slot. It is important to preclude any contamination of the transgenic DNA with plasmid sequences.

5. Alternative methods for extracting the DNA from agarose include the use of QIAEX or QIAquick columns. However, we obtained a higher frequency of transgenic founders when the microinjected DNA was purified by electroelution.

6. Four to six founders should be generated for each construct. Each founder is unique owing to the randomly integrated transgene. The position of the transgene in the genome may influence the expression level and sometimes also the tissue-specific expression pattern, despite the use of tissue-specific promoters. In addition, some founders might not transmit the transgene to the pups because of mosaicism.

7. The efficiency of a microinjection experiment is higher when one is using fertilized eggs from outbred rats such as Sprague-Dawley compared with inbred rats. However, in contrast to outbred strains, inbred strains provide better controls for the transgenic rats when a homozygous transgenic line is developed. We successfully used the inbred strain F344 as an alternative donor to Sprague-Dawley rats. In that case, the number of donors and stud males per experimental day should be increased up to 10–12 each.

8. In contrast to mice, the age of immature donors at the time of hormonally induced superovulation is very important and should be determined individually for each strain (the age just before the vagina opens spontaneously). In F344 females, we start PMSG injection at the age of 33–35 d and obtain 36.8 ± 13 eggs per rat. Superovulation can also be induced in adult females. Therefore, 40 μg LHRH-a are applied subcutaneously 50 h prior to the PMSG injection. Furthermore, instead of 25 IU PMSG, we inject 30 IU PMSG. The percentage of plugged females (65%) and the number of ovulated eggs (29.7 ± 9 eggs per female) is somewhat lower than in immature females. An alternative protocol for superovulation includes the continuous infusion of a mixture of 1.9 U highly purified FSH and 0.38 IU HCG over a 48-h period by means of an osmotic pump instead of using PMSG. The superovulatory response to this treatment is much higher (68.6 ± 18 eggs per female). The disadvantage is the high cost.

9. By selecting rats at random, 20 to 25% of the females may be in estrus at any given time since the mean duration of the estrous cycle is 4–5 d. Females tolerate copulation only when they are in the estrus stage. The appearance of a copulatory plug indicates successful mating. However, synchronization of the estrus cycle

in several individuals that are group-housed may cause considerable variation in the number obtained at any given time, Therefore, at least seven times more females should be mated than needed as foster mothers. To be 100% sure that we will obtain at least three successfully mated females, we place 35–40 females to 15 vasectomized males. The highest rate of pregnancy after embryo transfer is obtained if young stud females of a strain with good reproductive performance (e.g., Sprague-Dawley) are used as foster mothers (80 to 90%). If the females are older than 12 wk or become overweight, the rate of pregnancy is decreased (up to 60%).

10. The eggs should be exposed to hyaluronidase for no more than 5 min, since hyaluronidase may break down the zona pellucida.

11. The shape of the injection pipet can be decisive for the success of microinjection. Change the pipet immediately if you feel that the embryos die during injection.

12. You can use plasmid DNA as a positive control in PCR. However, it is always preferable to use genomic DNA for this purpose since impurities in DNA preparation can inhibit the PCR even if the plasmid DNA shows a positive signal. Once you have identified a positive founder, use DNA from this animal as positive control.

Acknowledgments

Thomas Krause and Hidenori Urata have contributed to the development of the transgenic rat overexpressing hAT_1 in the heart. The author thanks Dr. T. Inagami for providing the cDNA for the human AT_1 receptor. This study was supported by a grant from the European Commission (ERB-CHBGCT940725) and by Alexander von Humboldt grant IVI-7121.

References

1. Allen, A. M., Zhuo, J., and Mendelsohn, F. A. (2000) Localization and function of angiotensin AT_1 receptors. *Am. J. Hypertens.* **13,** 31S–38S.

2. Hollenberg, N. K. and Sever, P. S. (2000) The past, present and future of hypertension management: a potential role for AT(1)-receptor antagonists. *J. Renin. Angiotensin. Aldosterone. Syst.* **1,** 5–10.

3. Bader, M., Peters, J., Baltatu, O., Muller, D. N., Luft, F. C., and Ganten, D. (2001) Tissue renin-angiotensin systems: new insights from experimental animal models in hypertension research. *J. Mol. Med.* **79,** 76–102.

4. Urata, H., Hoffmann, S., and Ganten, D. (1994) Tissue angiotensin II system in the human heart. *Eur. Heart J.* **15,** 68–78.

5. Matsusaka, T., Hymes, J., and Ichikawa, I. (1996) Angiotensin in progressive renal diseases: theory and practice. *J. Am. Soc. Nephrol.* **7,** 2025–2043.

6. Baltatu, O. and Bader, M. (2003) Brain Renin-Angiotensin System. Lessons from Functional Genomics. *Neuroendocrinology* **78,** 253–259.

7. Bader, M. (2002) Role of the local renin-angiotensin system in cardiac damage: a minireview focussing on transgenic animal models. *J. Mol. Cell. Cardiol.* **34,** 1455–1462.

8. Paul, M., Wagner, J., Hoffmann, S., Urata, H., and Ganten, D. (1994) Transgenic rats: new experimental models for the study of candidate genes in hypertension research. *Annu. Rev. Physiol.* **56,** 811–829.
9. Paradis, P., Dali-Youcef, N., Paradis, F. W, Thibault G., and Nemer, M. (2000) Overexpression of angiotensin II type I receptor in cardiomyocytes induces cardiac hypertrophy and remodeling. *Proc. Natl. Acad. Sci. USA* **97,** 931–936.
10. Hein, L., Stevens, M. E., Barsh, G. S., Pratt, R. E., Kobilka, B. K., and Dzau, V. J. (1997) Overexpression of angiotensin AT$_1$ receptor transgene in the mouse myocardium produces a lethal phenotype associated with myocyte hyperplasia and heart block. *Proc. Natl. Acad. Sci. USA* **94,** 6391–6396.
11. Small, E. M. and Krieg, P. A. (2002) Molecular mechanisms of chamber-specific myocardial gene expression: transgenic analysis of the ANF promoter. *Cold Spring Harb. Symp. Quant. Biol.* **67,** 71–79.
12. Small, E. M. and Krieg, P. A. (2003) Transgenic analysis of the atrialnatriuretic factor (ANF) promoter: Nkx2-5 and GATA-4 binding sites are required for atrial specific expression of ANF. *Dev. Biol.* **261,** 116–131.
13. Chen, L. Y., Li, P., He, Q., Jiang, L. Q., Cui, C. J., Xu, L., and Liu, L. S. (2002) Transgenic study of the function of chymase in heart remodeling. *J. Hypertens.* **20,** 2047–2055.
14. Hoffmann, S., Krause, T., van Geel, P. P., et al. (2001) Overexpression of the human angiotensin II type 1 receptor in the rat heart augments load induced cardiac hypertrophy. *J. Mol. Med.* **79,** 601–608.
15. Hammes, A., Oberdorf-Maass, S., Rother, T., et al. (1998) Overexpression of the sarcolemmal calcium pump in the myocardium of transgenic rats. *Circ. Res.* **83,** 877–888.
16. Mahdavi, V., Chambers, A. P., and Nadal-Ginard, B. (1984) Cardiac alpha- and beta-myosin heavy chain genes are organized in tandem. *Proc. Natl. Acad. Sci. USA* **81,** 2626–2630.
17. Furuta, H., Guo, D. F., and Inagami, T. (1992) Molecular cloning and sequencing of the gene encoding human angiotensin II type 1 receptor. *Biochem. Biophys. Res. Commun.* **183,** 8–13.
18. Ausubel, F. M., Brent, R., Kingston, R. E., et al. (2000) *Current Protocols in Molecular Biology.* (Chanda, V. B., ed.), John Wiley, Massachusetts General Hospital, Havard Medical School.
19. Hogan, B., Costantini, F., and Lacy, E. (1986) *Manipulating the Mouse Embryo. A Laboratory Manual.* Cold Spring Harbor Laboratory, Cold Spring Harbor Laboratory Presss, New York.
20. Murphy, D. and Carter, D. A. (1993) *Transgenesis Techniques, Principles and Protocols, in Methods in Molecular Biology*, vol. 18. (Walker, J. M., ed.), Humana, Totowa, NJ, p. 467.

Index